30 DAY KICK START PLAN

Joe ♡

ONE OF A LIMITED EDITION
SIGNED BY JOE

30 DAY KICK START PLAN

JOE WICKS
THE BODY COACH

First published 2020 by Bluebird
an imprint of Pan Macmillan
The Smithson, 6 Briset Street, London EC1M 5NR

Associated companies throughout the world
www.panmacmillan.com

ISBN 978-1-5098-5618-3

1 3 5 7 9 8 6 4 2
A CIP catalogue record for this book is available from the British Library.
Printed and bound in Italy.

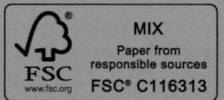

Publisher Carole Tonkinson
Managing Editor Martha Burley
Senior Production Controller Sarah Badhan
Art Direction Nikki Dupin, Nic&Lou
Art Direction and Design Emma Wells, Nic&Lou
Food Styling Natalie Thomson
Prop Styling Charlie Phillips

Visit www.panmacmillan.com to read more about all our books
and to buy them. You will also find features, author interviews and
news of any author events, and you can sign up for e-newsletters
so that you're always first to hear about our new releases.

CONTENTS

HELLO

I'm **Joe Wicks**, aka **The Body Coach**, and I've dedicated the past 10 years of my life to helping people get fitter, stronger and healthier. I started as a young and ambitious personal trainer, working with clients one-to-one and running my own outdoor boot camps. I then took all my passion and energy for motivating and inspiring people, and put it into my books, social media and, most recently, my new The Body Coach fitness app. Nothing makes me happier than knowing I've helped someone on their journey to become healthier and happier. It's the driving force behind everything I do – and really, I believe it to be my purpose in life.

When I started out, success in the fitness industry was predominantly about physical transformation and those impressive 'before and after' images you see on social media. Those images are still what many want to see, because they are inspirational and can spark change in people's lives. They motivate a lot of people to get up and start working out. In those days, the language I used on social media and in my early books emphasized the promise of 'fat loss' and 'gaining lean muscle', and how my plan would make you look. I rarely spoke about how regular exercise and healthy food could make you feel!

Having worked with hundreds of thousands of people, I've come to realize that the things you can't see are actually more important and powerful than the things you can. Exercise isn't just about looking good; it's about feeling good, mentally strong, energized, optimistic, confident and in control. Exercise can play a huge part in helping people manage anxiety, depression, low self-esteem and stress. The more people I help, the more I understand that it's this inner transformation that I need to be talking about. I'm changing the narrative and shining a light on the wellbeing and mental-health benefits of exercise because I know that focusing on how you feel is the fastest way to living a healthy and happy life.

When you shift your goal from meeting a particular body image to achieving a good state of being (in which you're both emotionally balanced and mentally strong), that's when you find true motivation. That's when you want to take action, gain momentum and sustain a positive lifestyle. When you do that for long enough and have a strong mindset as a result, you will also be naturally burning body fat, building muscle and transforming your body physically.

I've been on my own personal journey with health and fitness over the years. In my teenage years, I was very motivated by a desire to get stronger, build muscle and change the way I felt about my skinny body. I wasn't confident and was concerned about how other people perceived how I looked. This state of

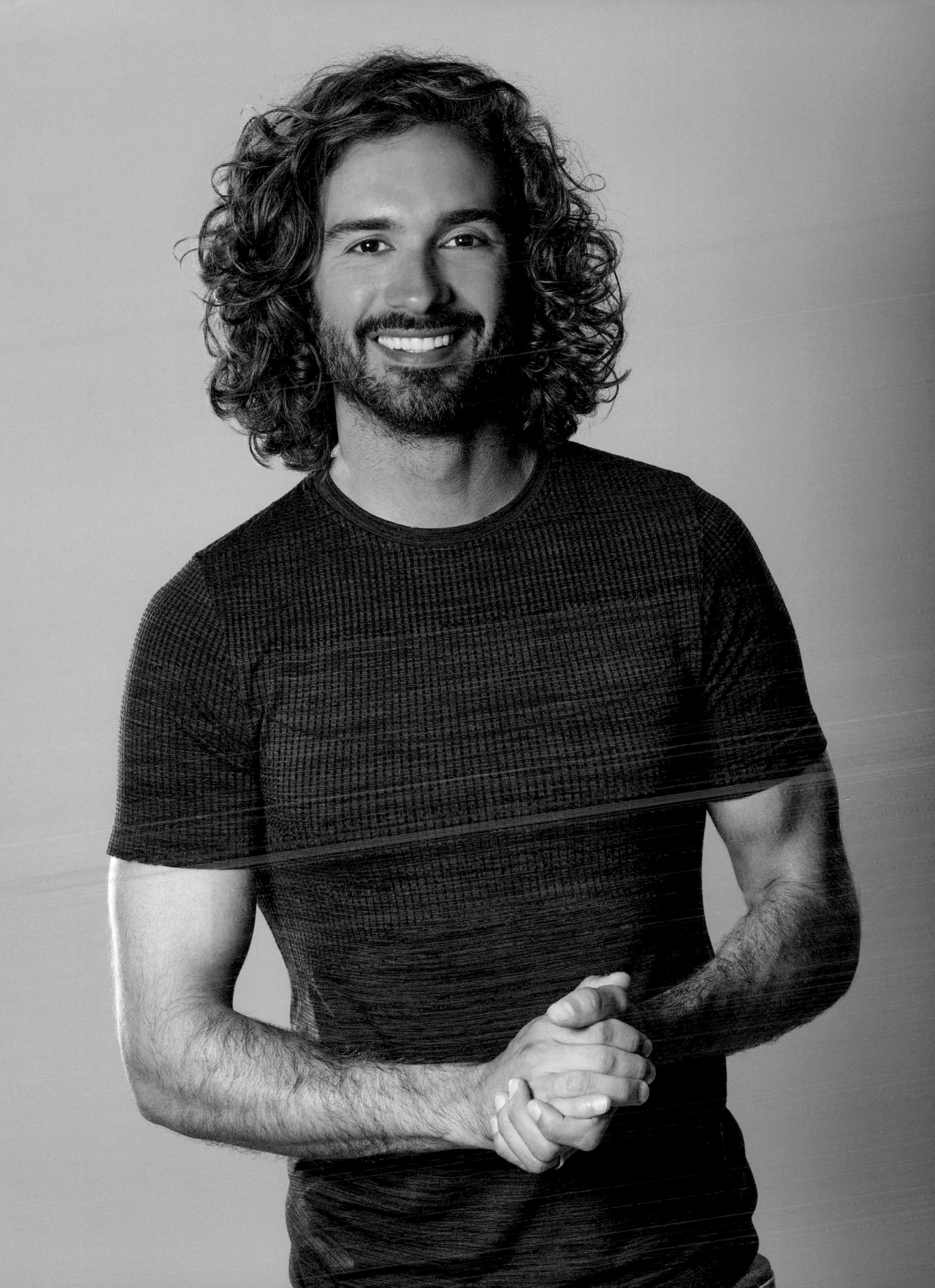

mind lasted into my early 20s. Now, at 34 and as a dad of two young kids, my motivation to exercise has changed completely. I don't worry about what other people think and I don't exercise just to look a certain way. I exercise to feel happy and positive every day, and I eat healthy food to feel energized.

I'm often asked what inspires me to exercise all year round – even on holiday, during the winter months or when I'm not getting much sleep. The answer is always the same: I exercise because it makes me feel happy. I need it in my life. It's not optional for me: it's essential, because it makes me a better person. I sleep better. I'm more productive, more energized, more ambitious. I'm more patient with my kids and I'm a better husband; I'm less stressed, calmer and nicer to be around. So for me, exercise is a daily ritual I can't go without.

With our modern lifestyles, it's now even easier to be sedentary and put on extra weight. And it seems more people than ever are becoming stressed, anxious and depressed. If you feel that way, it's time to take action. Now is the time to take the small steps to overcome what's holding you back, to allow you to live your life to the fullest. It's time for you to feel happy, strong and confident.

30 Day Kick Start Plan is going to do just that. It's going to kick start a new life for you, building healthy habits and daily routines to ensure you can succeed in the long term.

Give me just 30 days and follow this plan. Commit to it and you will feel the benefits. You are quickly going to feel more energized, happier, calmer and more motivated, and you will sleep better. This is not an extreme plan, and it's not unrealistic or unsustainable. It's a simple and achievable lifestyle change. You can tailor it according to your experience and lifestyle, whether you're new to fitness and healthy living or you've recently fallen out of your positive routine. It's about really quick and tasty home-cooked food and regular home workouts. Many people believe it takes 21 days to form a new habit, so with 30 days, you can not only form great healthy-living habits but also start to cement them for the long term. If you really stick to the **30 Day Kick Start Plan**, you will have the tools in place to unlock your happiness, control your energy and generally kick ass and feel like a winner. Are you ready to kick start your life? Are you ready to own it and be in control? Let's do it. Let's light it up. When you lose the excuses, you will find your success.

Good luck. Enjoy the journey. It's just 30 days. One day at a time.

Love, Joe

WHY 30 DAYS?

When I first started my online fitness business, I launched my 90 Day Plan, split into three cycles of 30 days each. It consists of home workouts and a tailored meal plan, and gets incredible results for those who fully commit and see it through, but I'd be lying if I said everyone who signs up goes on to complete all three cycles. These are the biggest challenges people face: motivation and consistency!

I've always offered support to get everyone who signs up to complete the plan, but unfortunately, many people still lose motivation and drop off after the first month. I've always asked myself, why does this happen? How come some people commit to it, smash it and stick it out, while others fall off the wagon right away? How can I help people change their habits and implement new ones that stick?

I made the plan 90 days because I don't believe in crash diets and quick fixes. I wanted to create a sustainable long-term plan that would get great results. Three months seemed like a manageable timeframe for people to get stuck in and not feel overwhelmed. I don't think many people would have signed up to the 'Forever Plan', even though that's what I personally see the plan as. Fitness and strength can be gained over 90 days, but in order to keep that progress and maintain it, you have to be working on it all year round, and this takes a lot of effort.

What I realize now is that motivation is strongest during the first 30 days, which is why I've decided to create this **30 Day Kick Start Plan**. During the first 30 days, people feel motivated and inspired – spurred on by the initial weight loss and increased energy as they switch from a sedentary lifestyle to an active one.

Long-term behavioural change is one of the hardest things to achieve, especially when it comes to fitness and nutrition. Years of unhealthy eating habits or neglecting regular exercise can make changes seem overwhelming. That's why I'm sharing my strategies to help keep you motivated – not just at the start of the plan but all year round (see page 26).

There are also many emotional and psychological barriers to contend with. When we are stressed, anxious, depressed or tired, our food choices can often be unhealthy. People can overeat or under-eat as a coping mechanism. We also live in an environment where there is temptation and food to grab on every corner.

Over the next 30 days, I want to unlock the potential in you. I'm not promising a radical fat-loss transformation, but that's not my gauge of success here. I'm promising that you will sleep better and have more energy, and that you'll feel happier, less stressed and more motivated every day. I want this plan to launch you into a new way of life and get you so lit that you don't want to stop. I know that you can succeed if you choose to. So, do you choose to? Are you fed up of feeling the way you do? Are you willing to work for your goals? Are you ready to commit for 30 days and not give up? Let's do it. You can change and transform your life.

LET'S GET INTO THE PSYCHOLOGY OF THINGS

I believe that in order to transform yourself physically, you need to understand yourself mentally and emotionally. It's important for you to understand what is driving you to change, what motivates you – and also what demotivates you and causes you to give up. When you understand what holds you back, you can start to acknowledge these things sooner and put strategies in place to avoid them.

I want to start by asking you a series of questions to help you dive into your motivation and learn a little bit about your psychology. It's not a test; it's just a useful and insightful exercise to help you understand yourself better. You may find it easy, or you may find it difficult and quite an emotional thing to do. Try to open up and be honest with yourself. Let any emotions and feelings surface and then you can let go of them. This exercise can help you release any negativity holding you back and allow your mind to set new, positive belief systems.

Find the questions over the page, and write down your answers in a notebook. If you prefer, you can use notes or voice notes on your phone or you can just answer the questions in your mind. All you need is 15 to 30 minutes of uninterrupted quiet time to explore the reasons why you're ready to kick start new habits.

I really hope exercise helps you think differently about your future. Change and transformation is possible with the right mindset. The answer to the last question is probably the most important of all: the answer you gave is the result you will achieve.

66 I ALWAYS FIND THIS HELPS ME TO GET ON TRACK AND I HOPE IT HELPS YOU! 99

"

I have been a yo-yo dieter
and have struggled with
anxiety and depression over
the years. But now I feel so
much stronger, happier and
healthier and I don't care
what the scales say.

The food is delicious and
I never feel like I'm missing
out. When I do have a 'treat
meal' I think your recipes are
far tastier than takeaways.
Being healthy and strong
and setting a good example
for my son is amazing.

"

DANIELLE, 31

1	Why did you pick up this book?
2	What is it you want to change in your life?
3	How long have you been wanting to change?
4	In the past, what or who has stopped you from succeeding?
5	What emotions or situations (if any) lead you to binge on food?
6	What emotions or situations (if any) lead to you under-eating or neglecting your food intake?
7	What events or experiences in your life have affected your physical or mental health?
8	Do you have any memories or negative thoughts you want to let go of?
9	When do you feel motivated?
10	What makes you feel demotivated?

11 How do you feel about your current levels of fitness?

12 How do you feel after you exercise?

13 How do you feel about your current diet?

14 What does a successful day look like to you?

15 What does an unsuccessful day look like to you?

16 How confident do you feel right now?

17 When was the last time you felt fit, happy and confident?

18 What would make you feel more confident?

19 What do you want to achieve with 30 Day Kick Start Plan?

20 Do you believe you can succeed?

WHAT DOES THE PLAN INVOLVE?

30 Day Kick Start Plan consists of four main pillars which I've found to be fundamental to success in my physical and mental health. Each pillar will be used to lay the foundations for your new lifestyle, and they are equally important. For example, poor-quality sleep or not enough sleep will affect your motivation to set goals, prepare healthy food and exercise, so putting effort into all of the following is key.

1 NUTRITION
You will have a flexible, simple, structured meal plan to follow.

2 FITNESS
You will have an exercise plan to follow at home.

3 SLEEP
You will focus on improving the quality of your sleep, which is absolutely essential to success.

4 GOAL SETTING
You will set small daily and weekly goals and learn strategies to achieve and maintain a winner's mindset each day.

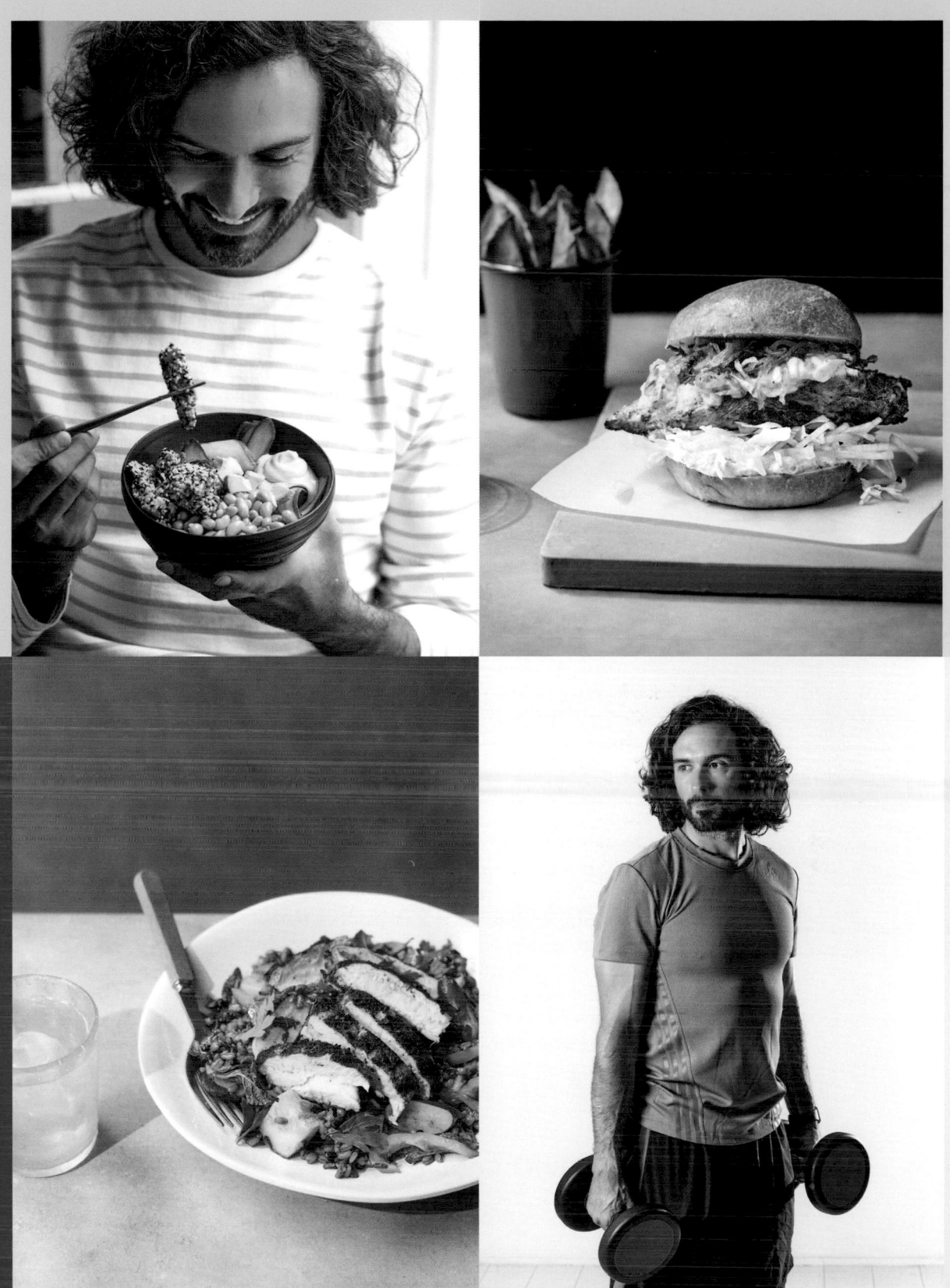

NUTRITION

Here are the fundamentals of nutrition to help you understand the rationale behind the plan. There is so much information online and it's difficult to know what is fact, so I'm sharing some simple science to explain where we get our energy from and how we burn body fat.

WHERE DO WE GET ENERGY FROM AND HOW DO WE EXPEND IT?

The human body gets its energy from three main sources: fat, protein and carbohydrates. These are called macronutrients, and each category serves an important function in the human body. A good balance of these macronutrients is optimal for health, as you'll see within the recipes in this book (see pages 30–221).

The human body expends energy through all movement and physical activity, whether you're walking, standing, carrying objects, dancing or working out. This is known as daily energy expenditure and it differs each day, in line with your activity. The majority of the energy used by the body actually goes towards maintaining essential functions such as breathing, digestion, cell production and blood transport. These are all involuntary actions which take place even at rest. This is known as basal energy expenditure.

The body must work hard to digest and process food. This is known as the thermic effect of food. Different food results in differing amounts of energy being used. Fat requires the least energy to process, followed by carbs, and protein requires the most energy to break down and utilize. This means it's a good idea to have a decent amount of protein in every meal.

WHAT CAUSES THE BODY TO GAIN OR LOSE FAT?

The human body can be seen as an engine which requires fuel to function. Our fuel is the food we eat. If you consume the same amount of energy as you expend, you will maintain the same body weight (this is known as energy maintenance). If you consume more energy than you are expending, your body will start to store excess energy as body fat (this is known as energy surplus). Finally, if you expend more energy than you consume, you will start to lose body fat, as your body will utilize stored fat for energy (this is known as energy deficit).

DO I NEED TO COUNT CALORIES?

This topic is often debated within the fitness and nutrition community and it's something I do get criticized about. I've never tracked or counted calories myself. I have no idea how much I consume each day, week or month. I do know that if I'm eating way more food than I need and not exercising consistently, I will have an energy surplus and start to gain body fat like anyone else.

This extra energy I consume has to go somewhere, and for me, it usually stores around my tummy and lower back. If I then decide I want to drop body fat, I do two things: I consume a bit less food and I expend a bit more energy through activity and exercise. This could mean skipping pudding, not drinking fizzy drinks or booze for a few weeks, snacking less in between meals and generally just focusing on healthy home cooking and smaller portion sizes at mealtimes.

I never do anything drastic. By simply removing some of those foods, I know when I increase my daily activity by going for walks, bike rides or putting 20% more effort into my workouts, I will start to tip those energy balance scales into a deficit. As a result, over time, I start to get leaner.

Of course you can lose weight by calorie counting, but you can also do it by changing your lifestyle. It comes down to your personality and what motivates you as an individual. If you are target driven, maybe calorie counting motivates you. If you already find it a challenge to balance food shopping, cooking, avoiding junk food and exercising regularly, then perhaps you could do without calorie counting. Your focus should be on daily lifestyle changes and consistency. As a by product, over time you will start to feel how much food is too much or too little for you.

HOW WILL I KNOW I'M IN AN ENERGY DEFICIT?

I believe we should eat to feel energized and eat intuitively based on our energy demands. There will be days when you're more active, and there will be days you eat more food, so the reality is you may not be in an energy deficit each day, but that's okay. Try to think about creating a small energy deficit over a week or month. This allows much more flexibility and reflects real life. Just keep it simple. If you find you are exercising consistently and using this meal plan but you're still not losing body fat, then you are not quite in an energy deficit yet. If that's the case, you can make small adjustments. Don't panic and cut things in half for a quick result because it won't be sustainable. If you feel like the portions are too large, my advice is just to reduce them a bit and see how your body responds after a week or two. Or if the portions feel too small and you feel hungry and low on energy, simply increase the portions slightly or have an extra snack during the day.

The main factor in sustainable fat loss and creating that energy deficit is simple: consistency. Consistently exercise and focus on sensible portions of home-cooked food while reducing heavily processed foods, fizzy drinks, fast food and alcohol.

HOW WILL I EAT WHILE I'M FOLLOWING THIS PLAN?

The plan breaks down into three sections: Reduced-carb meals (page 30), Post-workout meals (page 144) and Snacks (page 132). On an exercise day aim to eat two reduced-carb meals, one post-workout carb refuel meal and two snacks. On a rest day aim to eat three reduced-carb meals and two snacks.

A snack could be something from the snack section of this book, or it could be something like a piece of fruit, a handful of nuts or olives, or some peanut butter, Greek yoghurt, hummus or guacamole. I think fat-based snacks are ideal as they keep you feeling fuller for longer – and they can help stabilize blood sugar levels so you will start to lose those cravings for sugary snacks in between meals.

If at any point you feel like you need more carbs, either on your training day or your rest day, just add some more to a meal or swap a reduced-carb meal for a carb refuel meal. It's very important that you feel energized and happy with the food, so listen to your body and see how you feel day by day.

WHAT SHOULD I DO IF I HAVE A WOBBLE OR BLOWOUT?

If you do have a day where you lose all motivation, skip the exercise and just eat everything and anything in sight, know that you have not failed. You are not losing. You are just human. I have days where I feel stressed or emotional and I go on a blowout with fizzy drinks, crisps, ice cream, marmalade on toast, and burgers and chips. Trust me – when I go hard, I go hard! Afterwards, I always feel exhausted, bloated and lethargic because junk food does not make me feel good. But one thing I don't ever do is feel guilty about it. It's so important you do not let a blowout make you feel guilty or ashamed. Just acknowledge it as a day when your emotions changed, and you chose to eat more food than normal.

I never let a bad day of eating become a bad week of eating. Get back in the kitchen to prep your breakfast and lunch for the next day. Wake up and exercise, lift your energy, change your mood and move forward.

I CAN'T SEEM TO STICK TO A DIET. I ALWAYS GIVE UP.

The majority of diets focus heavily on restricting calories in order to get quick results. This is done by completely cutting out carbs or reducing fat, which may work in the short term, but for many people it soon proves to be unenjoyable and therefore unsustainable. Most diets focus on food intake but rarely emphasize the relationship between physical activity and energy expenditure, and how important it is to create that energy deficit that allows the body to burn fat.

I encourage you to enjoy generous portions of food that leave you feeling full and satisfied. I want you to fuel your body, not deprive it. I want you to eat the foods you love. I want you to enjoy treats and not feel guilty or upset with yourself. Alongside this healthier and more flexible approach to eating, I also encourage you to exercise. To walk more, to be active, to workout at home and to lift your mood each day. By being more active you will expend more energy and you will feel happier, and if you do this consistently for weeks and months, you will achieve the transformation you want. The key is to change your mindset around dieting as there is no quick solution. Extend your horizon and have a long-term vision of how you will feel in 6 months or a year if you continue to follow these principles. The only thing that guarantees results is a combination of consistency, patience and discipline.

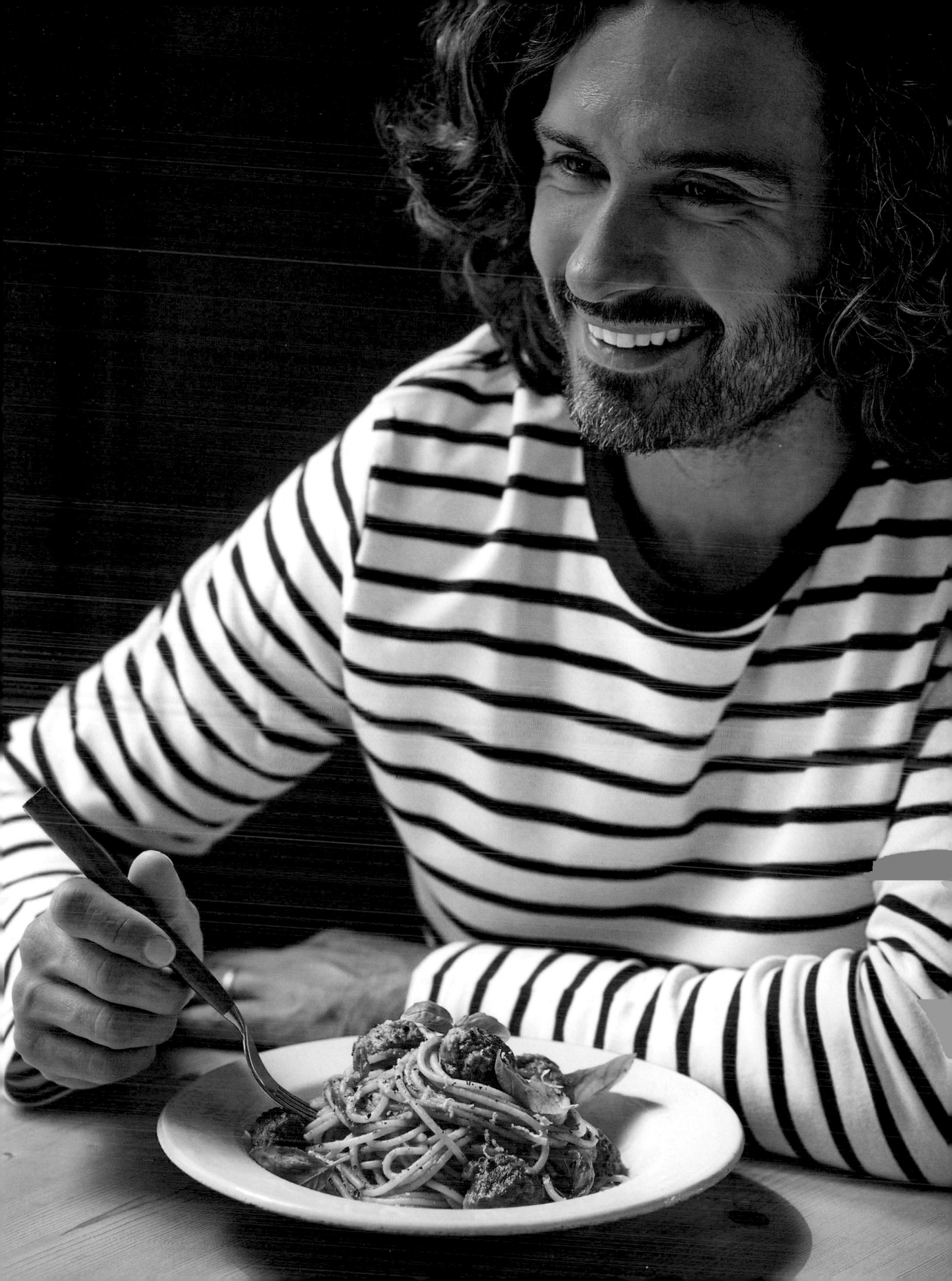

FITNESS

There are many ways you can start to increase your daily activity and energy expenditure. One thing I've learned over time is that, just like dieting, there is no perfect one-size-fits-all approach to exercise.

I've always been a huge fan of high-intensity interval training (HIIT) sessions and provide lots of these short workouts on my YouTube channel (TheBodyCoachTV). It is an effective way of getting maximum results in the shortest time possible, so it's perfect for busy people who are short on time.

What I know now is that many people don't enjoy HIIT training or are unable to do it for various reasons. HIIT is intense, sweaty, out of breath, heart-pounding exercise. Some people love it and just have it in their DNA to push themselves to the physical limits, while others find this very hard and unenjoyable.

It is more important than anything that you enjoy exercise and the feelings it gives you after you've completed it. Exercise doesn't need to be extreme to be effective. Remember all movement requires energy, so all forms of exercise are beneficial. I personally enjoy a combination of resistance training, HIIT cardio and low-intensity steady state cardio for my all-round fitness and mental health.

WHAT EXERCISE IS RIGHT FOR ME?

This plan includes a variety of options so you can pick and choose what works best for you and figure out what fits into your lifestyle. You may find that going on a long one-hour run just isn't feasible due to your work or family commitments, but doing 25 minutes of HIIT at home is possible. Your exercise method should be easy to fit into your day, accessible, enjoyable and rewarding.

HOW OFTEN SHOULD I EXERCISE?

I exercise 5 days per week and take 2 full rest days. It is very important to let the body recover and repair after training, so rest days are just as important to your overall health. My advice would be to aim for 4–5 exercise sessions per week, but if you can't always manage that, it's not a problem: do what you can. Plan your sessions into your week and block out that time. I believe 15 minutes is better than nothing, so if one day you can't do a full workout, do what you can.

THE TRAINING PLAN

I've included six home workouts in the back of the book (see page 222). There are two beginner workouts, two intermediate and two advanced. You might want to progress through them or you might prefer to stay at one level for a while. Find what is right for you.

TYPES OF TRAINING

1	HIIT (HIGH-INTENSITY INTERVAL TRAINING)

HIIT (high-intensity interval training): This consists of short bursts of maximal effort, followed by a rest period and repeated multiple times. For example, 30 seconds doing mountain climbers and 30 seconds rest, repeated four times. The aim of this type of training is to push as hard as you can to elevate your heart rate as much as possible during the working sets. This workout should be at a high intensity throughout and would typically last from 15–30 minutes in total duration.

2	RESISTANCE (WEIGHT TRAINING)

Resistance (weight training): This form of training involves increasing your strength and lean muscle by loading the muscles with weight. This can be achieved by loading the muscles with just your own body weight, but to be most effective it's important to build the load progressively and challenge the muscles with weight. Equipment such as barbells, dumbbells, cable machines, kettle bells or resistance bands can all be used to add resistance.

3	LISS (LOW-INTENSITY STEADY STATE)

LISS (low-intensity steady state) cardio: This consists of less-intense, longer periods of continuous exercise. For example, walking, jogging, cycling, rowing or swimming for 30 minutes or more.

SLEEP

The moment my wife Rosie and I had our second baby, Marley, was the first time I truly felt the negative effects of sleep deprivation and broken sleep on my own physical health. In those early weeks I found it hard to train consistently and with the same intensity. I always made the effort to do something, even if only a 20-minute power walk to clear my mind, but I definitely found it harder to stay lean, fit and emotionally strong.

It's no surprise that 90% of people who suffer from depression also have poor sleep. The link between sleep, exercise and depression is clear, which means it's very important to work on the health of your sleep as well as your body.

If you can, keep a regular sleep routine and think about your sleeping environment. Is it as peaceful, relaxing and clutter free as it can be? Listening to guided meditations can be a great way to help you fall asleep. Turning off devices and winding down earlier in the evening can make a huge difference to your day and week. You could also try using an app that dims the brightness of your phone or laptop screen at certain times in the evening to minimize blue light, which will give your eyes a rest and help you get ready for a peaceful night's sleep.

A good night's sleep means you wake up refreshed and energized, with the ability to exercise effectively. You will also have the energy to prepare your own food so you don't have to rely on processed foods to get you through the day. Your mood will improve, you will be more patient and understanding with others and it also allows you to be more productive at work. So sleep really is the magic ingredient after which all the other good stuff will follow.

GOAL SETTING

Goal setting is a powerful tool to help with your motivation. Even realizing the smallest of goals can result in a big sense of achievement, which only grows stronger each day and increases your motivation.

Having said that, it's very important to set achievable and realistic goals which are not just based on body image or weight. If goals are unrealistic and your expectations are too high, you're less likely to achieve them, which can be really detrimental to your progress. The last thing you want is to feel disheartened by not achieving something, as this could lead to you wanting to give up altogether.

A short-term achievable goal could be 'today I am not going to drink fizzy drinks or alcohol, I'll just drink water' or 'I am going to go to bed an hour earlier every night this week'. All of these little wins really do add up and make a massive difference over a month or year.

Goals become even more powerful and meaningful when you write them down or say them out loud. Use the notes or voice notes on your phone or go old school and write your daily and weekly goals on post-it notes around the house. Come back to them to remind yourself of what you want to achieve.

LIFESTYLE CHOICES TO GIVE YOU A BOOST

There are always going to be little choices you can make along the way to help you stick to the plan and avoid stepping backwards. Here are just a few pointers to consider.

ALCOHOL CONSUMPTION: IS IT HOLDING YOU BACK FROM SUCCEEDING?

This section may not apply to you if you don't drink alcohol but I think it's important to include for those who do. Alcohol is something people enjoy in different ways, quantities and frequencies. I love a gin and tonic myself! But if you are exercising and eating well, alcohol could be the one thing holding you back from getting lean and fit. Here's why.

Firstly, alcohol in any form contains calories and it's easy to consume a lot in a short period of time. Guilty as charged! The calories in alcohol offer no useful nutrition for the body so they can be described as empty calories.

The body is also unable to store alcohol, which means it has to convert it to energy and get rid of it immediately. During this time the body basically puts the brakes on burning fat and prioritizes the metabolism of alcohol until it's out of your system.

Alcohol also increases your appetite which means you consume far more food on the nights you drink. Does anyone else find themselves eating six crumpets with butter before bed after a night on the sauce? It also hugely dehydrates you and you wake up hungover, craving carbohydrates and as much junk you can get your hands on.

Alongside the obvious energy intake associated with a boozy night out, there are also the detrimental side effects on your energy output. When I'm hungover, I personally really struggle to move the next day and usually don't get back into full training until 2 days later. It also makes me feel awful and emotional and I lose all motivation to eat healthily and exercise. This means a weekend of alcohol can set you back massively and undo a whole week of hard work. So the question is, over this next 30 days, how much do you want to transform? How much do you want that drink? Do you want that hangover and to miss a couple of days training? Or do you want to give your body a chance to make progress and your mind a chance to wake up clear, focused and alert?

HYDRATION: WHY IS IT SO IMPORTANT?

Good hydration is essential for optimal health, digestion, fat loss and energy. Many people struggle to drink enough water throughout the day. My advice is to invest in a good reusable metal water bottle which keeps your water fresh and cold. By carrying it with you at all times you are far more likely to drink regularly and fill it up a few times each day.

A hydrated body is more efficient at burning body fat, so aim to drink 2–4 litres per day. Water can help suppress the urge to snack and graze – this is important as most of the time you are likely to be thirsty, not hungry. Another key thing to remember is that drinking more water means you are less likely to consume calories from other drinks such as coffee, milk, juice, sodas, alcohol and so on. This is a very good thing because you are trying to create an energy deficit, so it's better to eat your calories and feel full than drink your calories and still feel hungry afterwards.

Hydration also helps with your digestion, so when you drink plenty of water, you can feel less bloated and tired.

THE BENEFITS OF MEDITATION

Do you have a busy mind? Do thoughts, ideas and worries run through your head at a million miles per hour before bed or first thing when you wake up in the morning? That's what happens to me, and if you feel the same, I really believe meditation can help change your life.

For years, several people close to me tried to encourage me to meditate. I downloaded a few guided meditation apps and gave it a go, but I found It so difficult to sit and focus on the meditation that I always gave up. I told myself I couldn't be mindful. I thought I couldn't feel present, that I was no good at meditating and it wasn't for me. It took a chat with Russell Brand on his podcast 'Under The Skin' for me to give it a proper go. He said to me, 'Joe, I really think meditation could be wonderful and powerful for you if you give it a try.' So I committed to doing 20 minutes of guided meditation every day for 2 weeks – and no lie, it changed my life.

For the first time in years, I put my phone down, I slowed down, I breathed and I let myself go to a place of calm and peaceful presence I'd never been to before. I just searched '20-minute guided meditation' on YouTube and randomly chose a new one each day. Some talk you through learning to be present, to be positive, to feel gratitude or to let go of negativity. Meditating allowed me to slow my busy mind down for the first time ever and think about things I'd never thought about.

To be honest, I don't do it consistently, 7 days a week, and I don't always enjoy it. I do it about 3–4 days a week, which I feel is perfect for me. Some days I do it and I can't stand it, and I spend the whole time frustrated and wishing for it to finish. But other days, I'll learn something new about myself or feel more connected, and it's just amazing when you have those little breakthroughs and moments of growth.

I genuinely can't recommend it enough. It's one of those skills which you get better at over time – just like learning to cook or exercise. The more you do it, the more experience you get and the more you get out of it. It can help you let go of past memories, trauma or any negativity you feel about yourself or the world.

HOW TO GET STARTED

I like to follow apps or YouTube tutorials, but if you're a complete beginner, a really simple thing is to spend time focusing on your breath. It can instantly calm and release any tension you're holding in your body.

- **To give it a go, make yourself as comfortable as you can, whether you're sitting on a chair, on the floor or lying on your back.**

- **Relax your shoulders and let your hands hang loose at your sides, in your lap or on your knees.**

- **Close your eyes and start to deepen your breath, without forcing it. If you can, breathe in through your nose and out through your mouth, gently and regularly.**

- **Gradually start to lengthen your breath, counting to five on the inhale and five on the exhale. Try this for 3–5 minutes and see if you can focus your mind on the simple act of breathing.**

How do you feel afterwards? Did you manage to keep your mind clear of distractions? It might take practice to start with, but the more regularly you try it, the easier it will be and the more transformative it can feel.

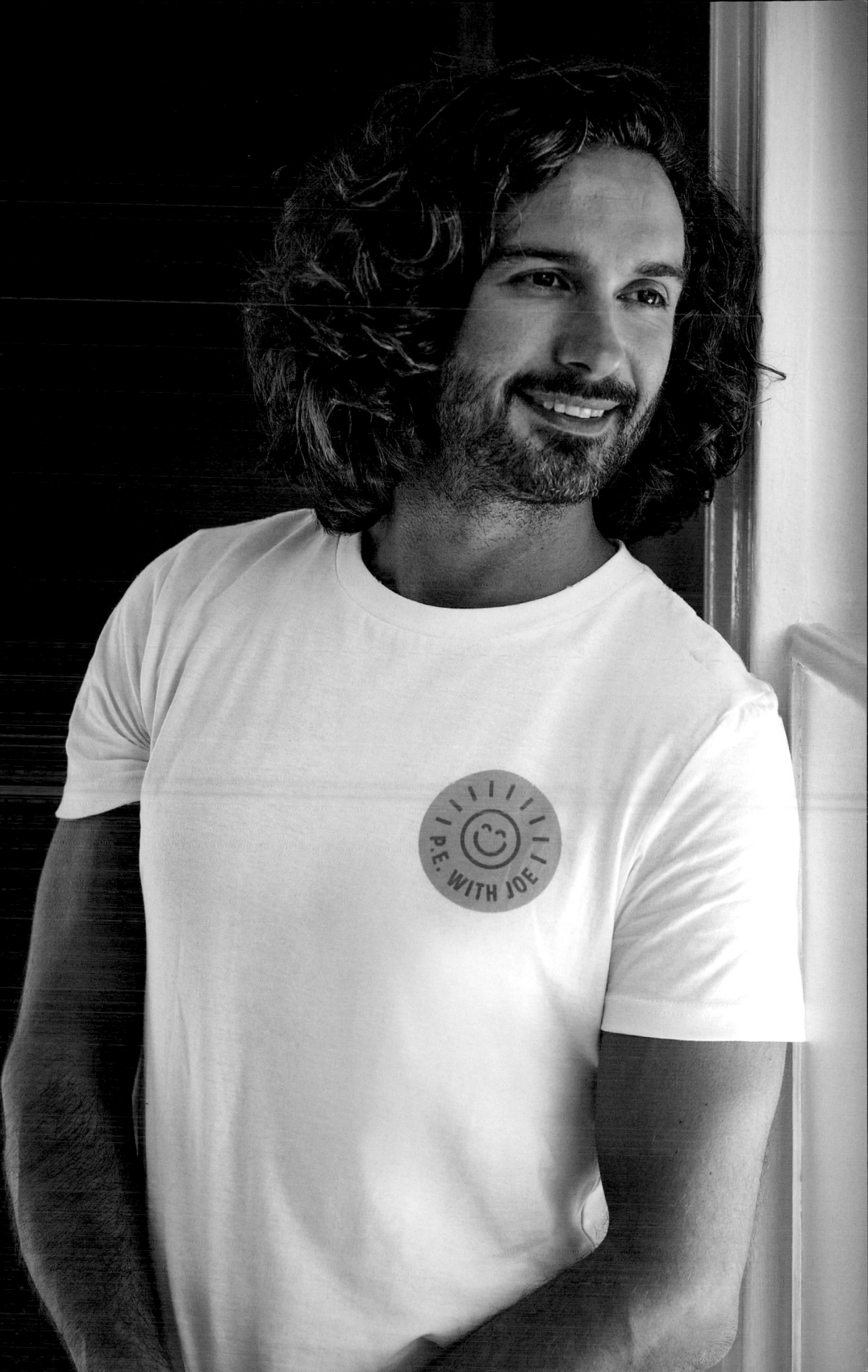

KEEPING MOTIVATED

Here are my tips for staying motivated and tracking progress on the plan. These techniques are key to keeping going and jumping back on the wagon even when the going gets tough.

1 | MIND OVER MATTER

There are two main types of messages I get from people on social media. The first is from someone who has completed one of my plans: they've achieved their goals and they're feeling great.

The second is from someone who is thinking about making a change, but they lack motivation. They believe they don't have the time to exercise or cook healthy meals. This is what some people tell themselves, but it's the first thing that has to change. It's a limiting belief: if that's your approach, you've already decided you can't make a change. Getting rid of that mental barrier will free you from this whole mindset. Instead of thinking 'I can't do it', begin by thinking 'I can, and I will'.

Lots of people know they want to change but lack the motivation to do it. If you're someone who struggles with motivation, don't sit around waiting for it to come – that day may never arrive. What you need to do is take action. Get up and commit yourself to a workout in the morning and see how you feel afterwards. Most people take the view that motivation leads to action. But I believe it's the opposite. Action leads to motivation, and that leads to more motivation!

2 | HEALTHY HABITS

Having some structure to your routine leads to habits forming. And when healthy habits become second nature, you're definitely on the right track. Because that's what this book is all about: we're going to start something new, and at the end of 30 days, you'll want to continue with it. Once you're in the habit of eating healthily, working out and getting enough sleep, you've got the key foundations of a healthier lifestyle that you'll stick with.

3 | KEEPING A JOURNAL

Lots of my clients say that keeping a journal can really help them stay motivated and accountable. Give it a go and see if it helps you. Take a few minutes at the end of every day to write down how your day went. What did you achieve and how did you do it? If you had a bad day, write about what went wrong and how you got through it. How do you feel at the end of your day? Are you proud that you've spent another day committing yourself to change? Are you re-energized by that workout you did? If you don't like writing, make a video diary or use voice notes on your phone.

Recording your daily progress gives you something to look back at when you're feeling demotivated or having a wobble. It also helps to acknowledge your wins and how they made you feel, as this changes your attitude towards exercising and eating more healthily.

4 | CHANGES THAT LAST

We all know that if you slip back into bad habits, all your progress will begin to unravel. That's why diets don't work. You starve yourself for a month, grit your teeth, carry on – and then you're free! All those bad habits return because you're just so grateful not to be miserable anymore. A few months down the line, you're back to where you started. But it's not supposed to be like that. It has to lead to permanent change.

By setting out your goals, you'll always know what you are aiming for. Getting into the right mindset lets you focus on what you can achieve. Putting that structure in place makes it easy for you to stay on the right path. Then, once the structure is set up, a routine begins to form, and healthy habits are made. When exercising and eating healthily becomes a habit, you've successfully built into your life the change you needed.

5 | MASTER YOUR MOTIVATION

I've always said that one of the best motivation tools is progress pictures. Those photos can't lie, but the mirror can. Take a picture of yourself, front and side on, at the beginning of your 30 days and then another at the end. Take a few more during the journey if you want, and don't get tempted to weigh yourself on the scales, or the 'sad step', as I call them.

The hardest part of getting fit is getting started and you'll never be more motivated than you are right now. Through these 30 days your motivation will go up and down. That's fine, it's only natural.

A good idea is to record a little video message on your phone. Lots of my clients do this and find it really helpful. Record a message to yourself and tell yourself a few things: why this was so important to you, why have you started this journey to a healthier life, and what the outcome means to you. Later, every time you feel a wobble coming on, pull out your phone and watch your own personal pep talk.

6 | BUDDY UP

Having others around who are going through the same thing always helps. You pick each other up when you're having a bad day and can celebrate together when you reach your milestones. It also gives you someone that you don't want to let down. You might find it harder to give up when you have to explain it to someone else.

Research has shown that motivation to exercise increases if you work out with others. Find out if your family want to join in. If you live by yourself, there might be a friend who also wants to kick start a change. There are also plenty of support groups out there, if you have a look for them online or at a local gym or leisure centre.

If you don't have someone in your house to exercise with, start a fitness WhatsApp group with some friends or family. You don't have to be together to exercise together. Set a time to start a workout, video call if you want, or just check in with them at the beginning and end of your workouts. You don't have to do this alone and there's power in doing it with others.

7 | TURNING SET BACKS INTO COME BACKS

We've all been there. You wake up, you just want to go back to sleep and all motivation has gone out the window. Every time you feel a wobble coming on, go back to that piece of paper or voice note with your daily or weekly goals on it (see page 21). Think again about the person you wanted to meet at the end of the 30 days. Remember why you started this plan in the first place. What was so important to you at that time? Has that changed now? I bet that the answer will be 'no'. It's time to get up and try a workout or a walk. All those lovely endorphins will help lift your mood and give you a great chance to turn your day around. Just focus on today, don't worry about next week. Get an early night if you can. When you wake up tomorrow, congratulate yourself on sticking with your commitment to make a change. Everyone has bad days. But what's important is to recognize each one for what it is: just a bad day.

We all need a social life as well. But don't let a night out end your chance to change. Your social life and fitness life should be in harmony. Maintain that balance and get back on track after a night out. You don't have to sacrifice one for the other.

8 | YOUR SUPER SUPPORT SYSTEM

What resources do you have to help you get started? You've got this book, but what else? If you have a good look around, you'll find other things as well. Look for supportive family members or friends, join an online group, write a journal or find an exercise buddy. Tell people about what you're planning on doing, share it on social media or blog about it if you can. Let people know that you've made a commitment to change. Update them on your progress and share your photos if you want. All this will help you keep on track. Sharing your decision to change, and the journey, will help you stay motivated and will make you less likely to veer off track. People will want to know how you're getting on, and by making a public commitment, you will strengthen your support system.

9 | PREP LIKE A BOSS

Another key to success is adding some structure to your day. Lots of my clients like to do their workouts in the morning, as then they know it's done for the day. I think training first thing in the morning can be truly transformative to your life. I find that training early wakes you up, gets you energized and helps you make better food choices throughout the day.

Last thing at night, set your alarm clock a bit earlier – I call it winners o'clock – and put your gym clothes out. You should feel your energy levels rising after the first few days and you'll be able to cope with an earlier start. If you're really struggling to get up in the morning, put your alarm on the other side of the room the night before (that way, you have to get up). If you can't train in the mornings or prefer evenings, that's fine. Aim to exercise at whatever time of day suits you, which should also be when you feel you have the most energy.

Decide which days are best for your workouts, and then you'll know what sort of meals you'll be eating each day. Take some time on a Sunday to choose what meals you're going to make the following week. Get your weekly shop sorted, so there's no chance of you being unable to make a meal. Block out a slot of time to prep your food, and batch-cook meals when you can. I've created the recipes so the meals are easy to make, and if you put the prep in, you won't be tempted to stray off plan during the week.

10 | KEEP LEARNING

For some of you, this might be the first time you've really thought about your fitness or health. For others, you may have achieved your goals in the past but want to set new ones. Whatever stage you're at, there is always more to learn. I spend a lot of time reading about new health and fitness studies that either strengthen what I knew before or lead me to ask more questions. You might find during these 30 days that you take a real interest in nutrition and want to know more about how the body's digestive system works, or what its daily requirements are. Or, you might decide you really like running and want to find out more about training for a 10k. Maybe you started to enjoy cooking and want to learn which flavours complement each other so you can start freestyling your meals when the 30 days are over. Whatever it is that pulls your attention, nurture it and let it become a passion – because the key to a long-term, healthy lifestyle is to enjoy what you are doing.

11 | STAY IN TOUCH

Don't forget to come back to these pages whenever you need a boost of encouragement or motivation. These are tools and ideas that can keep you on track and will help you beyond the first 30 days. Throughout the book, you will also find fantastic inspirational stories from members of my online community. I love nothing more than finding out how you're getting on, so please keep in touch and let me know how the first 30 days are going! Everything is so much easier when we support each other. You can do this!

INSTAGRAM @thebodycoach
TWITTER @thebodycoach
FACEBOOK @JoeWicksTheBodyCoach
YOUTUBE The Body Coach TV

REDUCED CARB

INGREDIENTS

2 large handfuls of mixed
    frozen berries
2 tbsp peanut butter
1 scoop (30g) vanilla protein
    powder
250ml almond milk

PBJ SMOOTHIE

Put all the ingredients in a blender and blitz until smooth. Add a splash of water if the smoothie is a little thick for your liking.

INGREDIENTS

1 medium ripe banana,
    roughly chopped
2 tbsp almond butter
250ml almond milk
1 pitted date
big pinch of cinnamon
big pinch of ginger

CHAI SPICED BANANA SMOOTHIE

 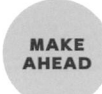

Put all the ingredients in a blender and blitz until smooth. Pour into a glass and top with a pinch more cinnamon and ginger.

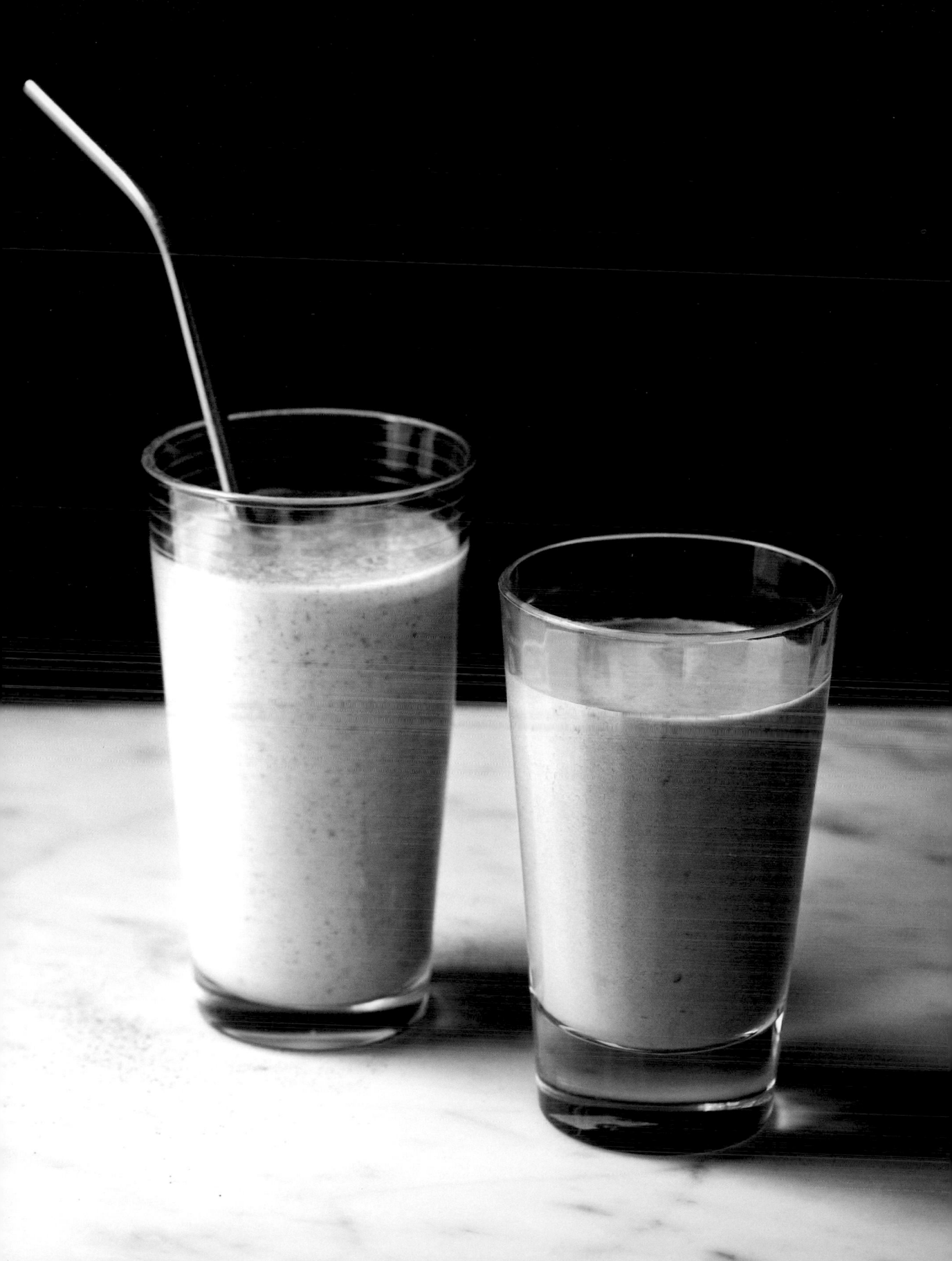

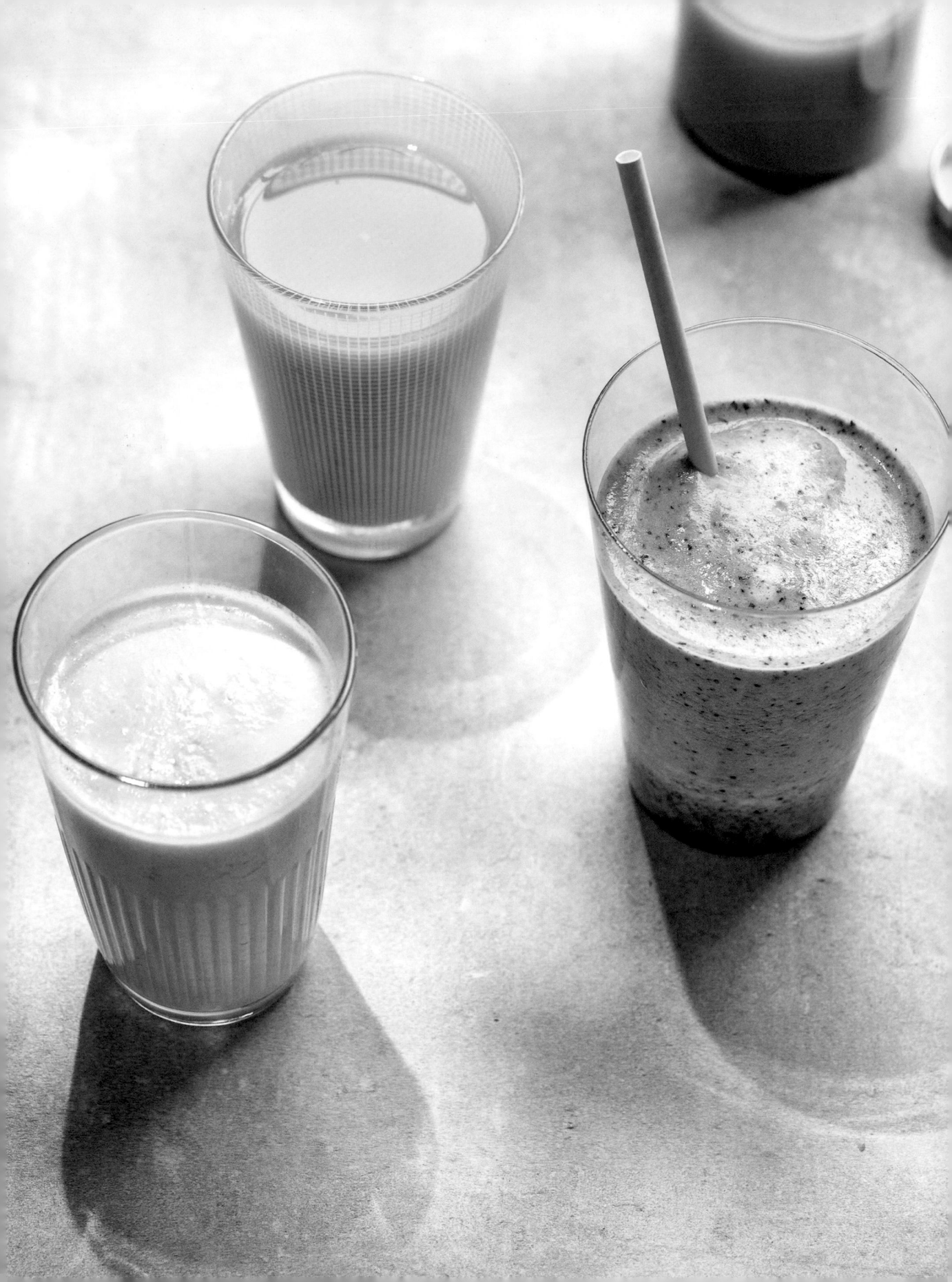

GOLDEN SMOOTHIE

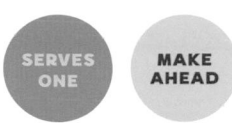

INGREDIENTS

1 medium ripe banana, roughly chopped
½ tsp ground turmeric
2 large handfuls of mango chunks
small piece of fresh ginger, peeled and roughly chopped
3 tbsp Greek yoghurt

Put all in the ingredients in a blender along with 200ml water and blitz until smooth.

BLUEBERRY SMOOTHIE

 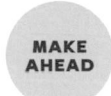

INGREDIENTS

2 large handfuls of frozen blueberries
handful of baby spinach leaves
½ avocado, de-stoned and flesh scooped out
squeeze of lemon juice
1 scoop (30g) vanilla protein powder
250ml almond milk

Put all the ingredients in a blender and blitz until smooth.

CARROT, ORANGE AND GINGER SMOOTHIE

 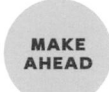

INGREDIENTS

1 medium ripe banana, roughly chopped
1 large carrot, peeled and sliced
small piece of fresh ginger, peeled and roughly chopped
big pinch of cayenne pepper
250ml orange juice

Put all the ingredients into a blender and blitz until smooth. Serve with a pinch of cayenne pepper sprinkled on top.

INGREDIENTS

4 rashers of streaky bacon
   (120g)
2 small ripe bananas
2 eggs
2 heaped tbsp peanut butter
½ tsp ground cinnamon
big pinch of baking powder
salt
10g butter
drizzle of maple syrup – optional

ELVIS PANCAKES

SERVES
ONE

1. Preheat your grill to maximum.

2. Lay the rashers of bacon on a baking tray lined with baking parchment. Slide under the hot grill. Cook for about 4 minutes on each side, or until done to your liking. I like my bacon crispy on the outside but still a little soft.

3. Meanwhile using a fork, mash the bananas in a bowl into a rough puree. Crack in the eggs, spoon in 1 tablespoon peanut butter, sprinkle in the cinnamon, baking powder and a pinch of salt. Give everything a good stir. Pancake batter sorted.

4. Melt the butter in a large non-stick frying pan over a low to medium heat. Once bubbling, spoon the batter into the pan to make 4–6 pancakes. Fry the pancakes without moving them for 3 minutes on the first side, or until the batter has set, then flip and fry the pancakes for a further minute on the second side.

5. While the pancakes are gently frying, mix the remaining peanut butter with ½ tablespoon water in a small bowl. This will loosen it, making it easier to drizzle on the pancakes.

6. Pile the banana pancakes onto a plate. Top with the bacon, drizzle over the peanut butter along with a little maple syrup, if you like. Gobble down, Elvis-style.

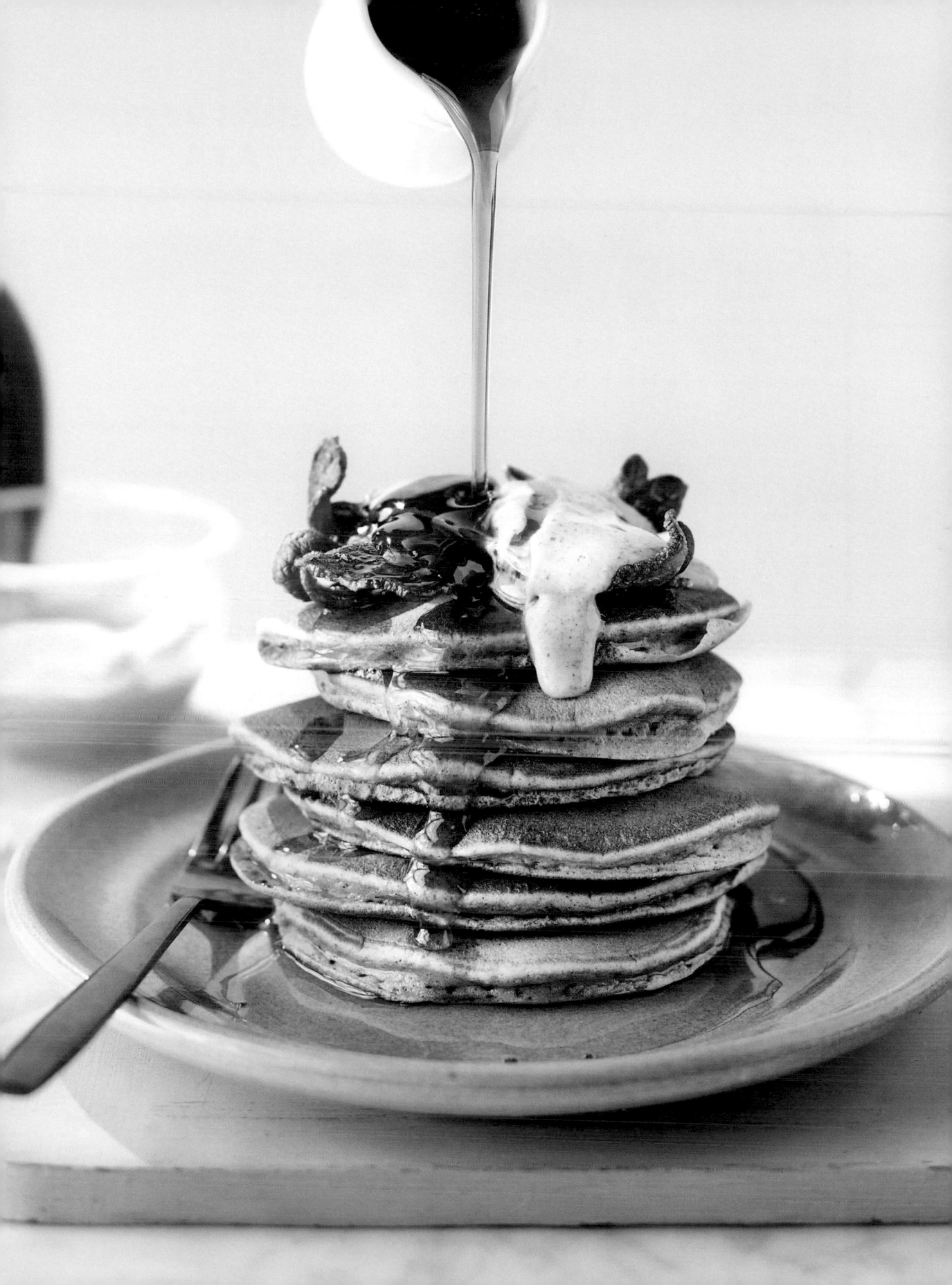

INGREDIENTS

1 red onion
20g butter
3 eggs
1 tbsp milk
salt and pepper
8 pitted mixed olives,
    roughly chopped
handful of parsley,
    roughly chopped
1 tbsp chilli jam, plus extra to
    serve – optional
30g manchego cheese, grated
rocket salad, to serve

*** YOU COULD DOUBLE THE RECIPE
AND KEEP THE SECOND COOLED
FRITTATA COVERED IN THE FRIDGE
FOR THE NEXT DAY.**

MANCHEGO, CHILLI JAM AND OLIVE FRITTATA

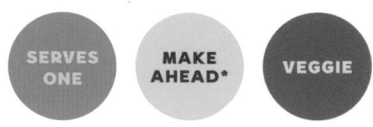

1. Preheat the grill to maximum.

2. Finely slice the red onion.

3. Melt the butter in a small non-stick ovenproof frying pan over a medium heat. Once bubbling, chuck in the sliced onion along with a pinch of salt. Cook, stirring occasionally, for 5 minutes until the onion is collapsed.

4. Crack the eggs into a jug. Whisk well with a fork until the white and yolk combine, pour in the milk and season with a generous pinch of salt and pepper. Whisk again.

5. Come back to the onion. Scrape the olives and parsley into the pan. Pour in the egg mixture and swirl the pan so that it coats the entire base. Dot in the chilli jam and scatter over the manchego cheese.

6. Cook for 3 minutes until the frittata is mostly set, then slide under the grill for 2–3 minutes until puffed up and golden. Serve with a rocket salad and more chilli jam, if you like.

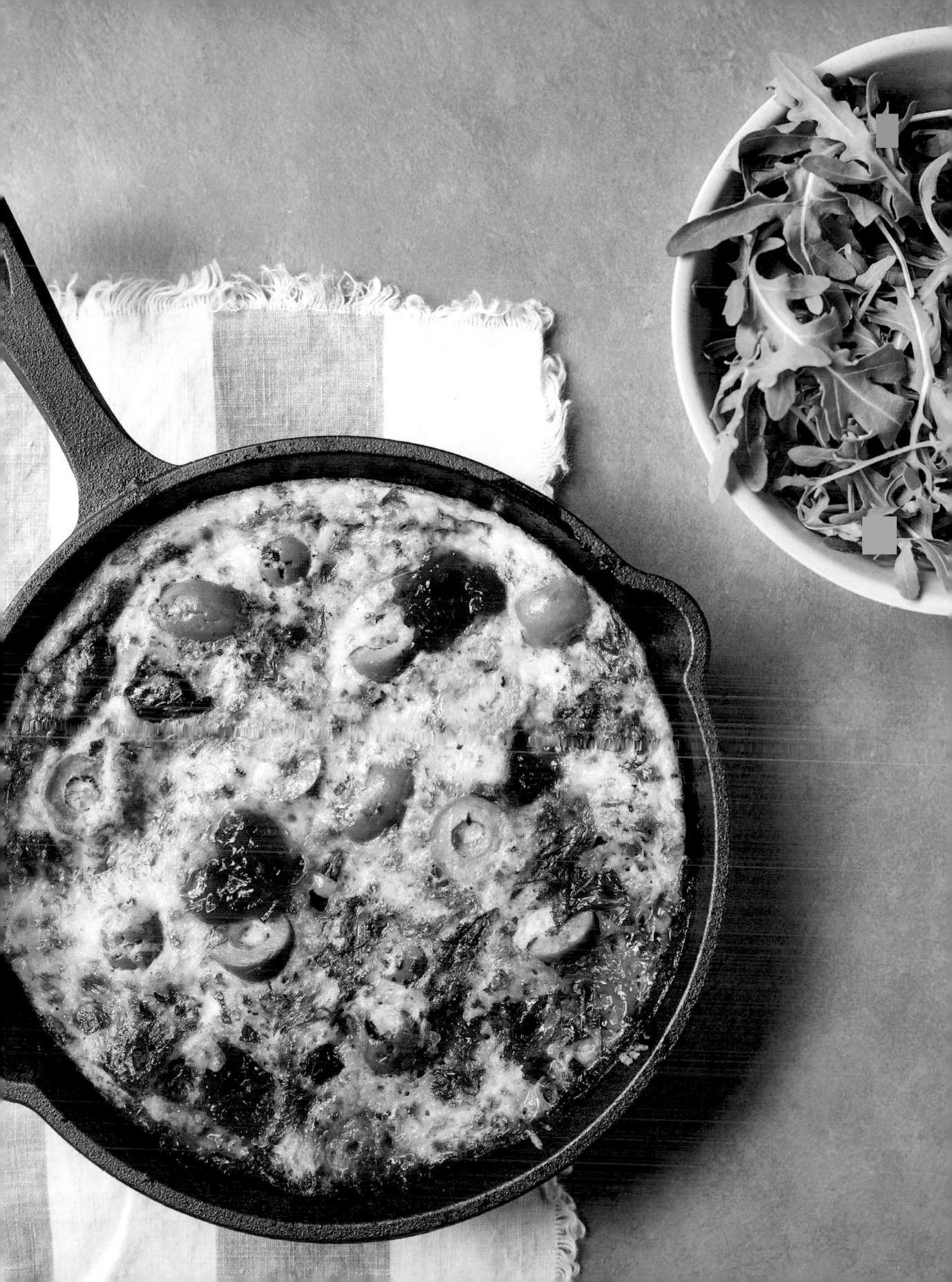

INGREDIENTS

1 small onion
1 green pepper
20g butter
2 medium ripe tomatoes
handful of parsley
3 eggs
salt and pepper
½ tsp smoked paprika
big pinch of dried oregano
½ tsp dried chilli flakes, plus
    extra to serve
30g feta
toasted pitta – optional

SPICY TURKISH SCRAMBLED EGGS

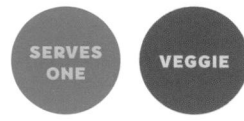

SERVES ONE

VEGGIE

1. Finely chop the onion and green pepper.

2. Melt the butter in a non-stick frying pan over a medium heat. Once bubbling, scrape in the onion and pepper. Cook for 5 minutes, stirring occasionally, until softened.

3. Meanwhile chop the tomatoes and parsley. Crack the eggs into a jug, whisk well with a fork until the white and yolk combine and season with a generous pinch of salt and pepper.

4. Come back to the onion and pepper. Chuck in the chopped tomatoes and most of the parsley along with the smoked paprika, dried oregano and chilli flakes. Cook for 2 minutes then pour in the eggs.

5. Softly scramble the eggs with the other ingredients, drawing the cooked egg from the edges into the middle until the egg is just cooked.

6. Dish up the eggs, crumble over the feta and remaining parsley. Scatter over a few chilli flakes to serve. If you are extra-hungry, eat with a toasted pitta for scooping.

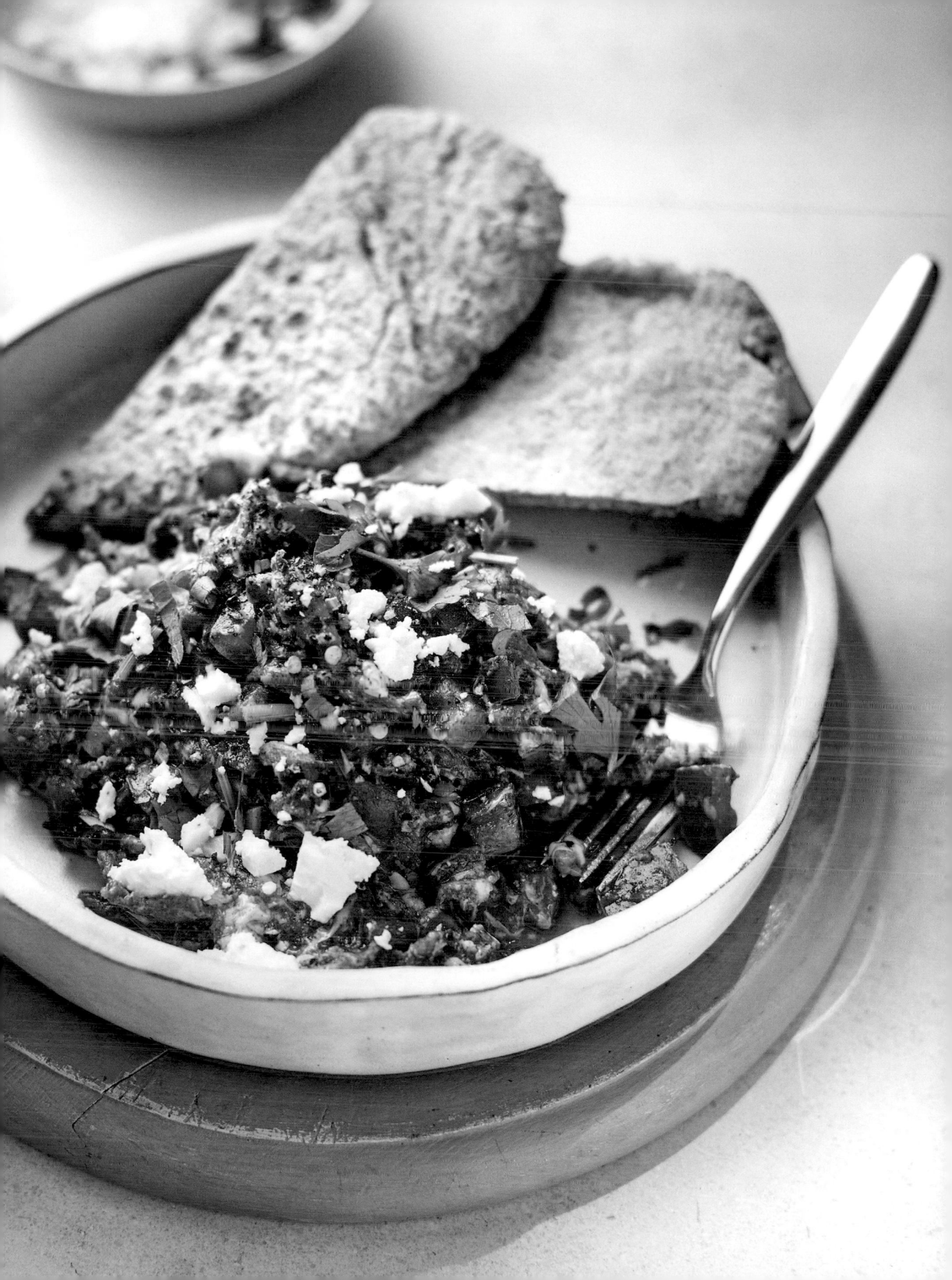

INGREDIENTS

1 x 200g skinless chicken
    breast fillet
drizzle of olive oil
salt and pepper
50g butter
small handful of sage
1 clove garlic
100g asparagus tips
100g frozen peas
pinch of dried chilli flakes
juice of ½ lemon
green salad, to serve

SAGE BUTTER CHICKEN WITH LEMONY SPRING GREENS

SERVES ONE

1. Place the chicken between two pieces of cling film or baking parchment on a chopping board. Using a rolling pin, meat mallet or any other blunt instrument, bash the chicken until it is about 1cm thick all over. Drizzle the chicken breast with a little olive oil, rubbing it into the flesh, and season with salt and pepper.

2. Melt 15g of the butter in a non-stick frying pan over a medium to high heat. When bubbling, carefully lay the chicken in the pan and fry for about 4 minutes.

3. Meanwhile pick the sage leaves and finely chop the garlic clove. When the chicken has had 4 minutes, flip it and fry for a further 4 minutes while you cook the greens.

4. Put the asparagus in a microwaveable bowl. Season with salt and pepper. Cover and zap on high for 2 minutes. Chuck in the peas and cook for a further 2 minutes until tender.

5. Come back to the chicken. Melt the remaining butter into the frying pan, add the sage leaves, chopped garlic and chilli flakes. Cook for 1 minute more, stirring, until the sage leaves are crisp. Take the pan off the heat; by now the chicken will be cooked through. Check by slicing into a thicker part to make sure the meat is white all the way through, with no raw pink bits left. Using a slotted spoon, remove the chicken and sage leaves onto a serving plate.

6. Put the frying pan back on a high heat. Chuck in the asparagus and peas. Cook for 30 seconds more until the veg is warmed through, then squeeze over the lemon juice. Pile the veg onto the plate alongside the chicken and spoon over all those unreal buttery juices. Serve with a green salad.

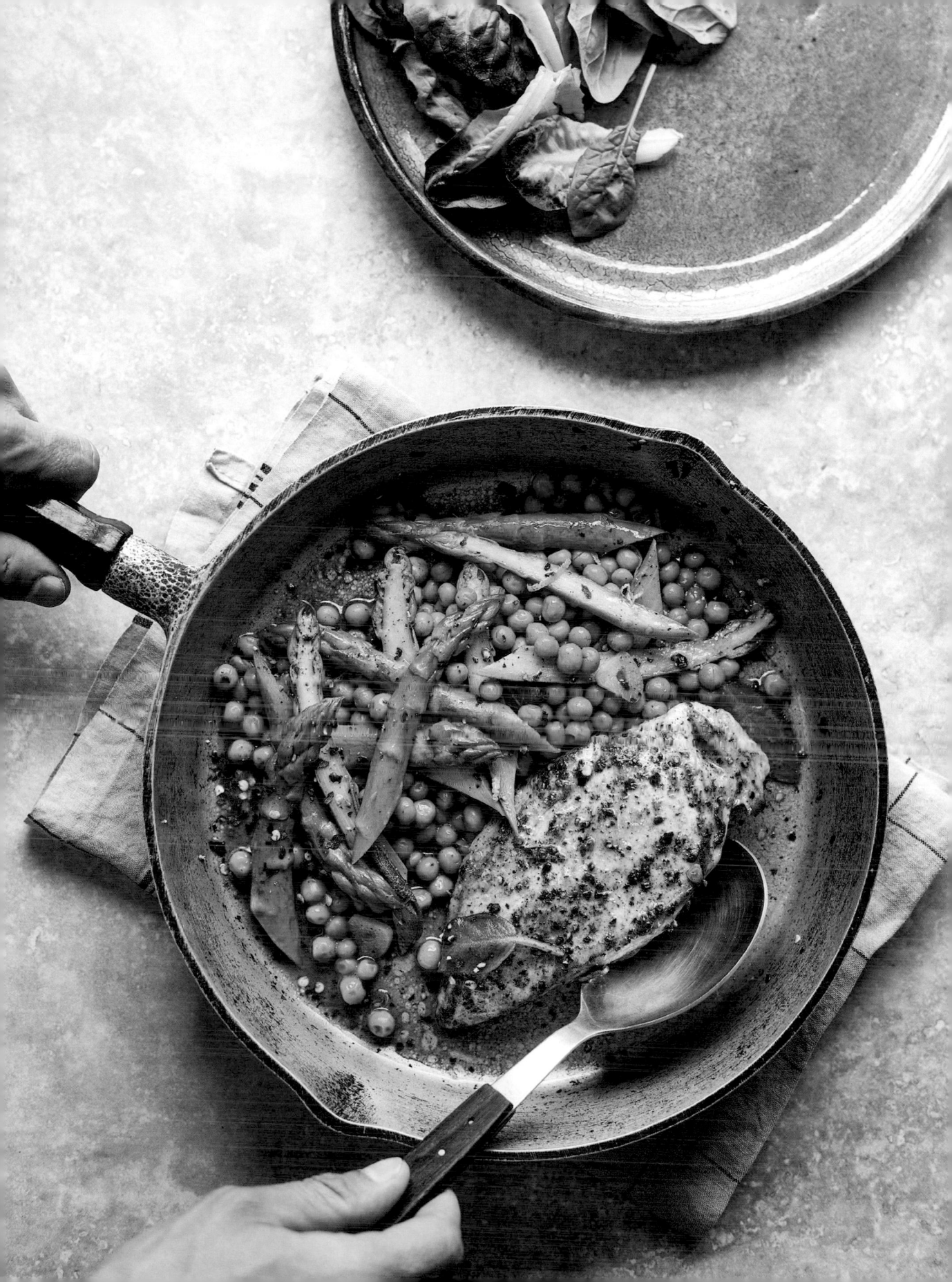

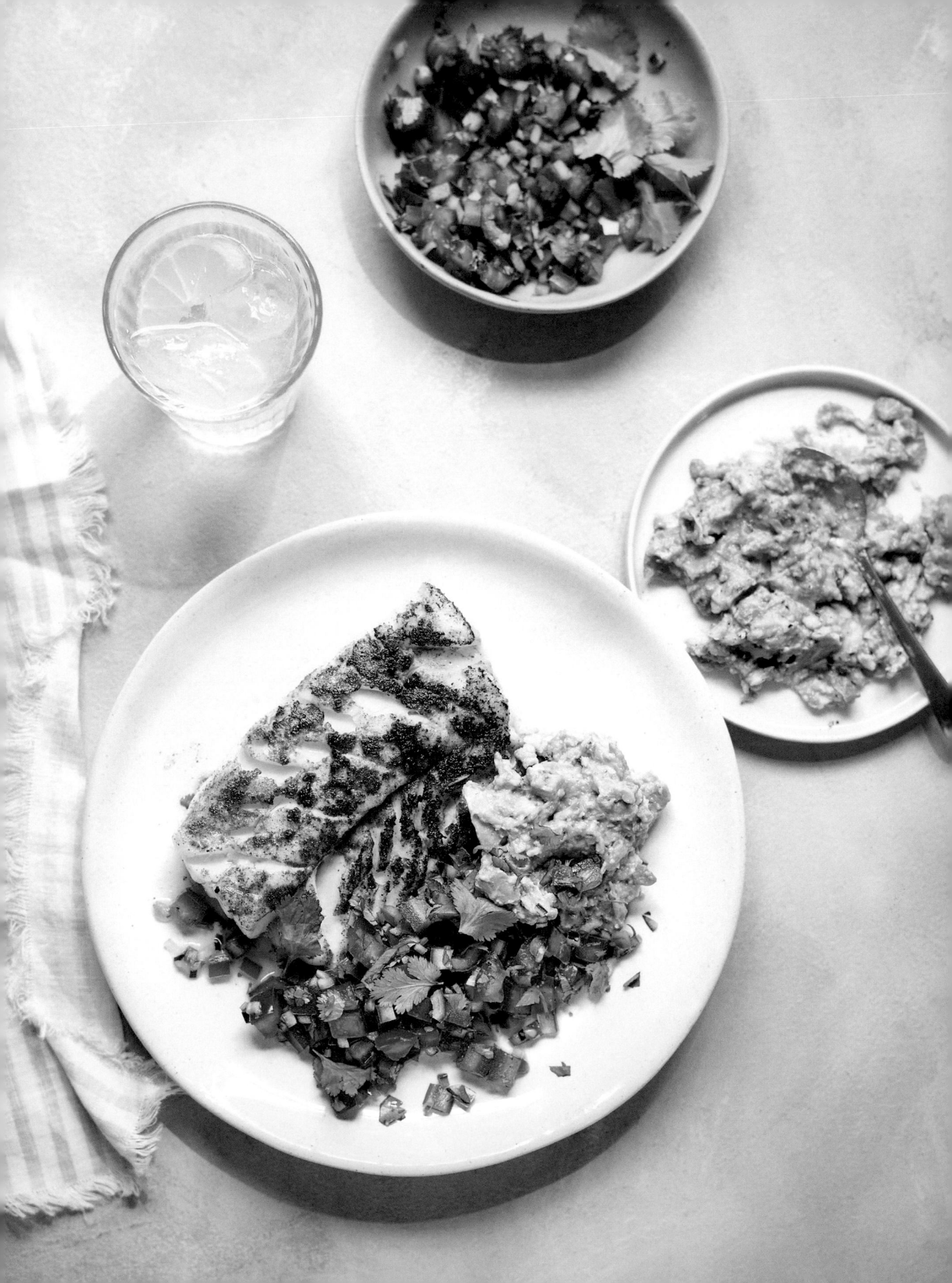

BLACKENED COD WITH PICO DE GALLO SALSA AND SMASHED AVO

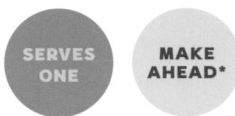

SERVES ONE

MAKE AHEAD*

INGREDIENTS

½ small red onion
handful of coriander (stalks and all)
1 large ripe tomato
½ jalapeño
juice of 1 lime
salt and pepper
1 tbsp coconut oil
1 x 200g skinless cod fillet
1 tbsp fajita seasoning
1 ripe avocado, de-stoned

* MAKE THE SALSA AND SMASHED AVOCADO BEFOREHAND, BUT COOK THE COD JUST BEFORE SERVING.

1. Make the salsa. Finely chop the red onion, most of the coriander, the tomato and the jalapeño – remove the seeds if you don't like it hot. Scrape into a bowl, squeeze in the juice of half the lime. Give everything a good mix and season with salt and pepper to taste.

2. Melt the coconut oil in a non-stick frying pan over a medium to high heat. Coat the cod in the fajita seasoning, then place into the hot pan. Cook for about 4 minutes on each side, carefully flipping halfway.

3. Meanwhile make the smashed avo. Scoop the avocado into a bowl, squeeze in the juice of the remaining lime half, season, then use your fork to roughly mash.

4. Come back to the cod, check that it is cooked through by cutting into one of the thicker parts to make sure it has turned from raw, pale flesh to cooked bright white.

5. Lay the blackened cod onto a plate, dish up the salsa and smashed avocado then scatter over the remaining coriander leaves.

INGREDIENTS

40g hazelnuts
200g green beans
1 jarred roasted red pepper, drained
½ tsp smoked paprika
1 tbsp olive oil
splash of sherry or red wine vinegar
salt and pepper
1 x 225g sirloin steak, trimmed of visible fat

* THE ROMESCO SAUCE WILL KEEP FOR UP TO 3 DAYS IN THE FRIDGE.

STEAK WITH HAZELNUT ROMESCO AND GREEN BEANS

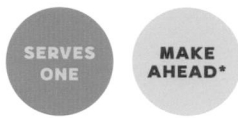

SERVES ONE

MAKE AHEAD*

1. Toast the hazelnuts in a dry frying pan over a medium heat until they smell nutty. Allow to cool while you trim the green beans. Set aside the frying pan to use later.

2. Tip most of the hazelnuts into a small food processor with the jarred red pepper, smoked paprika and ½ tablespoon of the olive oil. Blitz until smooth, adding vinegar, salt and pepper to taste.

3. Put the frying pan over the highest heat. Drizzle the remaining olive oil over the steak, rubbing it into the flesh, and season all over with salt and pepper. When the pan is searingly hot, carefully lay the steak in. Cook according to preference – I like my steaks medium rare, so 2½ minutes on each side, turning regularly – then leave to rest, covered, until you're ready to eat.

4. While the steak is cooking, put the green beans in a microwaveable bowl with 2 tablespoons water and some seasoning. Cover and zap on high for 3–4 minutes until vivid green and tender.

5. Spoon the romesco sauce onto your plate. Lay the steak on top and pile the green beans alongside. Roughly chop the remaining hazelnuts and scatter over. Dream food.

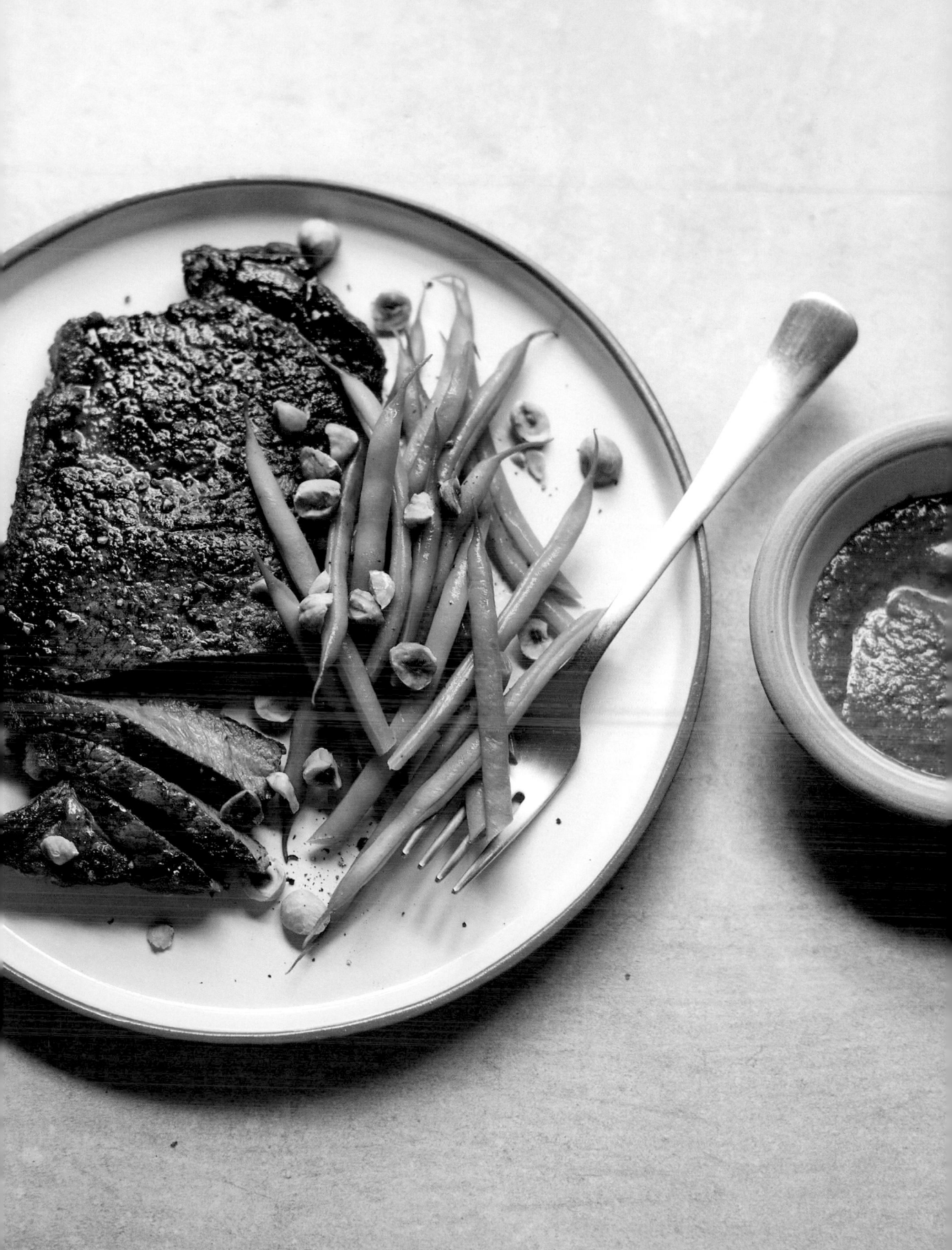

INGREDIENTS

½ small head of cauliflower,
    cut into quarters (leaves
    and stalks left on)
1 tbsp coconut oil
large handful of parsley
handful of mint leaves
½ tbsp medium curry powder
1 tbsp sesame seeds
salt and pepper
2 tbsp tahini
juice of ½ lemon
100g mange tout
2 tbsp pomegranate seeds

SESAME CAULIFLOWER, POMEGRANATE AND MIXED HERB SALAD WITH TAHINI DRESSING

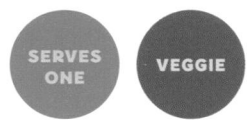

SERVES ONE   VEGGIE

1. Preheat your oven to 220°C (fan 200°/gas mark 7).

2. Put the cauliflower quarters into a microwaveable bowl with 1 tablespoon of water. Cover and zap on high for 4 minutes.

3. Meanwhile dollop the coconut oil into a roasting tray then place in the oven to melt. Roughly chop half the parsley and mint.

4. Carefully bring the hot roasting tray out of the oven. Tip in the cauliflower, sprinkle over the curry powder and sesame seeds, season with salt and pepper. Using tongs, coat the cauliflower in the spices and seeds then separate out into a single layer. Roast in the oven for 9–10 minutes.

5. Put the un-chopped parsley and mint into a blender. Add the tahini, lemon juice and 2 tablespoons of warm water. Blitz to a green, flecked dressing. Add a little more water if you need it – you want it a drizzling consistency. Season with salt and pepper to taste.

6. Roughly slice the mange tout. Pile into a bowl with most of the pomegranate seeds and chopped herbs. Come back to your roasted cauliflower, place it on top of the salad. Drizzle over the dressing and scatter over the remaining herbs and pomegranate seeds to serve.

Joe's Top Tip

This is very light so if you're extra hungry you could serve a toasted pitta bread on the side.

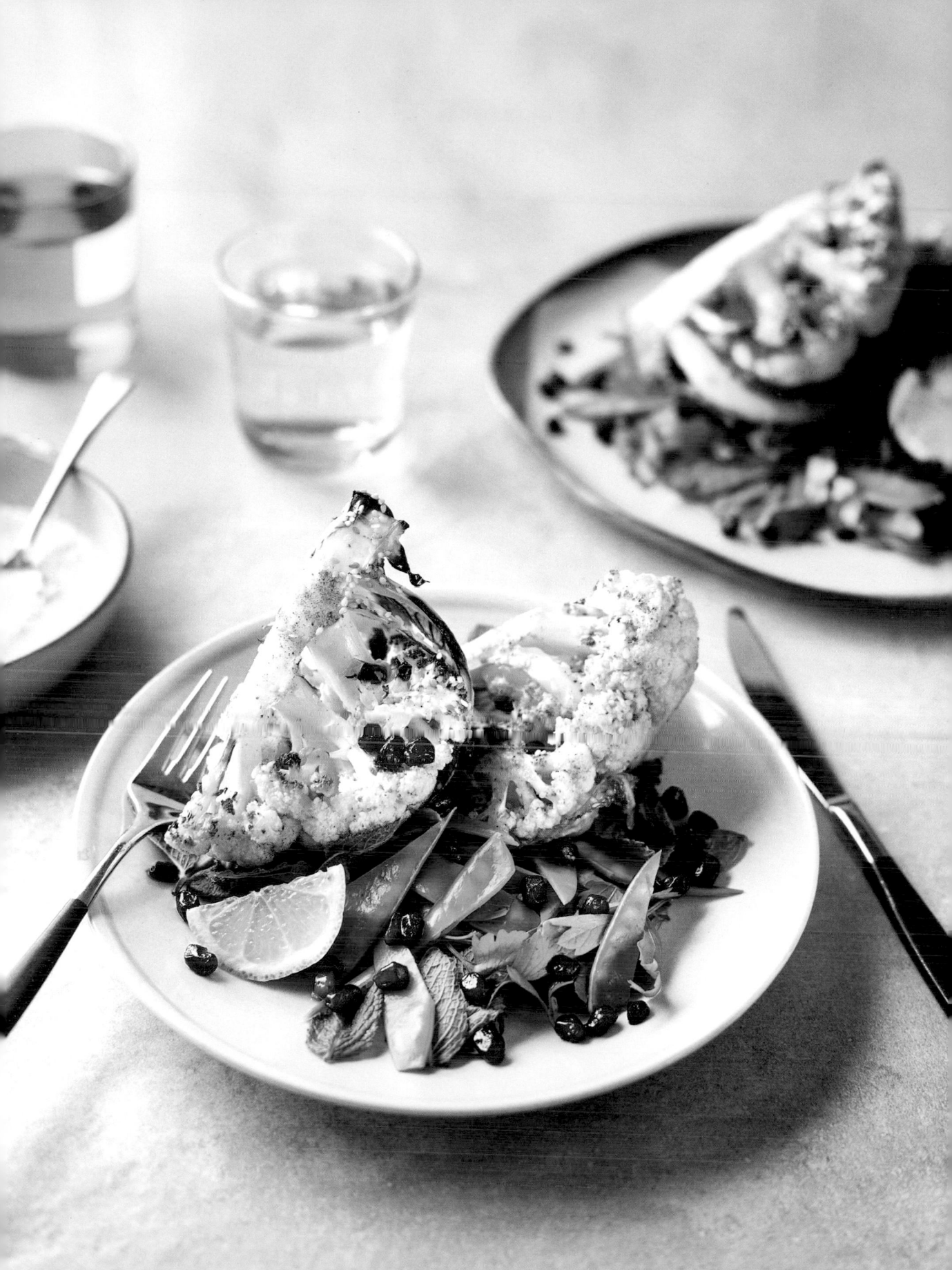

INGREDIENTS

½ cucumber
½ avocado, de-stoned
100g shelled frozen edamame
   beans
1 tbsp mayonnaise
1 tsp wasabi paste
1 tsp sesame oil
2 tsp soy sauce
2 tsp mirin
1 x 200g tuna steak
2 tbsp sesame seeds

WASABI TUNA MAYO 'POKE BOWL'

SERVES ONE

1. Bring a kettle of water to the boil.

2. Peel the cucumber into long ribbons. Scoop out the avocado and slice.

3. Pour the boiling water into a saucepan over a medium to high heat. Drop in the edamame beans and cook for 2 minutes until just tender. Meanwhile mix the mayonnaise with the wasabi paste in a small bowl.

4. Drain the edamame in a sieve or colander, then rinse under cold running water to cool. Shake off any excess water, then tip into a bowl. Add the cucumber ribbons, sesame oil, 1 teaspoon each of soy and mirin, toss together.

5. Cut the tuna into roughly 3cm strips. Pour over the remaining soy and mirin, rubbing the seasoning into the flesh. Spoon the sesame seeds onto a plate then roll the tuna in the seeds to coat.

6. Heat a dry non-stick frying pan over the highest heat. When the pan is searingly hot, carefully lay the tuna strips in, with enough space between each one so that they can fry evenly. Using tongs, sear the tuna for 10–20 seconds on each of the four sides – I like my tuna rare in the middle, cook it for longer if you like.

7. Pile the tuna into a bowl with the cucumber salad and sliced avocado. Spoon in the wasabi mayo.

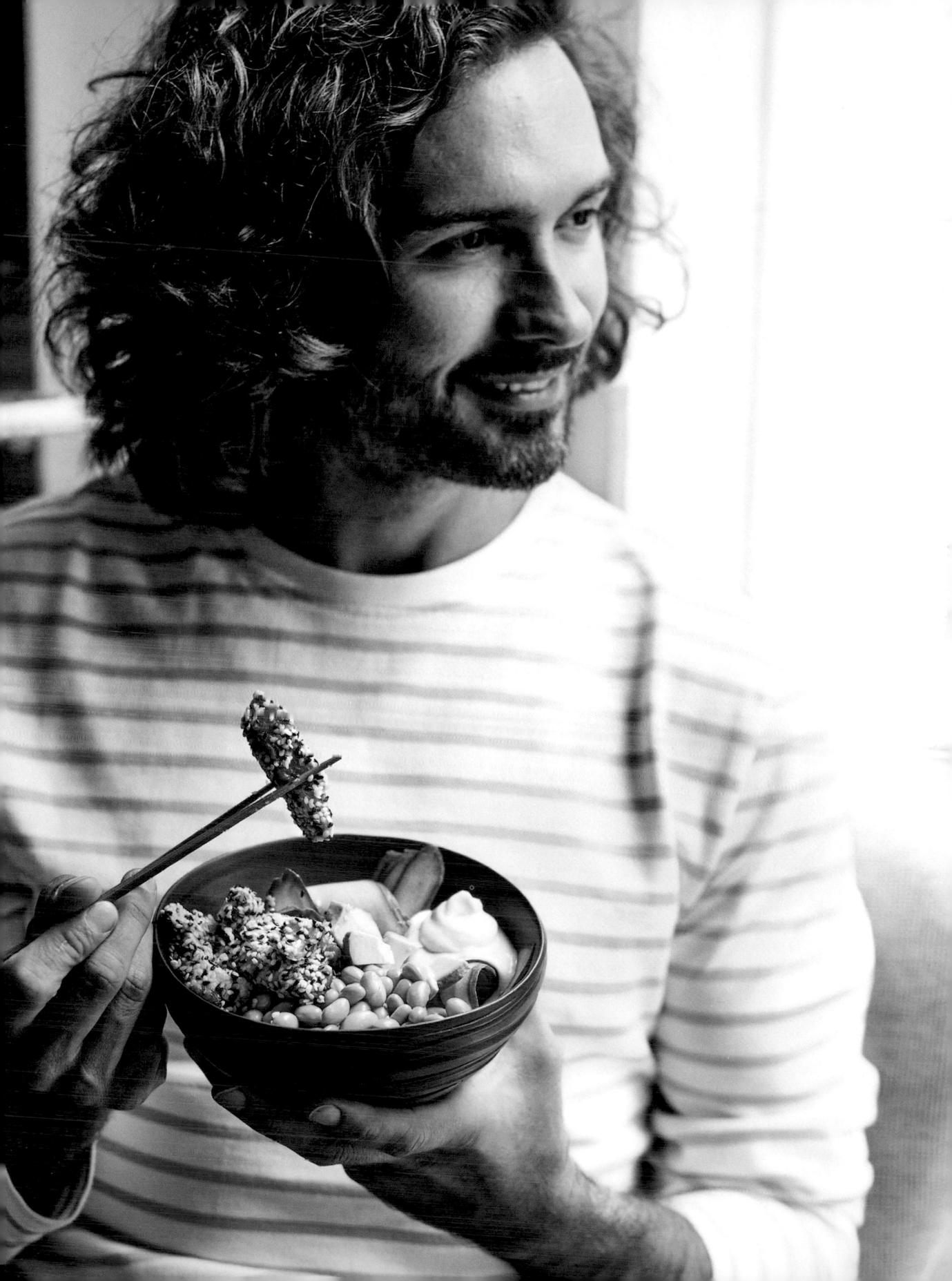

INGREDIENTS

30g feta
1½ tbsp olive oil
pinch of dried red chilli flakes
handful of parsley
1 tsp Dijon mustard
½ tbsp capers
1 tsp red wine vinegar,
    plus a drizzle
salt and pepper
1 x 200g tuna steak
1 clove garlic
100g cannellini or butter beans,
    drained and rinsed
2 handfuls of spinach

TUNA, WHITE BEAN, MARINATED FETA AND SALSA VERDE

SERVES
ONE

1. Cut the feta into rough cubes, put in a small bowl then pour over a little olive oil and sprinkle with chilli flakes. Leave to marinate.

2. Make the salsa verde. Put the parsley, stalks and all, into a small food processor. Blitz until finely chopped then spoon in the mustard, capers, 1 tablespoon of olive oil and the red wine vinegar. Blitz to a textured green sauce. Season to taste.

3. Heat a griddle pan over a super-high heat. Drizzle a little olive oil over the tuna steak, rubbing it into the flesh, and season all over with salt and pepper. When the pan is searingly hot, carefully lay the tuna in. Cook for 2 minutes on each side – I like my tuna rare in the middle, cook it for longer if you like.

4. Meanwhile melt the remaining olive oil in a saucepan over a medium heat. Crush in the garlic clove then drop in the cannellini or butterbeans along with the spinach. Cook for 1–2 minutes until the spinach is just wilted. Drizzle over a small splash of red wine vinegar and season to taste.

5. Pile the spinach and beans onto a plate. Lay the cooked tuna alongside and drizzle everything with the salsa verde. Scatter over the feta along with a few more chilli flakes, to finish.

Veggie Swap

Swap the tuna steak for 1 large courgette, sliced on a diagonal, drizzled with a little olive oil and griddled for 2–3 minutes on each side. Top with 2 tbsp toasted mixed seeds.

REDUCED CARB

52

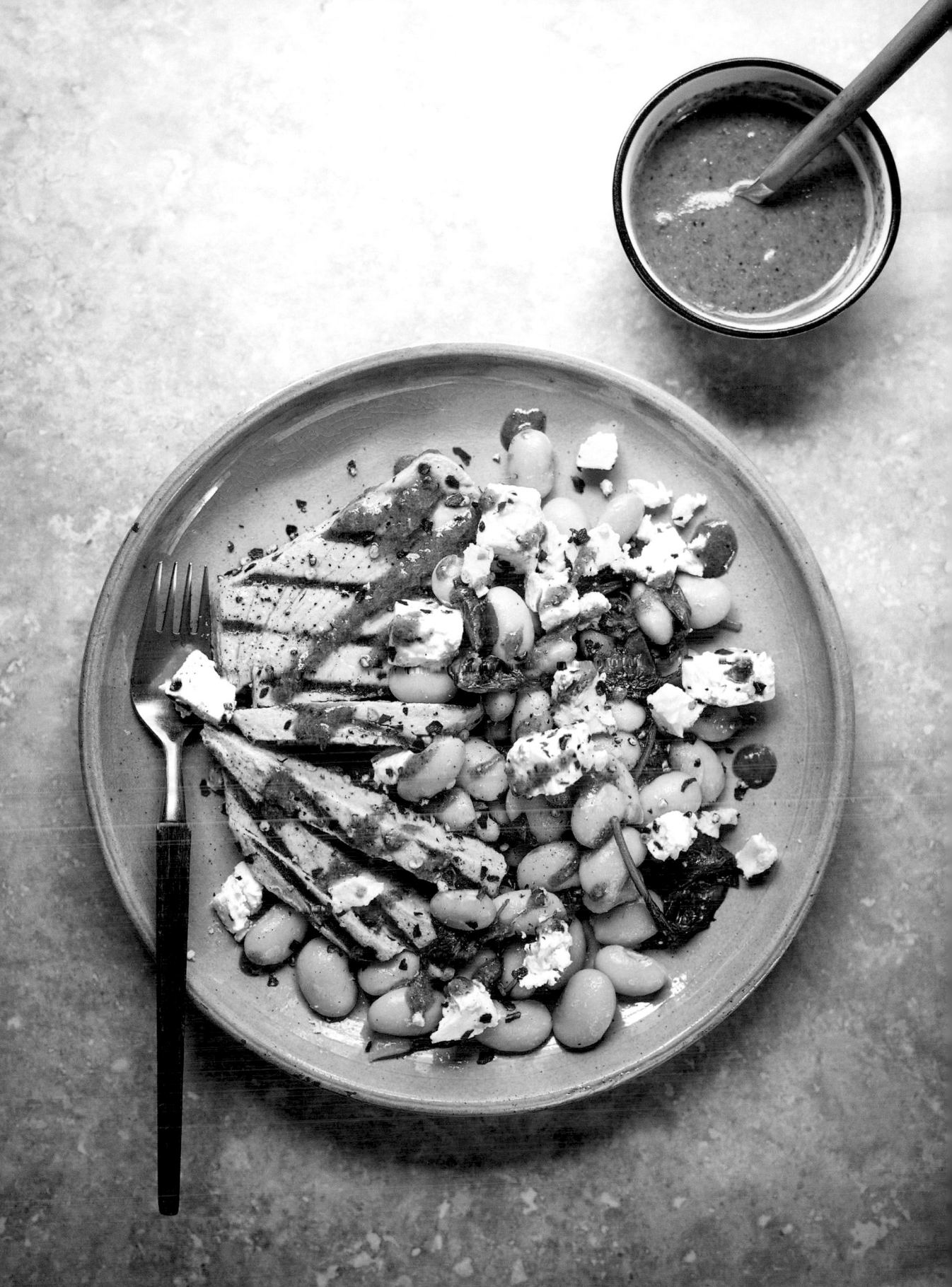

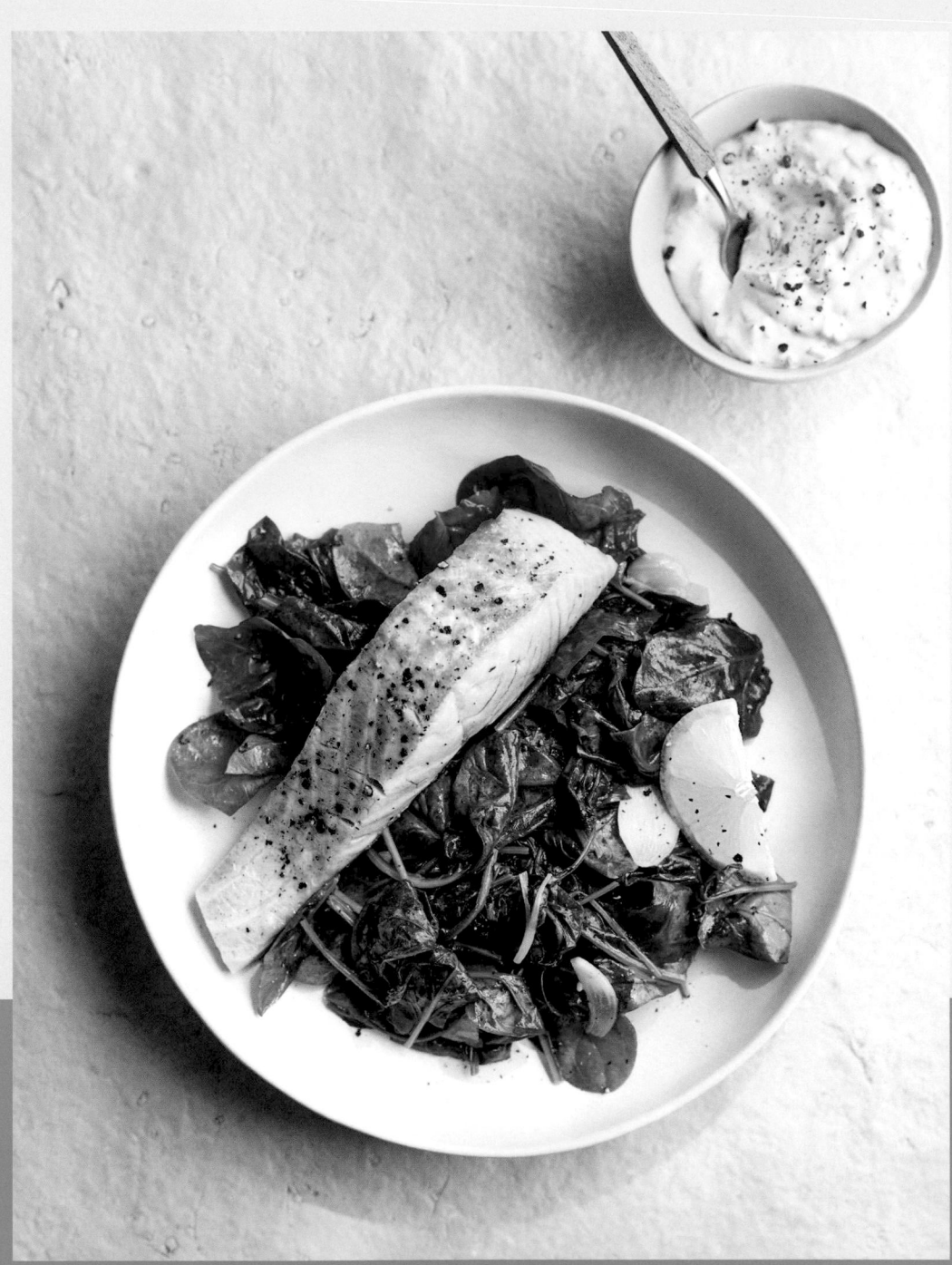

SALMON WITH TARRAGON CRÈME FRAICHE AND GARLICKY SPINACH

INGREDIENTS

1 lemon
handful of tarragon
1 x 200g skinless boneless
   salmon fillet
drizzle of olive oil
salt and pepper
2 tbsp crème fraiche
15g butter
1 large clove garlic
3 large handfuls of baby
   spinach leaves

* THE TARRAGON CRÈME FRAICHE WILL KEEP FOR 3 DAYS IN THE FRIDGE.

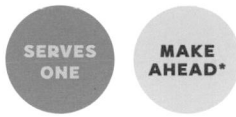

SERVES ONE **MAKE AHEAD***

1. Preheat your grill to maximum.

2. Cut the lemon in half, thinly slice one of the halves and cut the other half into two wedges. Strip the tarragon leaves away from the stalks, keeping both parts.

3. Put the lemon slices and tarragon stalks on the bottom of a baking tray. Cut the salmon fillet in half then place on top. Drizzle with a little olive oil and season with salt and pepper. Slide under the grill for 8 minutes.

4. Meanwhile finely chop the tarragon leaves. Scrape into a small bowl, add the crème fraiche. Stir together, adding salt, pepper and lemon juice to taste.

5. Melt the butter in a frying pan over a medium heat. When bubbling, crush in the garlic clove. Chuck in the spinach. Cook for 1–2 minutes, stirring, until the spinach has wilted.

6. By now the salmon should be cooked – you can check this by slicing into the thick end of one of the pieces to make sure the flesh has turned matt pink in colour.

7. Lay the salmon onto a plate, discarding the lemon slices and tarragon stalks. Pile the garlicky spinach alongside, spoon on the tarragon crème fraiche. Serve with the remaining lemon wedge, for squeezing.

INGREDIENTS

drizzle of olive oil
6–7 pork chipolatas (200g)
2 medium carrots
2 medium parsnips
½ chicken stock cube
1 tbsp caramelized onion chutney
½ tsp wholegrain mustard
40g butter, cut into cubes
salt and pepper

CHIPOLATAS IN ONION GRAVY WITH CARROT AND PARSNIP SMASH

SERVES ONE

1. Heat a frying pan over a medium to high heat. Drizzle in a little olive oil, add the chipolatas. Cook for about 7 minutes, turning regularly with tongs.

2. Meanwhile peel and roughly chop the carrots and parsnips. Put in a microwaveable bowl with 2 tablespoons of water. Cover and zap on high for 8 minutes until completely soft.

3. Bring a kettle of water to the boil. Put the chicken stock cube into a jug, measure in 150ml boiling water and whisk with a fork to dissolve.

4. Come back to the chipolatas. Make sure they are cooked through by cutting into one and checking there is no pink meat left. Turn down the heat and pour the chicken stock into the pan around the chipolatas. Spoon in the caramelized onion chutney and wholegrain mustard. Use a fork to whisk the chutney and mustard into the stock to create a gravy. Leave to bubble away while you finish the mash.

5. Carefully uncover the carrots and parsnips. Dump in the cubed butter along with a good pinch of salt and pepper, roughly mash.

6. Pile the mash onto a plate. Dish up the sausages and caramelized onion gravy. Proper comfort food.

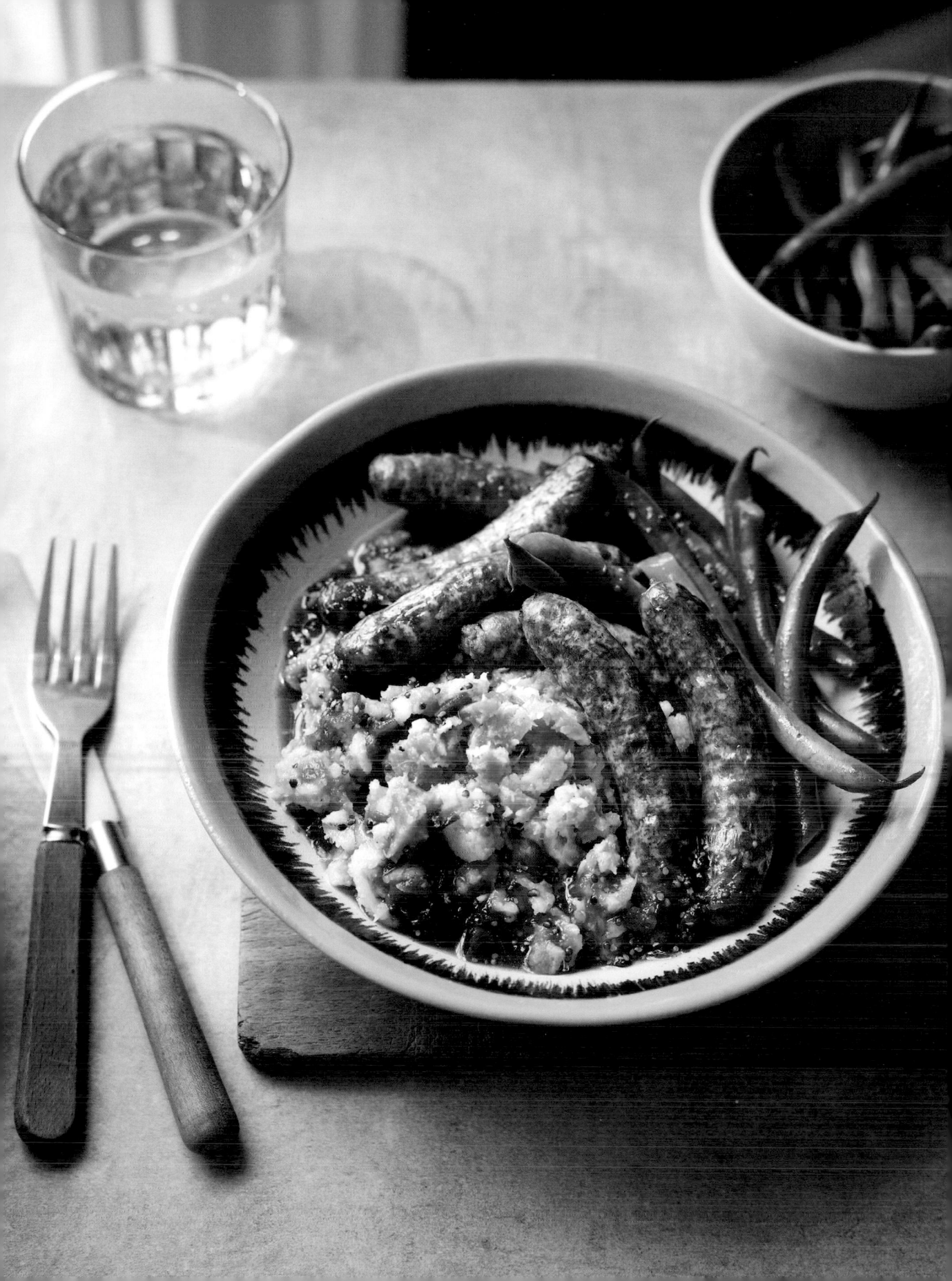

INGREDIENTS

handful of coriander

1 lemongrass stalk, tender white part only, roughly chopped

1 clove garlic

1 red chilli, halved – remove the seeds if you don't like it hot

small piece of ginger, peeled

50g creamed coconut

1 tbsp coconut oil

200g mange tout

200g raw king prawns

juice of ½ lime

splash of soy sauce

PRAWN AND LEMONGRASS COCONUT CURRY WITH MANGE TOUT

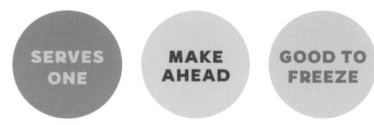

SERVES ONE

MAKE AHEAD

GOOD TO FREEZE

1. Bring a kettle of water to the boil.

2. Cut the coriander stalks away from the leaves. Put the stalks into a small food processor along with the lemongrass, garlic, red chilli, ginger and 1 tablespoon of water. Blitz to a finely chopped curry paste. Add a little more water if you need it.

3. Grab yourself a jug. Pour in 100ml boiling water then carefully drop in the creamed coconut. Use a fork to whisk the two together into a coconut milk. Don't worry if there are a few lumps remaining – they will dissolve in the saucepan.

4. Melt the coconut oil in a saucepan over a high heat. Scrape in the curry paste. Cook, stirring for 1–2 minutes, then lower the heat and pour in the coconut milk. Bring to a simmer then drop in the mange tout and raw king prawns. Cook for 2–3 minutes. The raw grey colour of the prawns will turn pink, which shows you they are cooked.

5. Take the pan off the heat. Squeeze in the lime juice and season with soy sauce to taste. Dish the curry into a bowl and tear over the coriander leaves, to serve.

Veggie Swap

Swap the prawns for 140g firm tofu, cut into cubes, and dropped into the curry instead of the prawns at step 4.

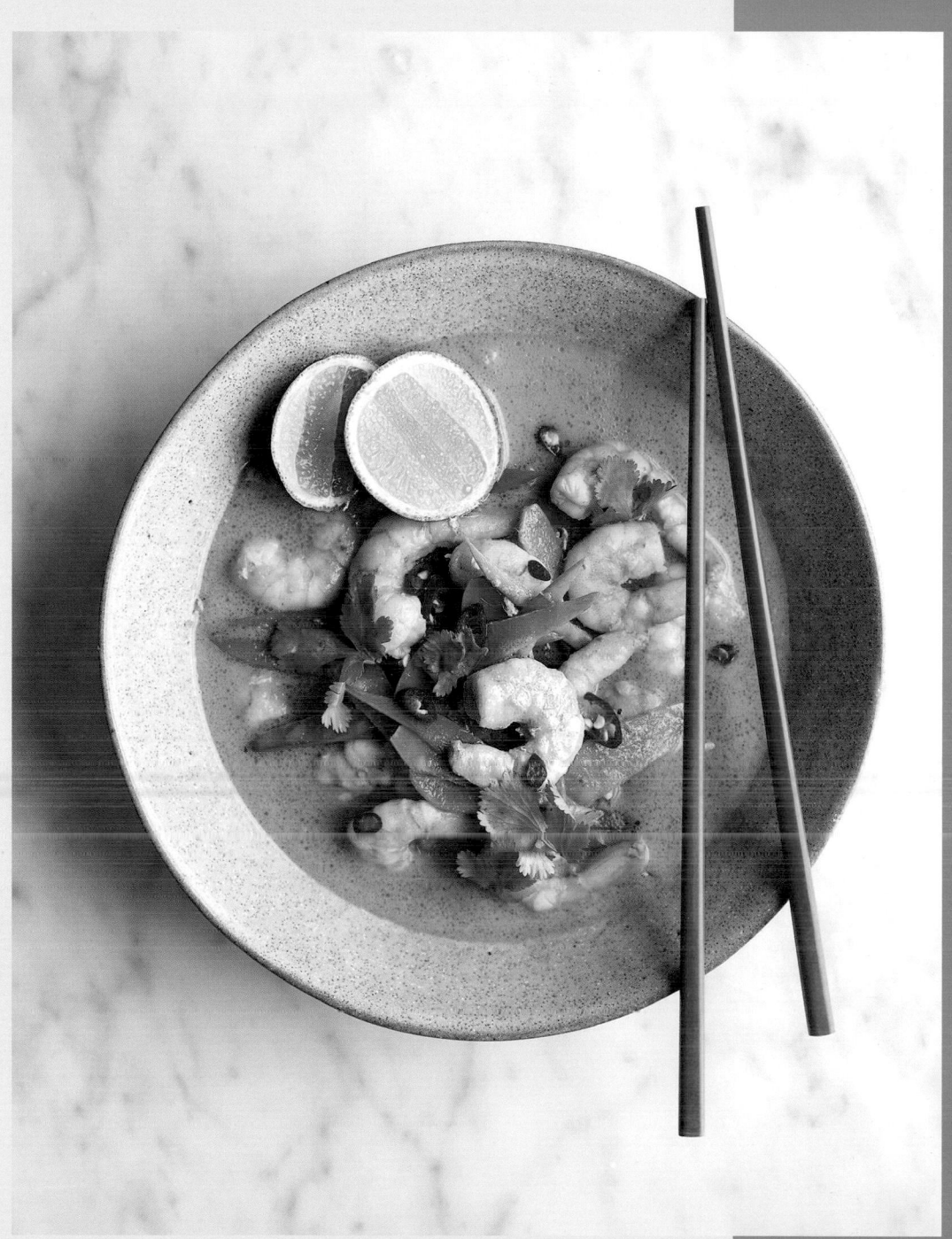

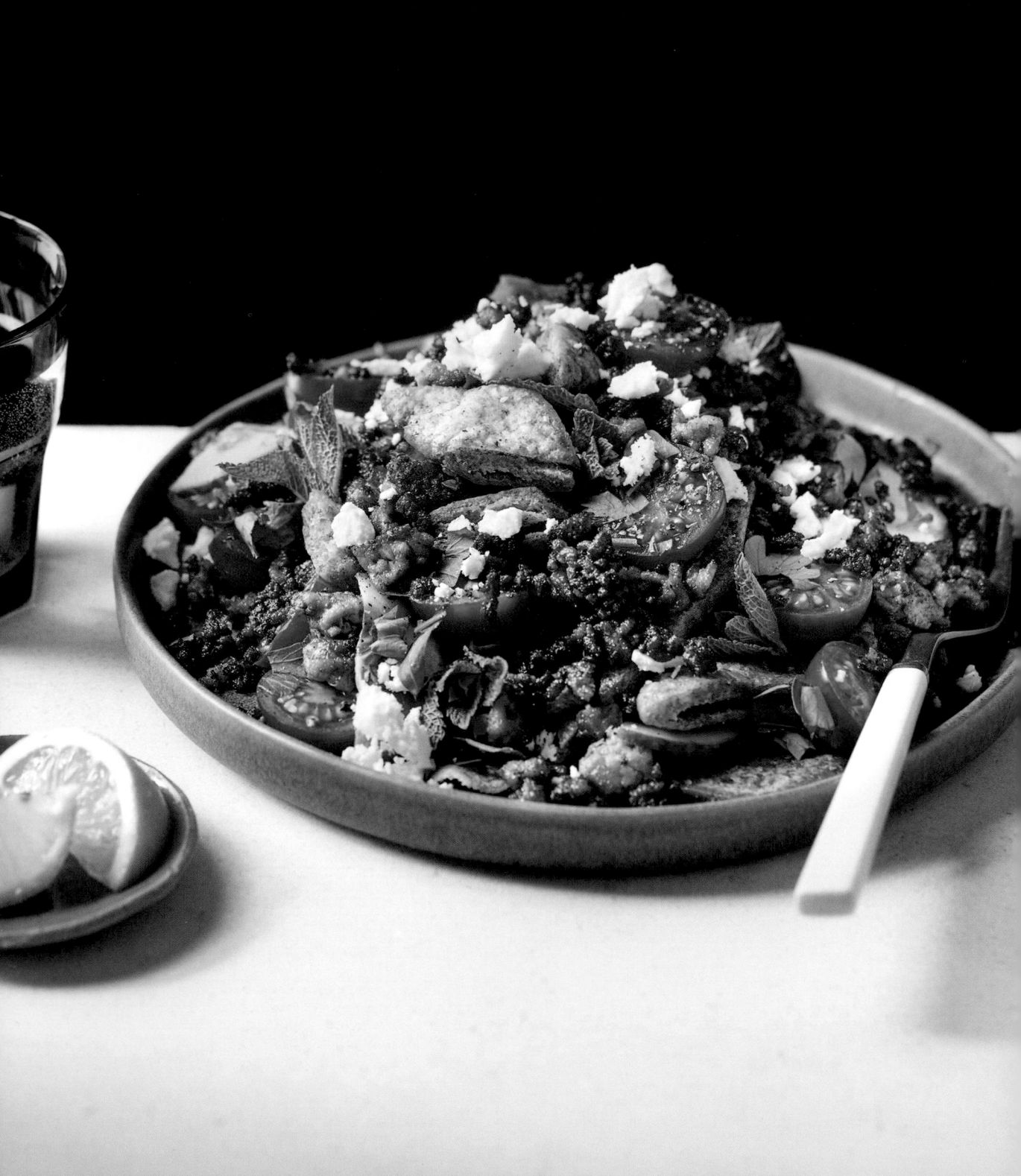

CUMIN-SPICED LAMB AND FETA FATTOUSH

SERVES
ONE

INGREDIENTS

1 pitta bread
1 tbsp olive oil
good pinch of smoked paprika
salt and pepper
200g reduced-fat lamb mince
2 tsp ground cumin
10 cherry tomatoes
¼ cucumber
handful of mint
large handful of parsley
juice of ½ lemon
30g feta

1. Preheat the oven to 200°C (fan 180°/gas mark 6).

2. Using scissors, cut the pitta into random shards. Transfer to a flat baking sheet then toss with 2 teaspoons of olive oil, a good pinch of smoked paprika and salt. Spread pitta out in a single layer and roast in the oven for 10 minutes, turning halfway until golden and crisp.

3. Meanwhile heat a frying pan or wok over a high heat. Drizzle in the remaining oil then tip the lamb mince into the pan. Add the ground cumin along with a pinch of salt and pepper. Use the back of a wooden spoon to break the mince into small pieces. Fry for 10 minutes. By this time it will be completely cooked through, deep brown and crisp.

4. While the lamb and pitta are cooking, make the salad. Halve the cherry tomatoes, slice the cucumber into half-moons, pick the mint leaves and chop the parsley (stalks and all). Scrape all these ingredients into a serving bowl, squeeze in the lemon juice. Mix well to combine.

5. Get your pitta out of the oven and mix it through the salad along with the cumin crispy lamb, which will be cooked by now. Crumble over the feta to serve.

Joe's Top Tip

For softer herbs such as parsley, I always chop up the stalks and chuck them into recipes with the leaves. They are full of flavour!

INGREDIENTS

1 x 225g sirloin steak,
   trimmed of visible fat
1 tbsp olive oil
salt and pepper
1 tsp Dijon mustard
1 ripe pear
½ tbsp balsamic vinegar
2 large handfuls of watercress
30g blue cheese

SEARED STEAK, BLUE CHEESE, PEAR AND WATERCRESS

SERVES
ONE

1. Heat a griddle pan over a high heat. Drizzle the steak with a little olive oil, rubbing it into the flesh, and season all over with salt and pepper. When the pan is searingly hot, carefully lay the steak in. Cook according to preference – I like my steaks medium rare, so 2½ minutes on each side, turning regularly.

2. Once the steak has finished cooking, dollop the mustard onto a plate. Transfer the steak to the plate, and using some tongs, turn the steak so that it gets coated on both sides in the mustard – then leave to rest, covered, until you're ready to eat.

3. While the steak is resting, core and slice the pear. Using a fork, whisk the remaining olive oil together with the balsamic vinegar in a small bowl. Pour the resting juices from the steak into the bowl for a big whack of flavour in the dressing.

4. Slice the mustardy steak on an angle. Pile the watercress onto a plate along with the sliced pear and steak. Pour over the dressing and toss everything together with your hands. Finish by crumbling over the blue cheese and cracking over some black pepper, then get stuck in.

Veggie Swap

Omit the steak and mix 3 pre-cooked beetroots, cut into wedges, and 30g toasted pecans through the rest of the ingredients.

POACHED SALMON WITH CREAM CHEESE AND CHIVE SCRAMBLED EGGS

INGREDIENTS

½ lemon
1 x 140g skinless boneless
    salmon fillet
salt and pepper
2 eggs
1 tbsp cream cheese
20g butter
small handful of chives
tabasco, to serve – optional

SERVES ONE

1. Slice ½ lemon into rounds. Season the salmon fillet on both sides with salt and pepper.

2. Heat a small dry frying pan over a low to medium heat. Place the lemon slices in the pan and pour in 250ml water. Once the water is just simmering, lay the salmon fillet into the pan – it should be just covered by water – if it needs a little more, top it up. Put on a lid and gently poach the salmon for around 7 minutes.

3. While the salmon is cooking, crack the eggs into a jug. Dollop in the cream cheese, whisk well with a fork until the white and yolk combine, then season with a generous pinch of salt and pepper.

4. Come back to the salmon, which by now should be cooked. Check by slicing into the thick end of the fillet to make sure the flesh has turned matt pink in colour. Take the pan off the heat, drain away all the water then keep the salmon in the pan with the lid on to stay warm.

5. Melt the butter in a small non-stick frying pan over a medium heat. Once bubbling, pour in the beaten cream cheese and eggs. Softly scramble the eggs, drawing the cooked egg from the edges into the middle until the egg is just cooked.

6. Dish up the scrambled eggs. Flake the poached salmon on top, then using scissors, snip over a few chives. I like to eat this with a few drops of tabasco.

Veggie Swap

Swap the salmon for 200g asparagus tips, poached in the same method as the salmon but for only 3 minutes.

REDUCED CARB

63

INGREDIENTS

120g frozen peas
1 baby gem lettuce
2 cornichons or 2 tsp capers
   plus 1 tsp pickling juice
2 tbsp natural yoghurt
handful of mint leaves
½ lemon
salt and pepper
1 x 200g skinless pollock fillet
2 pinches of cayenne pepper
1 tbsp olive oil

CAYENNE POLLOCK WITH MINTED PEA YOGHURT SAUCE AND BABY GEM

SERVES ONE

1. Bring a kettle of water to the boil.

2. Measure the frozen peas into a bowl. Pour over the boiling water and leave to defrost while you separate the baby gem lettuce leaves and chop the cornichons.

3. Drain the peas in a sieve or colander then rinse under cold running water. Shake off any excess water then tip the peas into a small food processor. Blitz until roughly chopped then add the natural yoghurt, mint leaves and a squeeze of lemon juice. Blitz again to a vivid green sauce. Season to taste.

4. Heat a non-stick frying pan over a high heat. Season the pollock on both sides with salt and pepper, then sprinkle the top with the cayenne.

5. When the pan is searingly hot, drizzle in ½ tablespoon of olive oil then carefully lay the pollock into the pan. Cook for about 4 minutes on each side, flipping halfway.

6. While the pollock is cooking, assemble the salad on your plate. Mix the baby gem lettuce with the chopped cornichons or capers, 1 teaspoon pickling juice from their jar, remaining olive oil, salt and pepper. Spoon the minted pea yoghurt sauce alongside.

7. Come back to the pollock. Check it is cooked through by cutting into one of the thicker parts to make sure it has turned from raw, pale flesh to cooked bright white. Once you're happy, place the pollock onto the plate. Serve with the remaining lemon for squeezing.

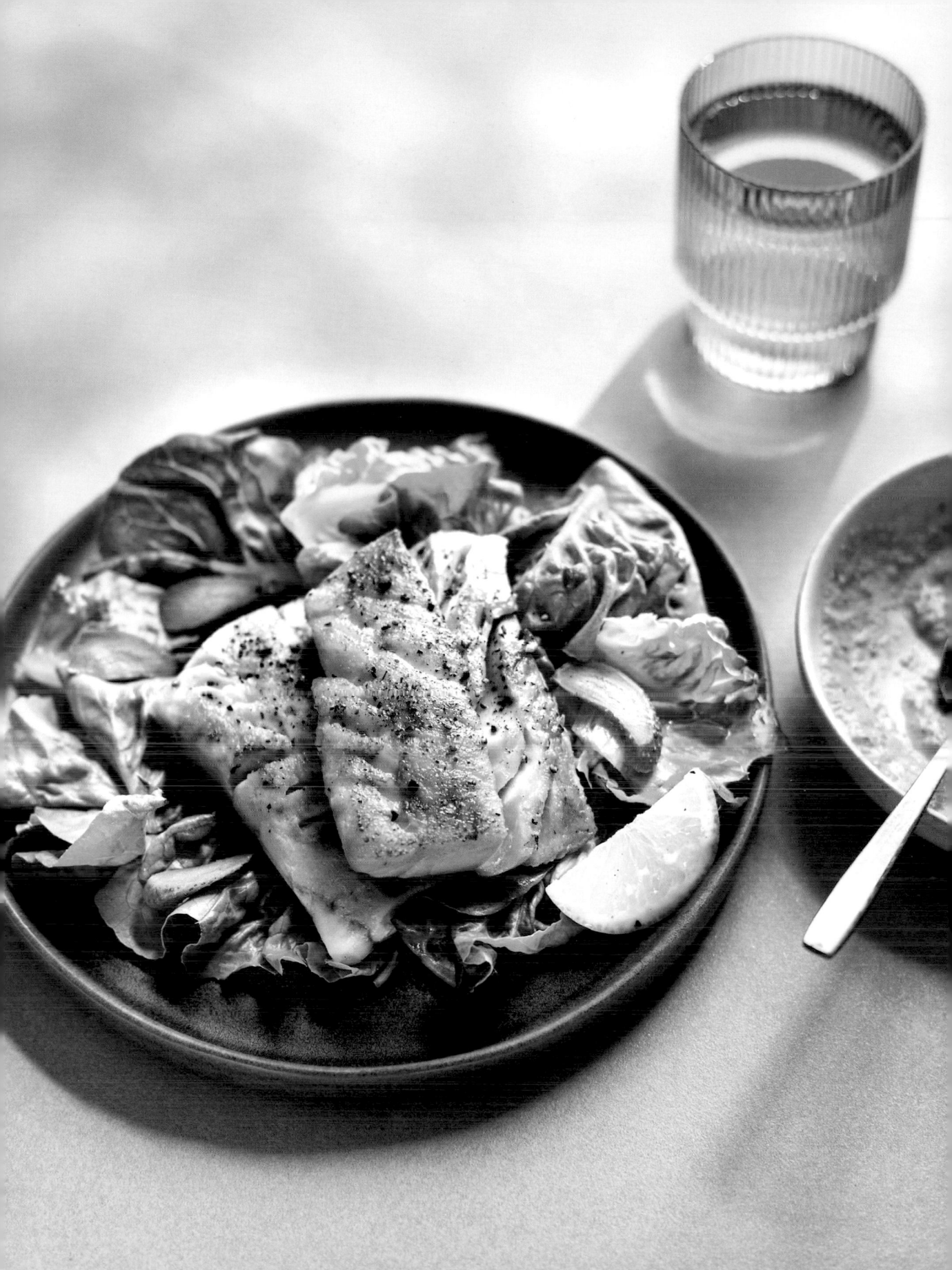

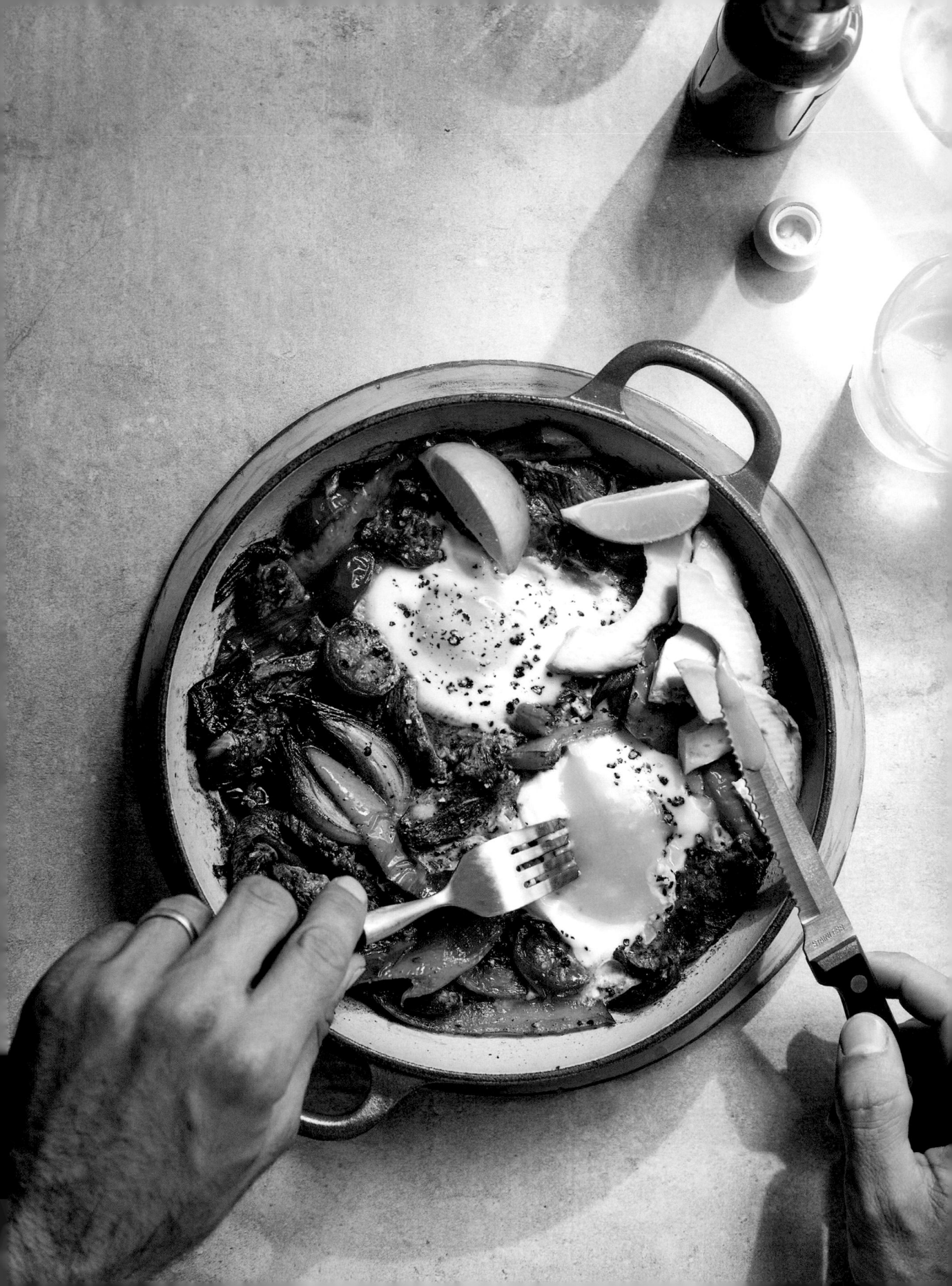

STEAK FAJITA FRIED EGGS

SERVES ONE

INGREDIENTS

1 tbsp coconut oil
1 red onion, sliced
1 orange or yellow pepper, sliced
salt and pepper
5 cherry tomatoes, cut in half
140g beef medallion steaks,
    sliced into 1cm strips
1 tbsp fajita seasoning
2 eggs
juice of ½ lime
½ ripe avocado, de-stoned
    and sliced
hot sauce, to serve – optional

1. Melt the coconut oil in a large non-stick frying pan over
   a medium to high heat. Chuck in the sliced red onion and
   pepper with a pinch of salt. Fry for 5 minutes, until the onion
   has collapsed and is nearly soft.

2. Drop in the tomatoes and sliced steak. Spoon over the fajita
   seasoning then give everything a good mix to coat with the
   spices. Using a wooden spoon, create two holes in the fajita
   mix. Crack in the eggs then crank up the heat.

3. Place a lid on the pan and cook for a further 2–3 minutes
   until the egg whites are set and the yolks are still runny.
   By this point the steak will also be cooked – I like mine just
   a little pink on the inside.

4. Take the pan off the heat. Remove the lid, squeeze over
   the lime juice and top with the sliced avocado. Drizzle over
   some hot sauce if you like. If you're like me, you'll eat this
   one straight out the pan.

Veggie Swap

Swap the steak for 4 slices
of halloumi, fried in the same
way as the steak.

REDUCED CARB

INGREDIENTS

2 new potatoes
½ fish stock cube
10g butter
1 clove garlic
1 tbsp plain flour
1 tsp smoked paprika
1 x 200g tin of sweetcorn,
    drained
200g raw king prawns
2 tbsp double cream
20g cheddar, grated
salt and pepper
handful of chives

PAPRIKA PRAWN, CORN AND CHEDDAR CHOWDER

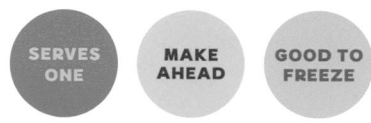

SERVES ONE   MAKE AHEAD   GOOD TO FREEZE

1. Bring a kettle of water to the boil.

2. Meanwhile quarter the new potatoes, leaving the skin on.
    Put in a microwaveable bowl with 1 tablespoon of water,
    cover and zap on high for 5 minutes.

3. Put the fish stock cube into a jug, measure in 300ml of
    boiling water and whisk with a fork to dissolve.

4. Melt the butter in a saucepan over a medium heat. When
    bubbling, crush in the garlic clove. Cook for 30 seconds,
    stirring almost constantly, then sprinkle in the flour and
    smoked paprika. Cook for 1 minute more then, while still
    stirring, pour in a big splash of fish stock. Once the fish
    stock has combined with the flour and butter, pour the rest
    in and bring up to the boil.

5. Come back to the potatoes, carefully uncover then add
    them to the saucepan along with the sweetcorn and raw king
    prawns. Cook for 2–3 minutes. The raw grey colour of the
    prawns will turn pink, which shows you they are cooked.

6. Once the prawns are cooked, turn down the heat to low and
    add the double cream and grated cheddar to the chowder.
    Cook for 1 minute more until the cheese has melted then
    season the chowder to taste.

7. Ladle into a large bowl. Using scissors, snip over some chives
    to finish.

GRILLED CHICKEN COBB SALAD

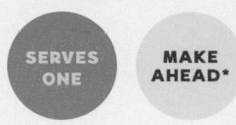

SERVES ONE

MAKE AHEAD*

INGREDIENTS

1 x 160g skinless chicken
   breast fillet
drizzle of olive oil
salt and pepper
1 egg
1 ripe avocado, de-stoned
1 tsp Dijon mustard
2 tsp white wine vinegar
1 large ripe tomato
½ small romaine lettuce
30g blue cheese

* KEEP THE DRESSING SEPARATE.

1. Bring a kettle of water to the boil.

2. Place the chicken between two pieces of cling film or baking parchment on a chopping board. Using a rolling pin, meat mallet or any other blunt instrument, bash the chicken until it is about 1cm thick all over. Drizzle with olive oil, rubbing it into the flesh, and season all over with salt and pepper.

3. Heat a griddle pan over a high heat and pour the boiling water into a saucepan over a medium heat.

4. Once the griddle pan is searingly hot, carefully lay the chicken in. Cook for about 4 minutes on each side.

5. While the chicken is cooking, lower the heat on the saucepan, so the water is hissing rather than bubbling, then lower in your egg. Cook for 6½ minutes.

6. Meanwhile make the dressing. Scoop out half the avocado. Put into a small food processor with the Dijon mustard, white wine vinegar and a splash of water, then blitz to a smooth dressing. Add a little more water if you need it. Season to taste.

7. Slice the remaining avocado half, tomato and romaine lettuce. Put all these ingredients onto a plate.

8. Come back to your chicken. Check it is cooked by slicing into a thicker part to make sure the meat is white all the way through, with no raw pink bits left. Place the grilled chicken with the salad.

9. By now your egg should be cooked. Carefully drain in a sieve or colander then rinse under cold running water until cool. Peel then cut in half.

10. Place the egg on top of the salad, then crumble over the blue cheese. Finish by drizzling over the creamy avocado dressing.

REDUCED CARB

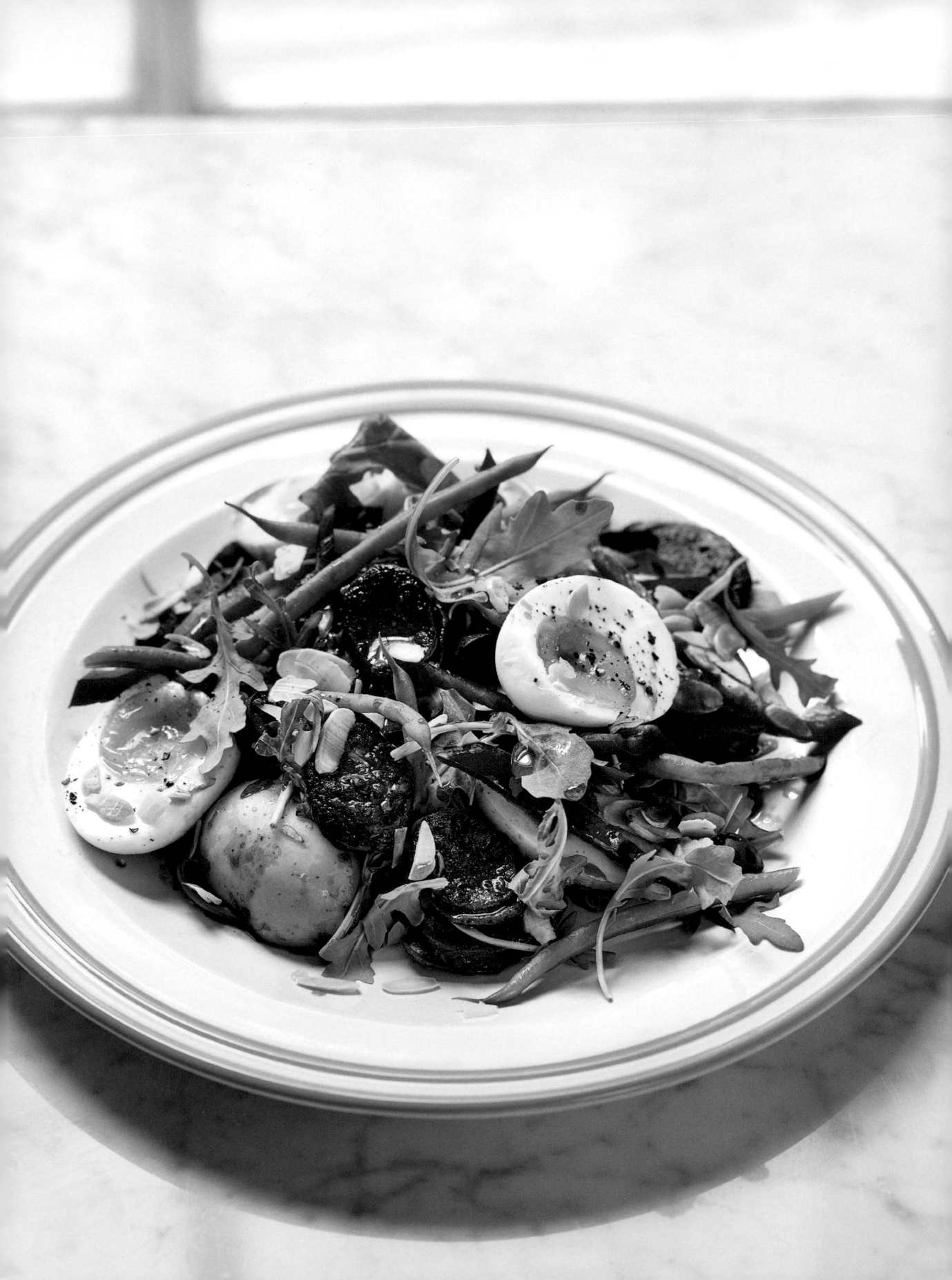

CHORIZO NIÇOISE SALAD

SERVES ONE

INGREDIENTS

2 new potatoes
2 eggs
1 tbsp olive oil
just over ½ chorizo ring (120g),
    sliced
100g green beans, trimmed
salt
½ tbsp sherry vinegar
2 handfuls of rocket
1 red pepper, sliced
5 pitted black olives
30g toasted flaked almonds

1. Bring a kettle of water to the boil.

2. Halve the new potatoes, leaving the skin on. Put in a microwaveable bowl with 1 tablespoon of water, cover and zap on high for 10 minutes until tender.

3. Pour the boiling water into a saucepan, adjust the heat so the water is hissing rather than bubbling, then lower in your eggs. Set a timer for 2½ minutes.

4. Meanwhile heat a frying pan over a medium heat. Add the olive oil along with the chorizo slices. Fry for around 4 minutes, turning occasionally, until crisp.

5. Come back to the eggs. Drop the green beans into the same pan of water along with a pinch of salt. Cook for 4 minutes more.

6. Once your chorizo is crisp, pour the sherry vinegar into the pan and give everything a good stir – you are making a warm dressing. Take the pan off the heat.

7. By now your eggs and beans should be cooked. Carefully drain in a sieve or colander then rinse under cold running water until cool. Peel then halve the eggs. Grab your new potatoes out of the microwave. Carefully uncover and drain.

8. Mix the potatoes with the rocket, sliced red pepper, olives, green beans, chorizo and its dressing on a serving plate. Top with the soft-boiled eggs and scatter over the flaked almonds.

INGREDIENTS

knob of fresh ginger, roughly
    chopped
1 clove garlic, roughly chopped
4 pineapple chunks, roughly
    chopped
1 tsp dried chilli flakes
1 tbsp soy sauce
1 x 225g sirloin steak, trimmed
    of visible fat, sliced into
    1cm strips
1 tbsp coconut oil
2 medium carrots, peeled and
    finely sliced
½ head of broccoli, stalk
    chopped, cut into
    medium florets
2 spring onions, finely sliced
    (green and white parts)
1 tbsp sesame seeds

BEEF BULGOGI

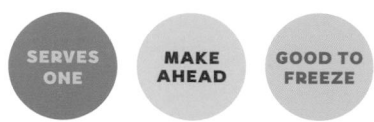

SERVES ONE   MAKE AHEAD   GOOD TO FREEZE

1. Put the fresh ginger, garlic, pineapple, chilli flakes and soy sauce into a small food processor with 1 tablespoon water. Blitz until finely chopped. Pour the marinade into a bowl. Add the steak strips and mix well to combine.

2. Melt the coconut oil in a wok or large frying pan over a high heat. Scrape in the carrot, broccoli and half the spring onion. Stir-fry for 4 minutes, then tip in the steak along with all the marinade – use a spatula to scrape it in, so you don't lose any of that flavour. Stir-fry for a further 2–3 minutes until the steak is cooked – I like mine just a little pink on the inside.

3. Dish up the beef bulgogi. Scatter over the remaining spring onion and sesame seeds.

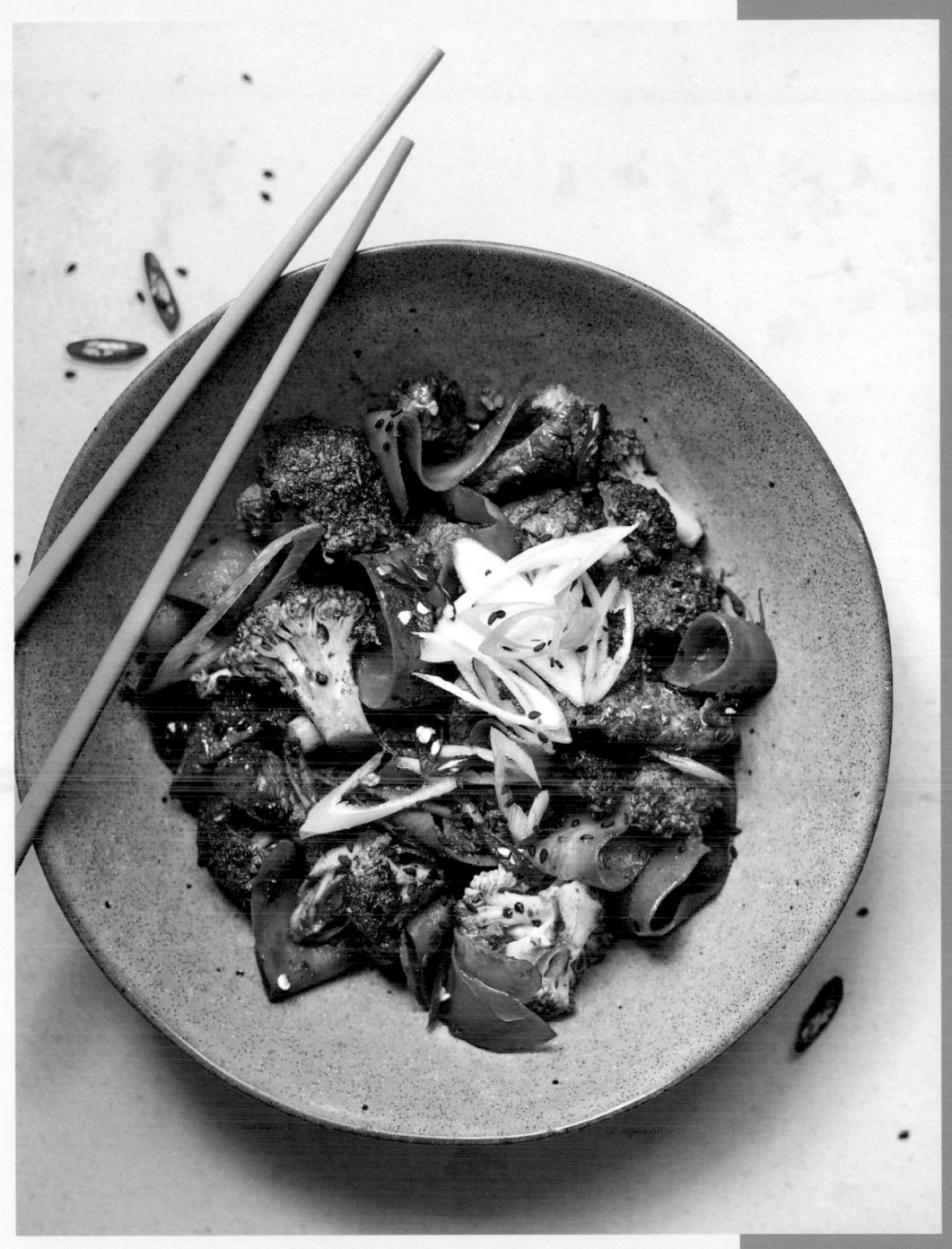

INGREDIENTS

½ tsp five spice
200g skinless, boneless
    chicken thighs, cut into
    large, bite-sized pieces
salt and pepper
1½ tbsp coconut oil
1 tbsp soy sauce
juice from 1 orange
small piece of ginger,
    finely sliced
200g little trees (tenderstem
    broccoli), any bigger stalks
    sliced in half lengthways
30g cashews
drizzle of honey

SOY, FIVE SPICE AND ORANGE CHICKEN WITH LITTLE TREES

SERVES ONE

1. Sprinkle the five spice over the pieces of chicken thigh, season with salt and pepper.

2. Melt 1 tablespoon coconut oil in a frying pan over a high heat. Lay the chicken pieces into the pan. Fry for 4 minutes, turning occasionally until nicely browned. Lower the heat, pour in the soy sauce and half the orange juice then place a lid on the pan. Cook for a further 4 minutes.

3. Meanwhile melt the remaining coconut oil in a separate frying pan over a medium to high heat. Chuck in the sliced ginger and little trees along with the remaining orange juice. Cover, so that the broccoli steams, and cook for 3 minutes, then take off the lid and add the cashews. Cook for a further 2–3 minutes uncovered, until all the orange juice has evaporated and the little trees are tender. Take the pan off the heat.

4. Come back to the chicken. Take off the lid and crank up the heat. Drizzle the chicken pieces with a little honey and cook for 1 minute more until the chicken is sticky and caramelized. Check the chicken is cooked by slicing into one of the larger pieces – the knife should cut through easily and the meat will have turned from pink to a whitish brown.

5. Dish up the chicken and little trees.

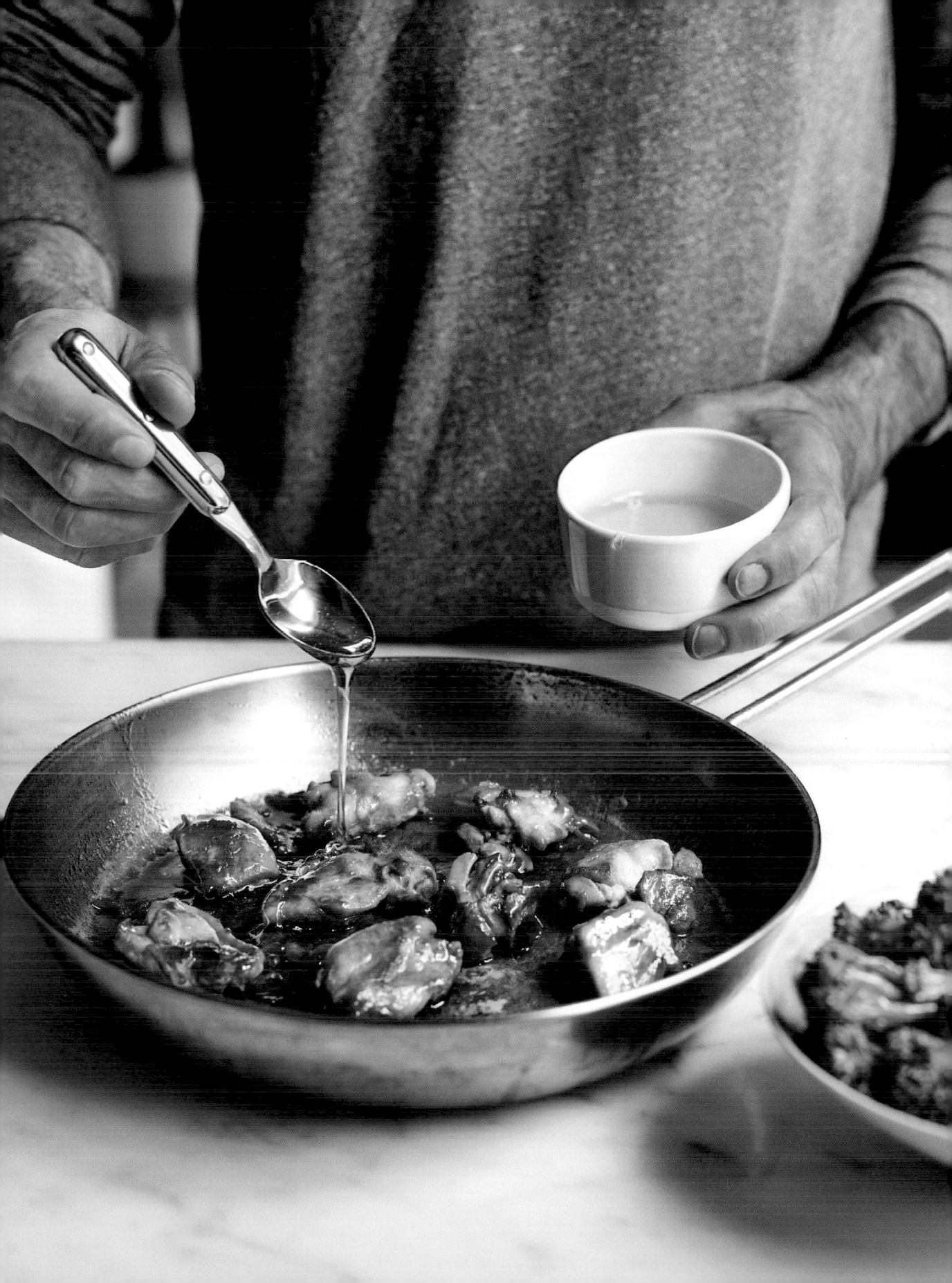

INGREDIENTS

2 tsp olive oil
2 small pork sausages (140g)
1 tsp ground coriander
salt and pepper
1 fat clove garlic
1 x 400g tin of cherry tomatoes
2 tsp harissa
2 eggs
20g feta
1 tbsp Greek yoghurt
handful of coriander

SAUSAGE SHAKSHUKA

SERVES ONE

1. Heat a frying pan over a medium heat. Add 1 teaspoon of olive oil then squeeze the sausages from their skins straight into the frying pan. Sprinkle in the ground coriander and some seasoning. Fry, stirring occasionally, for 5 minutes.

2. Meanwhile heat another small frying pan or saucepan over a medium heat. Add the remaining oil. Crush in the garlic clove. Cook for 30 seconds, stirring almost constantly, then chuck in the tin of cherry tomatoes and harissa. Give everything a good mix and season with salt and pepper. Bring to a simmer.

3. Using the back of your wooden spoon make two indents in the tomato sauce. Crack an egg into each then place a lid on top of the pan. Cook for 5–6 minutes or until the whites are cooked and the yolks are still runny.

4. While the eggs are cooking, crumble the feta into a small bowl. Spoon in the Greek yoghurt and mix together.

5. Come back to your sausages, which by now will be cooked through, brown and crisp. Take the pan off the heat.

6. Once the eggs are cooked to your liking, spoon over the crispy sausage, dollop on the feta yoghurt and tear over some coriander. I like to gobble it up straight from the pan.

Joe's Top Tip

For big taste, you can't beat tinned cherry tomatoes. They are a great way of boosting flavours in a dish when you're cooking quickly.

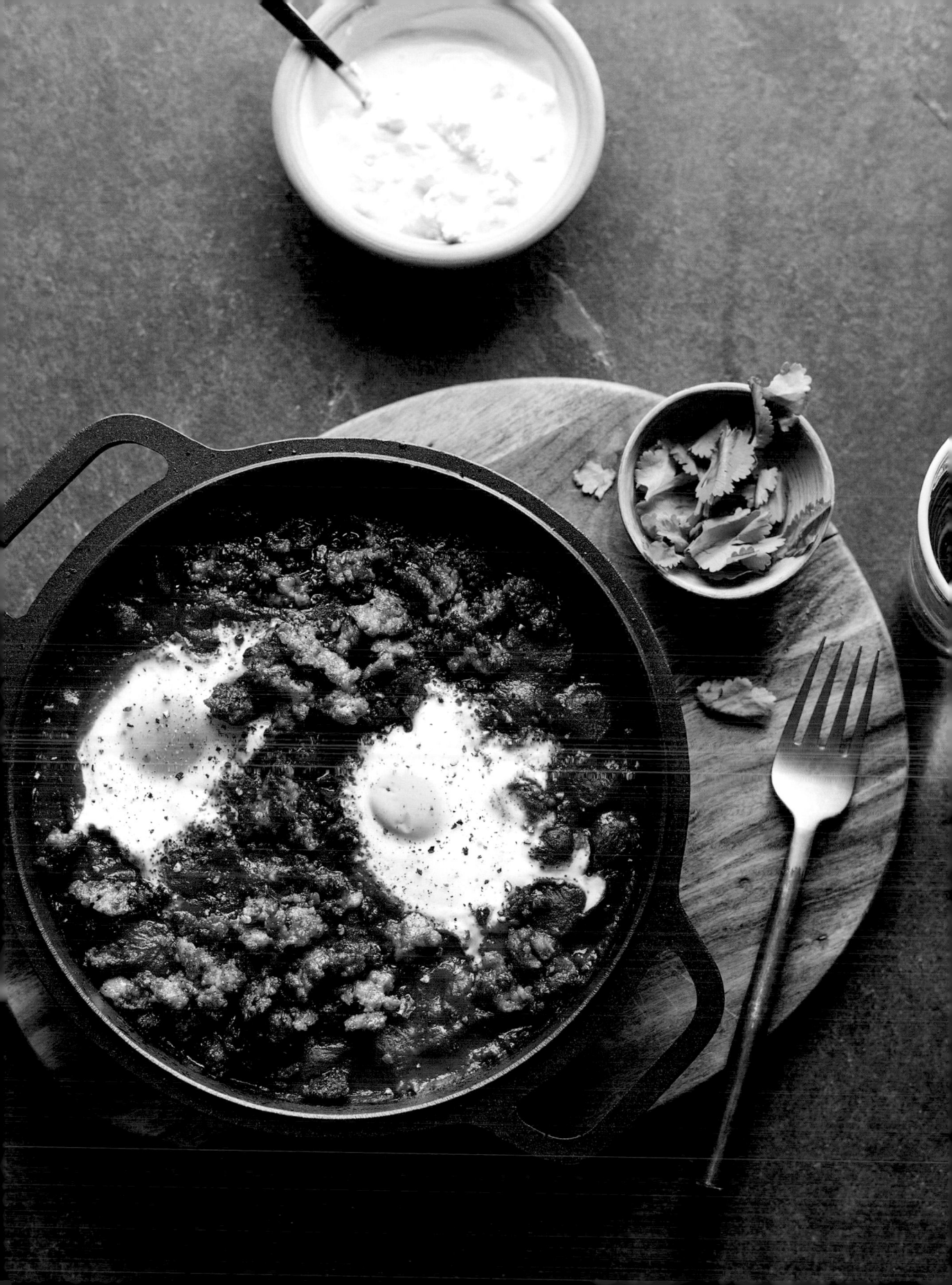

INGREDIENTS

1 medium parsnip

1 egg

zest and juice of ½ lemon

1 tbsp cornflour

salt and pepper

1 tbsp coconut oil

1–2 tsp creamed horseradish

1½ tbsp Greek yoghurt

small handful of parsley

160g smoked mackerel

* PARSNIP ROSTI ONLY.

SMOKED MACKEREL WITH HORSERADISH YOGHURT AND PARSNIP ROSTI

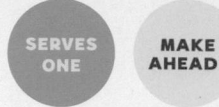

SERVES ONE   **MAKE AHEAD***

1. Grate the parsnip, skin and all, into a bowl. Crack in the egg, add the lemon zest, sprinkle in the cornflour and season with a generous pinch of salt and pepper. Mix everything together to make the rosti mixture.

2. Melt the coconut oil in a non-stick frying pan over a medium heat. Spoon the parsnip batter into the pan to make three rostis, using the back of your spoon to flatten them slightly. Fry for 3–4 minutes on each side, without moving the rostis around, until golden and crisp.

3. While the rostis are cooking, mix the creamed horseradish with the Greek yoghurt. Season with salt, pepper and lemon juice to taste. Roughly chop the parsley. Peel the skin away from the mackerel and discard, flake the mackerel into large pieces.

4. Come back to your rostis. Serve up onto a plate, dollop on the horseradish yoghurt and top with the smoked mackerel. Scatter over the chopped parsley to finish and serve with the remaining lemon for squeezing over.

Veggie Swap

Swap the smoked mackerel for 2 poached eggs. For my favourite way to poach an egg, check out p. 190.

CURRIED LAMB STEAKS WITH COCONUT YOGHURT AND CORIANDER CHUTNEY

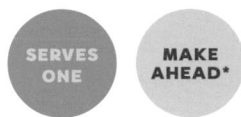

SERVES ONE   MAKE AHEAD*

INGREDIENTS

½ tbsp coconut oil

2 tsp garam masala

big pinch of ground turmeric

200g lamb steaks, trimmed of visible fat

salt and pepper

100g sugarsnap peas

handful of coriander

knob of fresh ginger, roughly chopped

½ green chilli – remove the seeds if you don't like it hot

juice of ½ lemon

2 tbsp coconut yoghurt

* REHEAT IN MICROWAVE OR HOT OVEN WHEN YOU'RE READY TO EAT.

1. Preheat the grill to maximum.

2. Ping the coconut oil in a microwaveable bowl to just melt. Stir in the garam masala and turmeric.

3. Lay the lamb steaks on a baking tray, season on both sides with salt and pepper then pour over the curried coconut oil. Rub the oil into both sides of the flesh, then slide under the hot grill. Cook for 3 minutes then flip the lamb over. Lay the sugarsnap peas around the lamb and cook for 3 minutes on the other side – I like my lamb a little pink in the middle, grill for an extra 2 minutes before flipping if you like yours well done.

4. Meanwhile put the coriander (stalks and all), ginger, green chilli and lemon juice into a small food processor. Blitz to a smooth chutney and season to taste.

5. Spoon the coconut yoghurt onto a plate. Lay the grilled lamb steaks and sugarsnaps on top, then drizzle over the coriander chutney.

Veggie Swap

Swap the lamb for 60g paneer cut into cubes, coated in the oil and spices then fried for 3–4 minutes, turning until all sides are golden and crisp. Microwave the sugarsnap peas with 100g trimmed green beans for 2 minutes with 1 tablespoon of water until tender.

REDUCED CARB

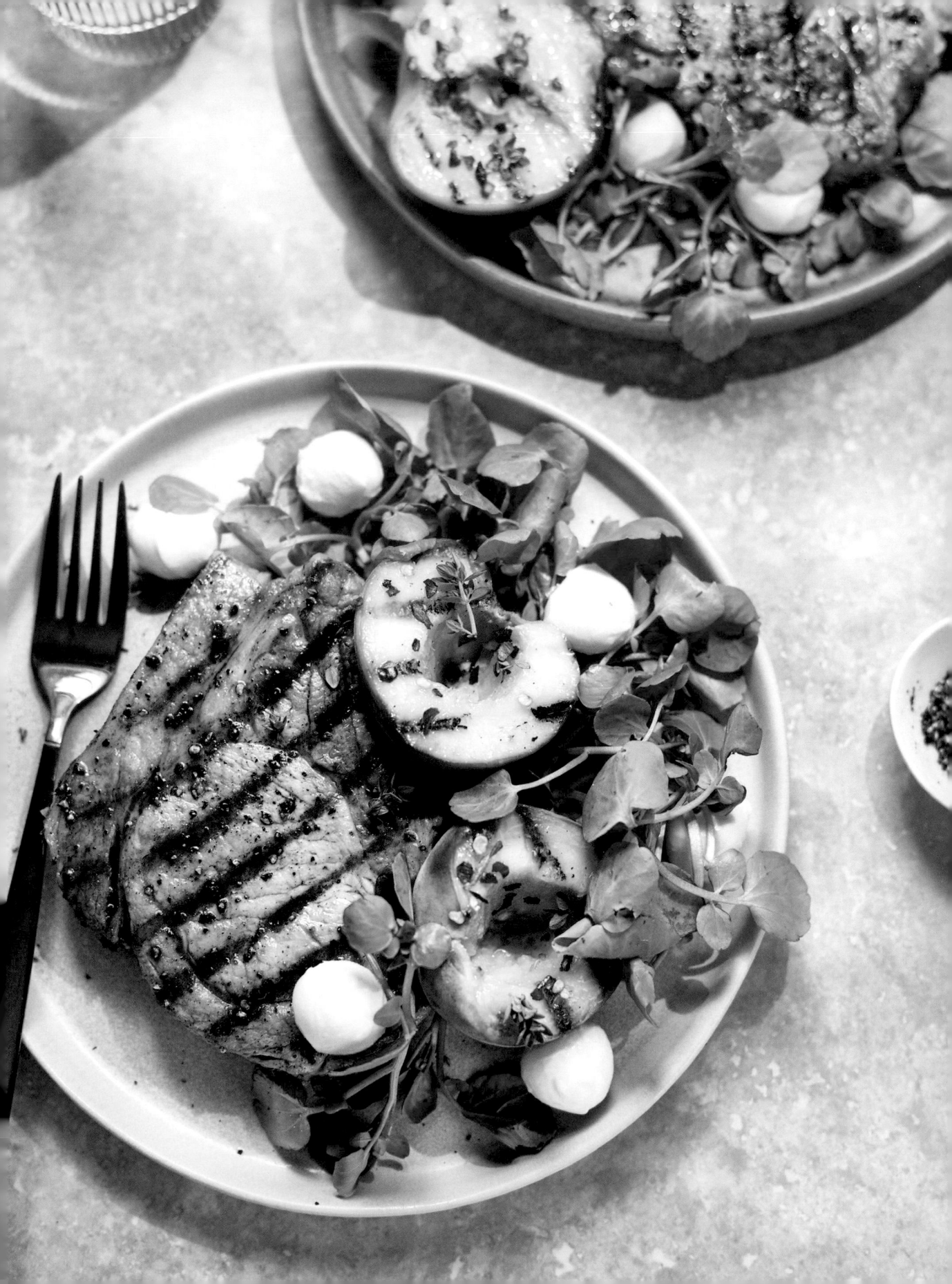

PORK CHOP WITH GRILLED PEACH, MOZZARELLA AND WATERCRESS

INGREDIENTS

1 x 200g boneless pork chop,
   trimmed of visible fat
1 tbsp olive oil
salt and pepper
1 peach or 2 apricots
2 sprigs of thyme
pinch of dried chilli flakes
2 handfuls of watercress
splash of white wine vinegar
40g mini mozzarella balls

SERVES ONE

1. Heat a griddle pan over a medium to high heat. Drizzle the pork chop with a little olive oil, rubbing it into the flesh, and season all over with salt and pepper. Once the griddle pan is hot, carefully lay the pork chop on one side of the pan. Cook for 6–7 minutes on each side.

2. Meanwhile cut the peach in half and de-stone. Pick the leaves from the sprigs of thyme. Drizzle the remaining oil over the peach, sprinkle over the thyme leaves and chilli flakes, using your fingers to massage them into the fruit.

3. Place the peach halves cut side down next to the pork chop. Grill for 1–2 minutes on each side until nicely caramelized. Transfer to a serving plate. Pile the watercress next to the peach, then drizzle a splash of white wine vinegar over both. Drop the mini mozzarella balls into the watercress salad.

4. Come back to the pork chop. Check it is cooked through by cutting into the thickest part to make sure there is no pink meat left.

5. Once you are happy with the meat, lay the pork on the plate next to the grilled peach halves and salad.

INGREDIENTS

60g butter
1 leek, finely sliced
2 medium carrots, finely chopped
2 celery sticks, finely chopped
salt and pepper
1 veggie stock cube
2 fat cloves garlic, finely
   chopped
knob of fresh ginger, finely
   chopped
1 tbsp medium curry powder
2 tsp cumin seeds
2 tbsp tomato puree
1 x 400g tin of green lentils,
   drained
1 head of cauliflower, cut into
   small florets
2 handfuls of frozen peas
30g cheddar, grated

*** ASSEMBLE THE COTTAGE PIE
COMPLETELY AND KEEP COVERED
IN THE FRIDGE. REHEAT IN A
HOT OVEN FOR 20 MINUTES
UNTIL BUBBLING, THEN GRILL FOR
5 MINUTES TO GET A CRISPY TOP.**

CURRIED COTTAGE PIE

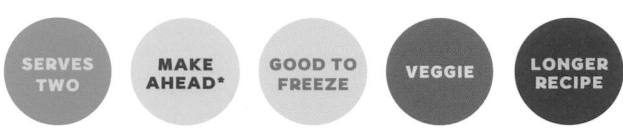

1. Melt 20g butter in a saucepan over a medium heat. Once bubbling, scrape in the chopped leek, carrots and celery along with a pinch of salt. Cook, stirring regularly, for 10 minutes until veg is completely soft.

2. Meanwhile bring a kettle of water to the boil. Put the veggie stock cube into a jug, measure in 150ml of boiling water and whisk with a fork to dissolve.

3. Come back to the saucepan, add the garlic and ginger. Cook for 1 minute more, sprinkle in the curry powder and cumin seeds, spoon in the tomato puree. Give everything a good mix and cook for 2 minutes more, then tip in the drained green lentils and the veggie stock.

4. Bring the pie mix to a simmer, turn down the heat to low and leave to gently bubble away while you make the mash.

5. Pour the remaining water from the kettle into a saucepan and re-boil. Salt the water and drop in the cauliflower florets. Cook for 10 minutes until completely tender. Drain into a sieve and leave to steam for a few minutes – this will stop you from having watery mash.

6. Preheat the grill to maximum.

7. Tip the cooked cauliflower into a food processor, add the remaining butter and some seasoning, blitz to a smooth mash. You can also do this with a stick blender.

8. Come back to your pie mix. Add the frozen peas and season to taste. Once the peas have defrosted, spoon the filling into an ovenproof dish. Spread the mash on top, then grate over the cheddar cheese. Slide under the grill for 5 minutes or until bubbling and golden with a crispy top. My low-carb cottage pie.

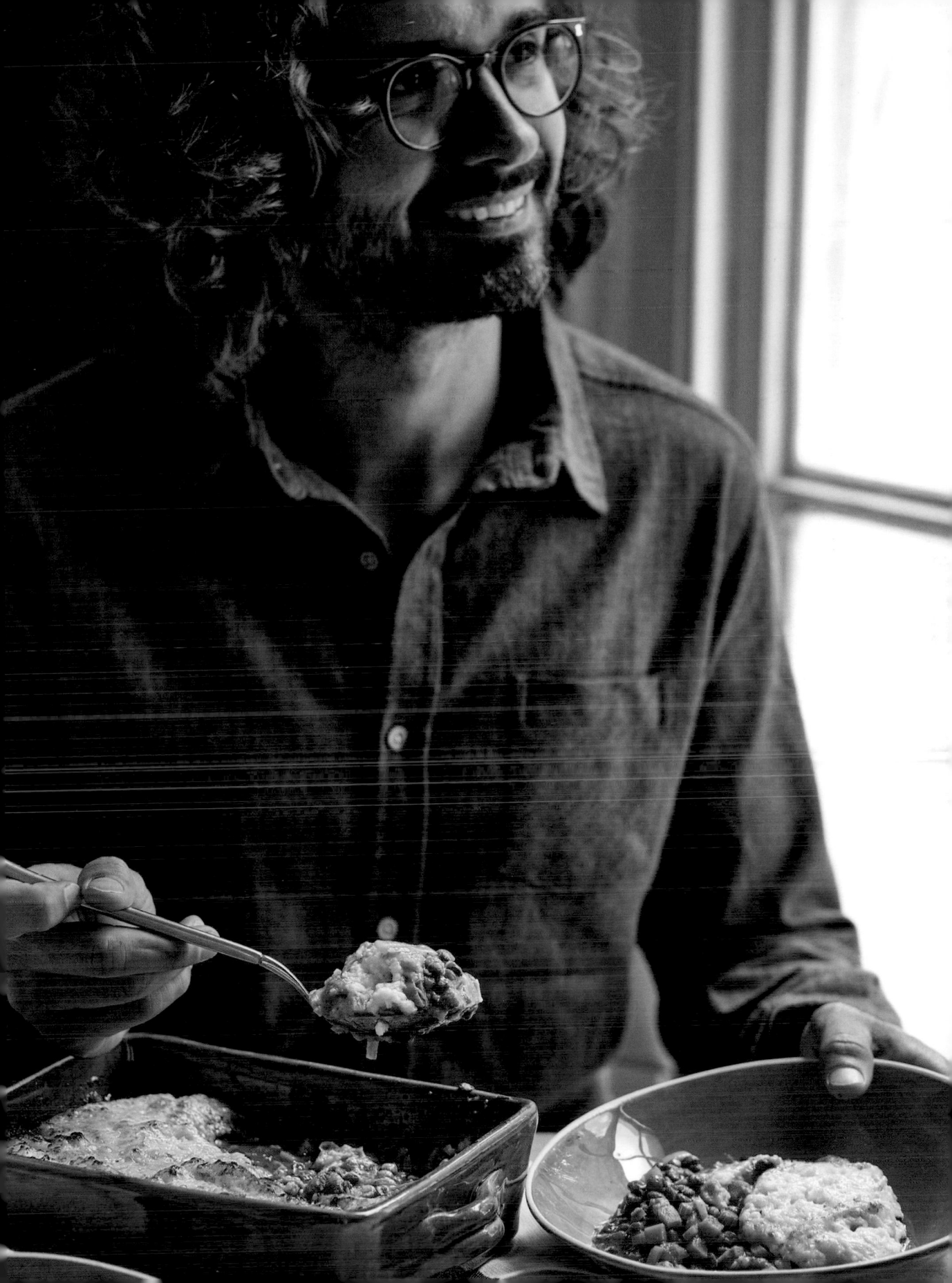

"

I'm a nurse so often work 12–13 hour shifts including lots of nights.

I can't believe the difference in energy levels and my mood since doing your workouts and learning about what foods I need to fuel my body correctly!

"

EMILY, 25

"

I really didn't exercise before, but you have changed that now.

Now I'm exercising regularly, I feel emotionally and physically great!

"

ANN, 61

INGREDIENTS

½ small red onion
juice of 1 lime
big pinch of sumac
salt and pepper
1 x 210g tin of chickpeas
1 small clove garlic
2–3 lamb chops (200g)
1 tbsp olive oil
small handful of parsley
20g pistachios
1 tbsp tahini

*** THE PICKLED RED ONIONS
WILL KEEP FOR 2 DAYS IN
THE FRIDGE.**

GRILLED LAMB CHOPS WITH WARM HUMMUS, QUICK PICKLED RED ONIONS AND PISTACHIOS

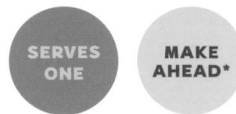

SERVES ONE · **MAKE AHEAD***

1. Slice the red onion as finely as you can. Scrape into a bowl, squeeze over the juice of half the lime, sprinkle with sumac, salt and black pepper. Use your hands to scrunch the onion with the lime juice – this will encourage it to soften. Leave to lightly pickle.

2. Empty the chickpeas along with their water into a microwaveable bowl. Add the garlic clove, cover and zap on high for 5 minutes.

3. Meanwhile heat a griddle pan over the highest heat. Drizzle the lamb chops with a little olive oil, rubbing it into the flesh, and season all over with salt and pepper. When the griddle pan is searingly hot, carefully lay the lamb chops in. Cook for 3 minutes on each side.

4. Roughly chop the parsley and pistachios, then come back to the chickpeas. Carefully uncover, then tip the chickpeas along with their water and garlic into a small food processor. Spoon in the tahini and remaining olive oil, blitz to a smooth hummus. Add a little more water if you need. Season with juice from the remaining lime half, salt and pepper to taste.

5. By now the lamb chops should be cooked. Check by cutting into one of the thicker parts – I like mine slightly pink in the centre.

6. Spoon the warm hummus onto a plate. Place the lamb chops on top then scatter over the lightly pickled onions, pistachios and parsley.

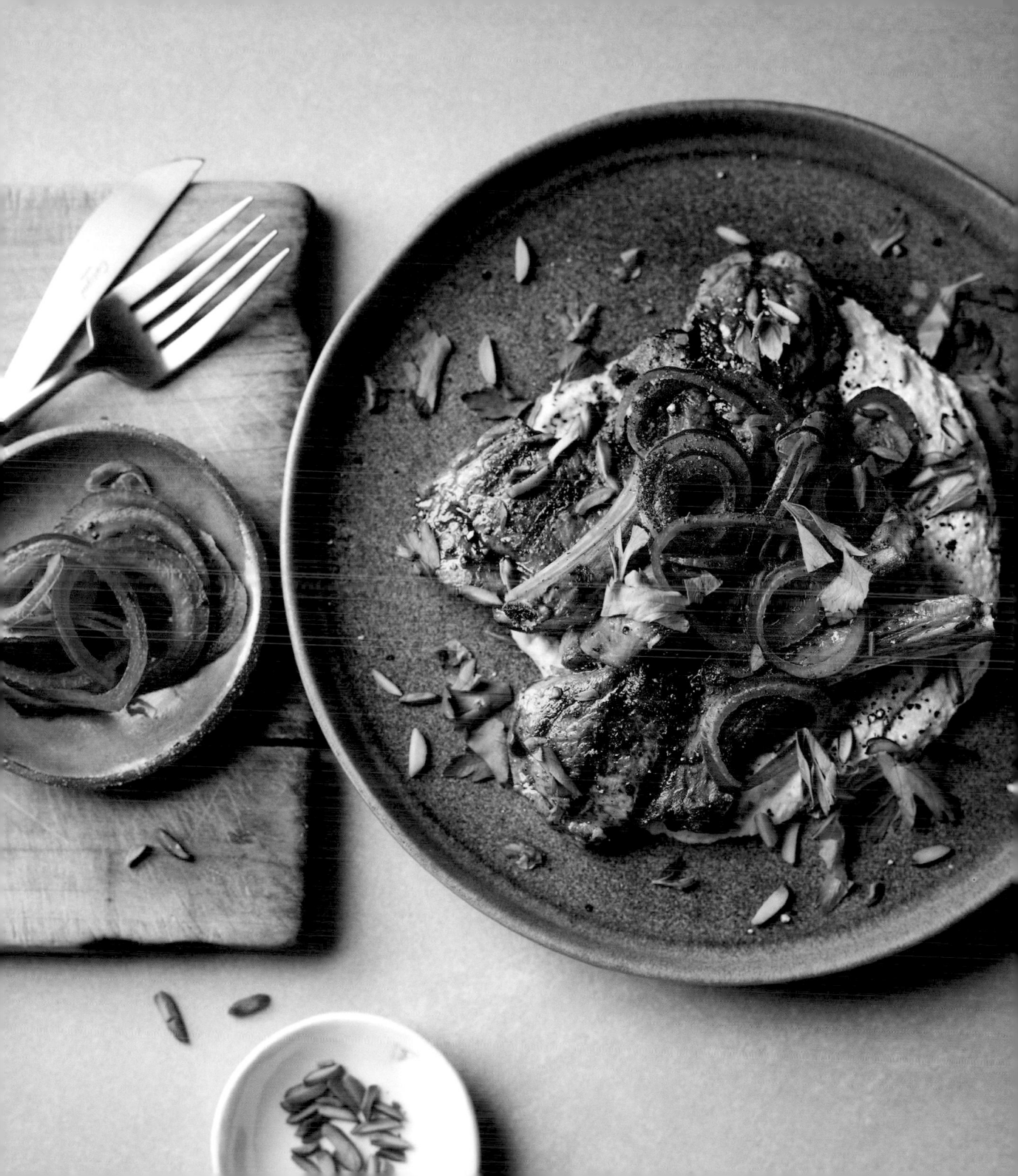

INGREDIENTS

1 x 225g sirloin steak, trimmed
of visible fat
drizzle of olive oil
salt and pepper
10 cherry tomatoes
2 large handfuls of rocket
juice of ½ lemon
15g butter
1 tbsp balsamic vinegar
30g goat's cheese

BALSAMIC STEAK WITH GOAT'S CHEESE, ROCKET AND CHERRY TOMATOES

SERVES
ONE

1. Heat a frying pan over the highest heat. Drizzle the steak with a little olive oil, rubbing it into the flesh, and season all over with salt and pepper. When the pan is searingly hot, carefully lay the steak in. Cook according to preference – I like my steaks medium rare, so 2½ minutes on each side, turning regularly – then leave to rest until you're ready to eat. Keep the frying pan to one side.

2. Meanwhile halve the cherry tomatoes. Pile the rocket onto a serving plate. Drop in the halved tomatoes and squeeze over the lemon juice.

3. Once the steak has rested, thinly slice the meat on an angle. Place the steak in with the rocket and tomatoes.

4. To finish, put the pan back on a medium heat (don't bother washing it – extra flavour). Melt in the butter. When bubbling, pour in the balsamic vinegar, stirring to combine. Once mixed together, pour the warm dressing over the steak. Crumble over the goat's cheese and crack over a good whack of black pepper before diving in.

REDUCED CARB

CREAMY TURKEY, MUSHROOM AND COURGETTE STROGANOFF

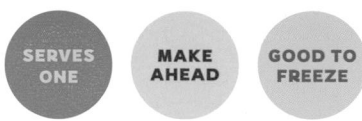

SERVES ONE MAKE AHEAD GOOD TO FREEZE

INGREDIENTS

20g butter
200g skinless turkey breast
    fillets, sliced into 1cm strips
100g button mushrooms, halved
1 medium courgette, sliced into
    half-moons
salt and pepper
1 clove garlic, finely chopped
big pinch of smoked paprika
2 tbsp sour cream
1 tsp Dijon mustard
3 cornichons, roughly
    chopped – optional
handful of parsley, chopped

1. Melt the butter in a non-stick frying pan over a high heat. When bubbling, chuck the turkey, mushrooms and courgette into the pan. Sprinkle everything with some salt and pepper. Fry, stirring regularly, for about 4 minutes until the turkey is nearly cooked through.

2. Lower the heat on the pan. Add the garlic and smoked paprika. Cook for 1 minute more then spoon in the sour cream, Dijon mustard and the cornichons, if you're using them. Pour in 75ml of water and give everything a good mix to create a super-creamy sauce.

3. Check the turkey is cooked by slicing into one of the larger pieces to make sure the meat is white all the way through, with no raw pink bits left.

4. Once you're happy with the meat, pile the creamy stroganoff into a bowl and scatter over the chopped parsley.

Veggie Swap

Swap the turkey for 200g sliced mushrooms of your choice, cooked in the same way as the turkey.

REDUCED CARB

INGREDIENTS

½ tbsp coconut oil
1 tbsp Thai green curry paste
200g reduced-fat pork mince
1 baby gem lettuce
30g salted roasted peanuts
small handful of mint leaves
small handful of coriander
    leaves
juice of ½ lime
splash of fish sauce
sliced red chilli, to serve –
    optional

THAI GREEN PORK LETTUCE CUPS

SERVES
ONE

1. Melt the coconut oil in a wok or frying pan over a high heat. Spoon in the curry paste and cook, stirring constantly, for 30 seconds until smelling amazing, then tip the pork mince into the pan. Use the back of a wooden spoon to break the mince into small pieces. Fry for 6–7 minutes.

2. Meanwhile separate the baby gem lettuce leaves onto a serving plate. Roughly chop the peanuts, mint and coriander leaves.

3. Come back to the pork mince. It should be cooked through but not too brown. Check this by making sure there are no pink bits left. Squeeze in the lime juice and a splash of fish sauce. Give everything a final stir then take the pan off the heat.

4. Pile the pork mince into each of the lettuce leaves, then scatter over the chopped peanuts, mint and coriander. Garnish with slices of red chilli if you like.

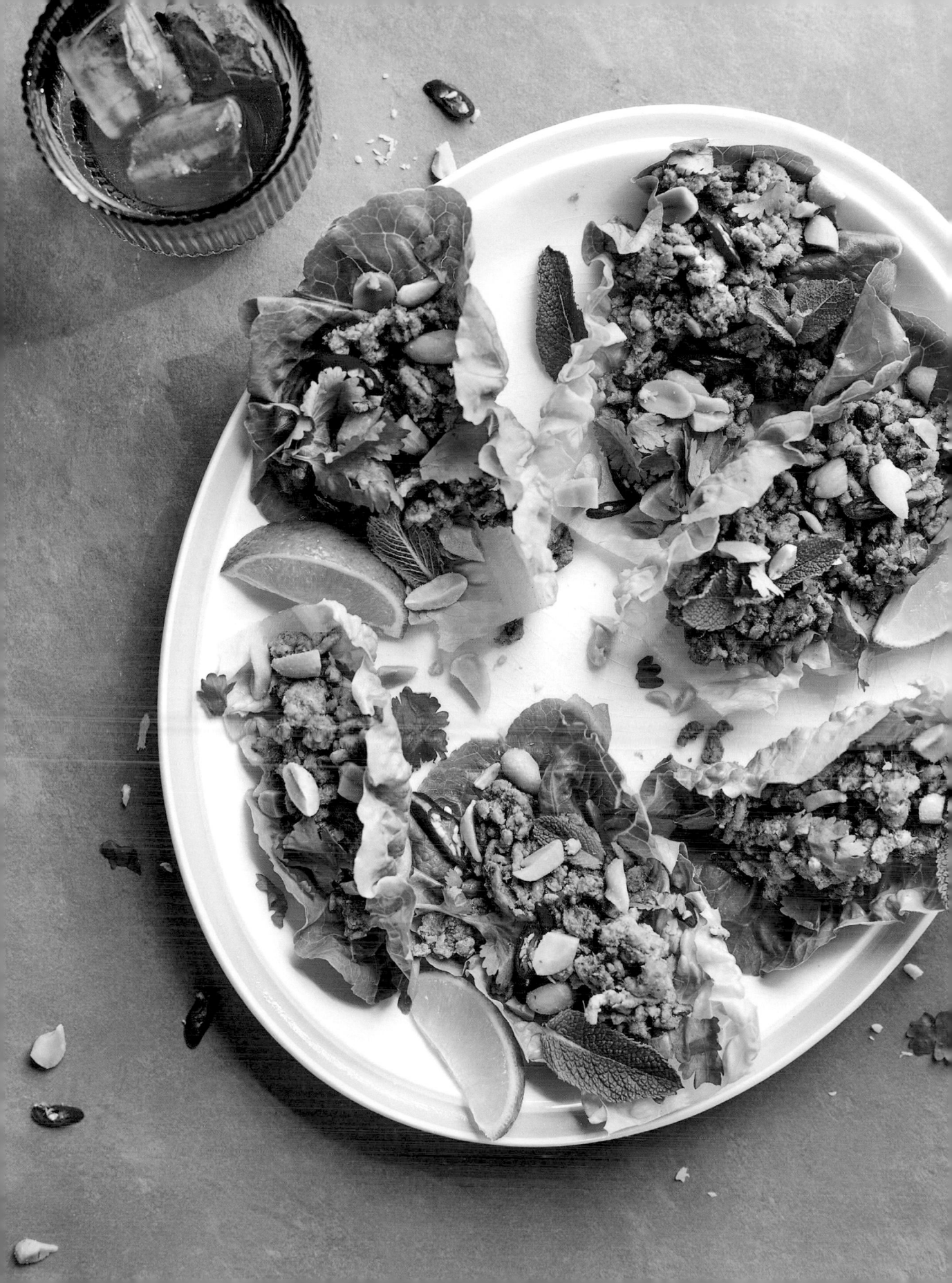

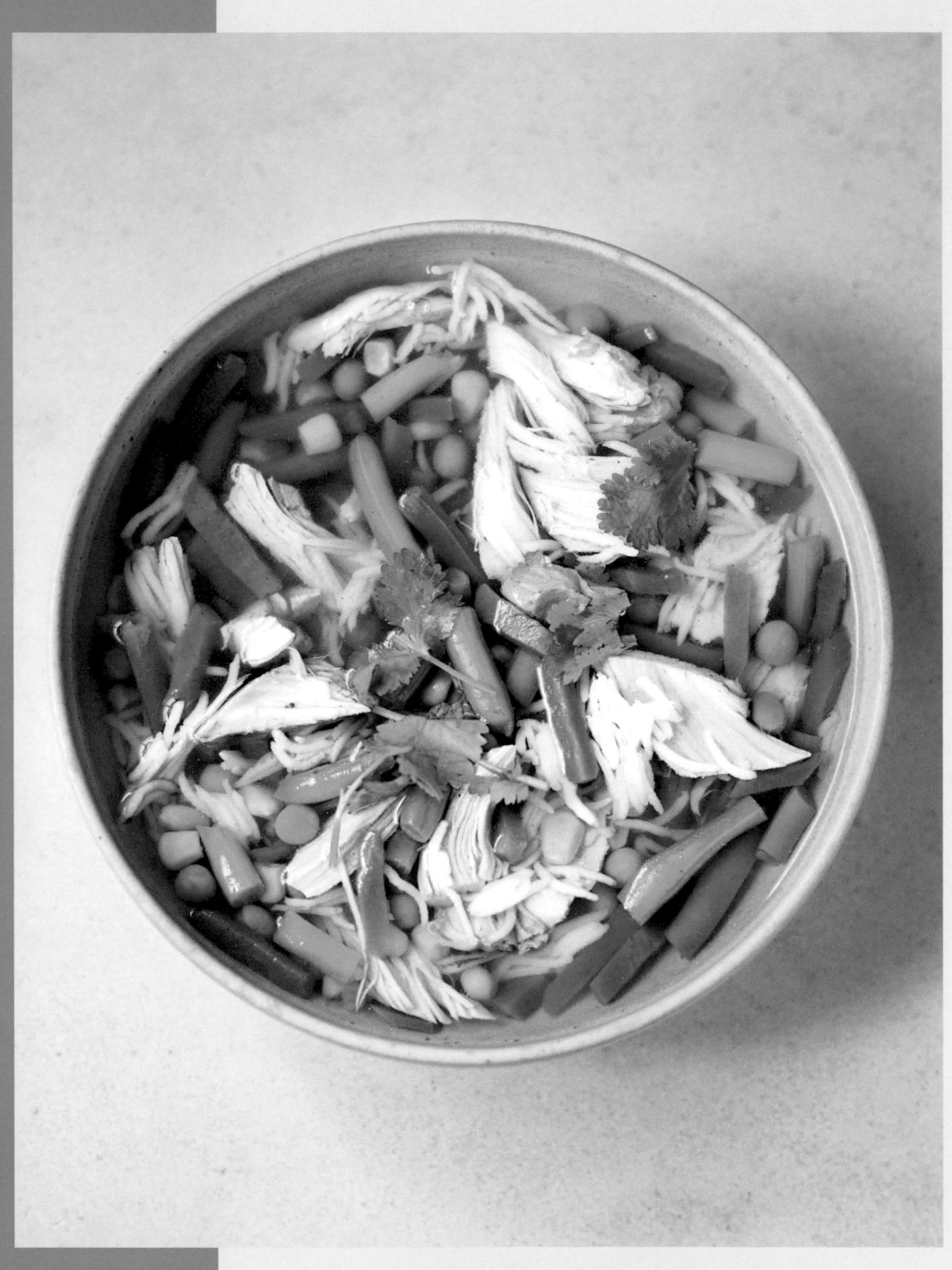

SPICY CHICKEN CURRY SOUP

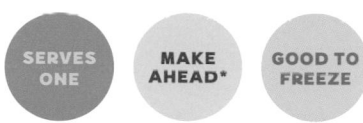

SERVES ONE   MAKE AHEAD*   GOOD TO FREEZE

INGREDIENTS

1 onion
1 tbsp coconut oil
1 tbsp medium curry powder
1 chicken stock cube
1 x 200g skinless chicken breast
   fillet, cut into quarters
salt and pepper
200g frozen mixed vegetables
60g pre-cooked rice (around
   ¼ rice pouch)
2 tbsp natural yoghurt
small handful of coriander

*** YOU COULD MULTIPLY THIS
RECIPE BY FOUR AND FREEZE OR
KEEP THE REMAINING PORTIONS
IN THE FRIDGE FOR UP TO 3 DAYS.**

1. Bring a kettle of water to the boil.

2. Grate the onion. Melt the coconut oil in a saucepan over a medium heat. Whack in the onion and sprinkle over the curry powder. Cook for 1 minute.

3. While the onion is cooking, put the chicken stock cube into a jug, measure in 300ml of boiling water and whisk with a fork to dissolve. Pour the chicken stock into the saucepan with the onion and curry powder.

4. Season the chicken breast pieces with salt and pepper then carefully drop them into the saucepan. Cover with a lid and cook for 8 minutes.

5. After 8 minutes the chicken should be cooked. Check by slicing into one of the pieces to make sure the meat is white all the way through, with no raw pink bits left. Once you're happy, using a slotted spoon lift the chicken onto a plate.

6. Add the frozen mixed vegetables and cooked rice to the saucepan, cook for 3 minutes more. Meanwhile, using two forks, shred the cooked chicken then put it back into the soup.

7. Season the soup to taste and spoon into a bowl. Dollop on the yoghurt and tear over some coriander to serve.

INGREDIENTS

½ small head of cauliflower

60g paneer (⅓ of the pack)

1 tbsp coconut oil

1 tsp ground turmeric

2 tsp garlic-ginger paste

½ tsp dried chilli flakes

2 large handfuls of baby
   spinach leaves

2 tsp garam masala

salt and pepper

juice of ½ lemon

SAAG PANEER WITH CAULIFLOWER 'RICE'

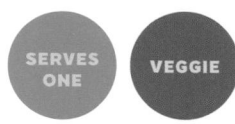

SERVES ONE   VEGGIE

1. Roughly chop the cauliflower then blitz in a food processor until it resembles rice. Keep to one side.

2. Cut the paneer into large cubes. Ping 1 teaspoon of coconut oil in a microwaveable bowl to melt. Stir in the ground turmeric, drop in the paneer cubes, toss to coat.

3. Heat a saucepan over a medium to high heat. Spoon in 1 teaspoon of coconut oil. Once melted, add the garlic-ginger paste and chilli flakes. Cook for 1 minute then dump the spinach into the pan. When wilted, keep the pan on a very low heat while you fry the paneer.

4. Heat a non-stick frying pan over a high heat. Lay the paneer in the pan, fry for 3–4 minutes, turning as each side becomes golden and crisp. Tip into the saucepan along with the spinach.

5. Put the frying pan back on the heat (don't bother washing it – extra flavour). Melt the remaining coconut oil. Tip in the cauliflower rice, sprinkle in the garam masala and a generous pinch of salt and black pepper. Fry for 2 minutes until the cauliflower is tender.

6. Dish up the cauliflower rice. Squeeze the lemon juice into the paneer and spinach, season to taste then pile on top of the 'rice'.

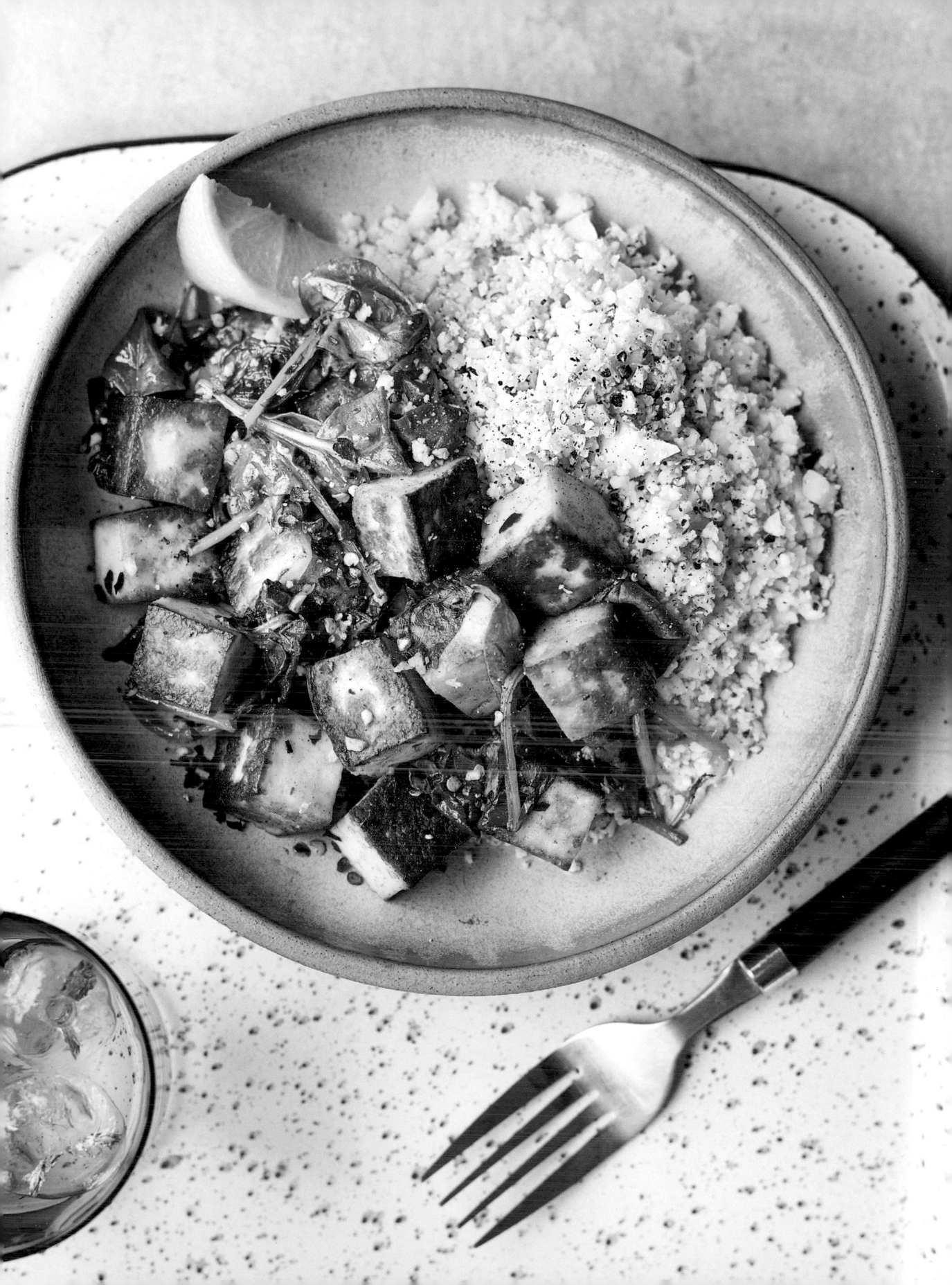

INGREDIENTS

30g hazelnuts
1 x 200g skinless chicken
    breast fillet
1 tbsp olive oil
salt and black pepper
1 tsp cumin seeds
1 small clove garlic
small handful of coriander
small handful of parsley
splash of sherry vinegar
2 large handfuls of rocket

CHARGRILLED CHICKEN WITH MOJO VERDE

SERVES
ONE

1. Toast the hazelnuts in a dry frying pan over a medium heat until they smell nutty. Take the pan off the heat and leave to cool.

2. Place the chicken between two pieces of cling film or baking parchment on a chopping board. Using a rolling pin, meat mallet or any other blunt instrument, bash the chicken until it is about 1cm thick all over. Drizzle with a little olive oil, rubbing it into the flesh, and season all over with salt and pepper.

3. Heat a griddle pan over a high heat. Once the pan is searingly hot, carefully lay the chicken in. Cook for about 4 minutes on each side.

4. While the chicken is cooking, tip the cooled hazelnuts out of the pan and roughly chop. Put the dry pan back over a medium heat. Sprinkle in the cumin seeds, cook for about 30 seconds or until you can just smell the spice. Carefully tip the cumin seeds into a small food processor.

5. Put the garlic, coriander and parsley (stalks and all) into the food processor along with the remaining olive oil and 1 tablespoon water. Blitz to a smooth green sauce. Season with sherry vinegar, salt and pepper to taste.

6. Come back to the chicken, which will now be cooked. Check by slicing into a thicker part to make sure the meat is white all the way through with no raw pink bits left. Place the grilled chicken onto a plate.

7. Spoon over the mojo verde sauce. Serve with a pile of rocket then scatter over the toasted hazelnuts.

Veggie Swap

Swap the chicken for 200g little trees (tenderstem broccoli), any bigger stalks sliced in half lengthways, cooked on a griddle pan in the same way as the chicken.

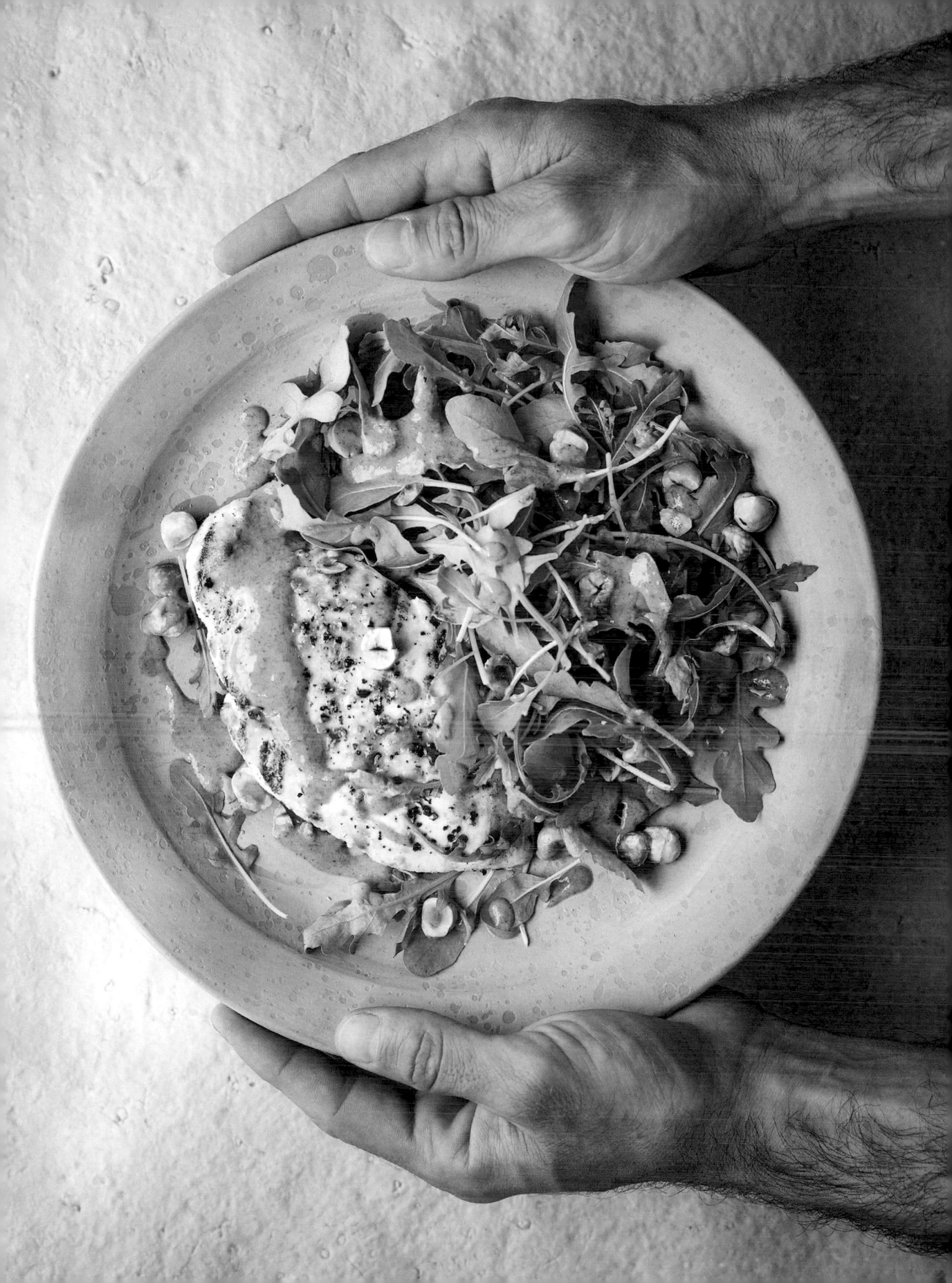

INGREDIENTS

2 tbsp almond butter

1 tsp soy sauce

juice of 1 lime

1 tbsp coconut oil

200g skinless, boneless
chicken thighs, cut into
large, bite-sized pieces

salt and pepper

⅛ small red cabbage

1 medium carrot, peeled

handful of coriander

½ red chilli

1 tbsp sesame seeds

*** REHEAT CHICKEN ONLY.
KEEP SLAW SEPARATE.**

ALMOND BUTTER SATAY CHICKEN WITH ASIAN SLAW

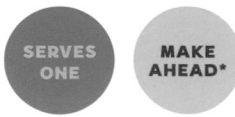

SERVES ONE

MAKE AHEAD*

1. First make the satay sauce. In a small bowl mix together the almond butter, soy sauce, juice of half the lime and 2 tablespoons of water.

2. Melt the coconut oil in a wok or frying pan over a high heat. Season the chicken thigh pieces with salt and pepper then put them into the pan. Fry for 6 minutes, turning occasionally.

3. Meanwhile grate the red cabbage and carrot into a bowl. Roughly chop the coriander and finely slice the red chilli – remove the seeds if you don't like it hot. Scrape the coriander and chilli into the cabbage bowl. Sprinkle in the sesame seeds and squeeze over the juice from the remaining lime half. Mix the slaw together, season to taste.

4. Come back to the chicken. Lower the heat, pour in the satay sauce. Bubble away, stirring for a couple of minutes, or until the chicken is cooked. Check by slicing into one of the larger pieces – the knife should cut through easily and the meat will have turned from pink to a whitish brown.

5. Pile the slaw onto a plate and dish up the satay chicken.

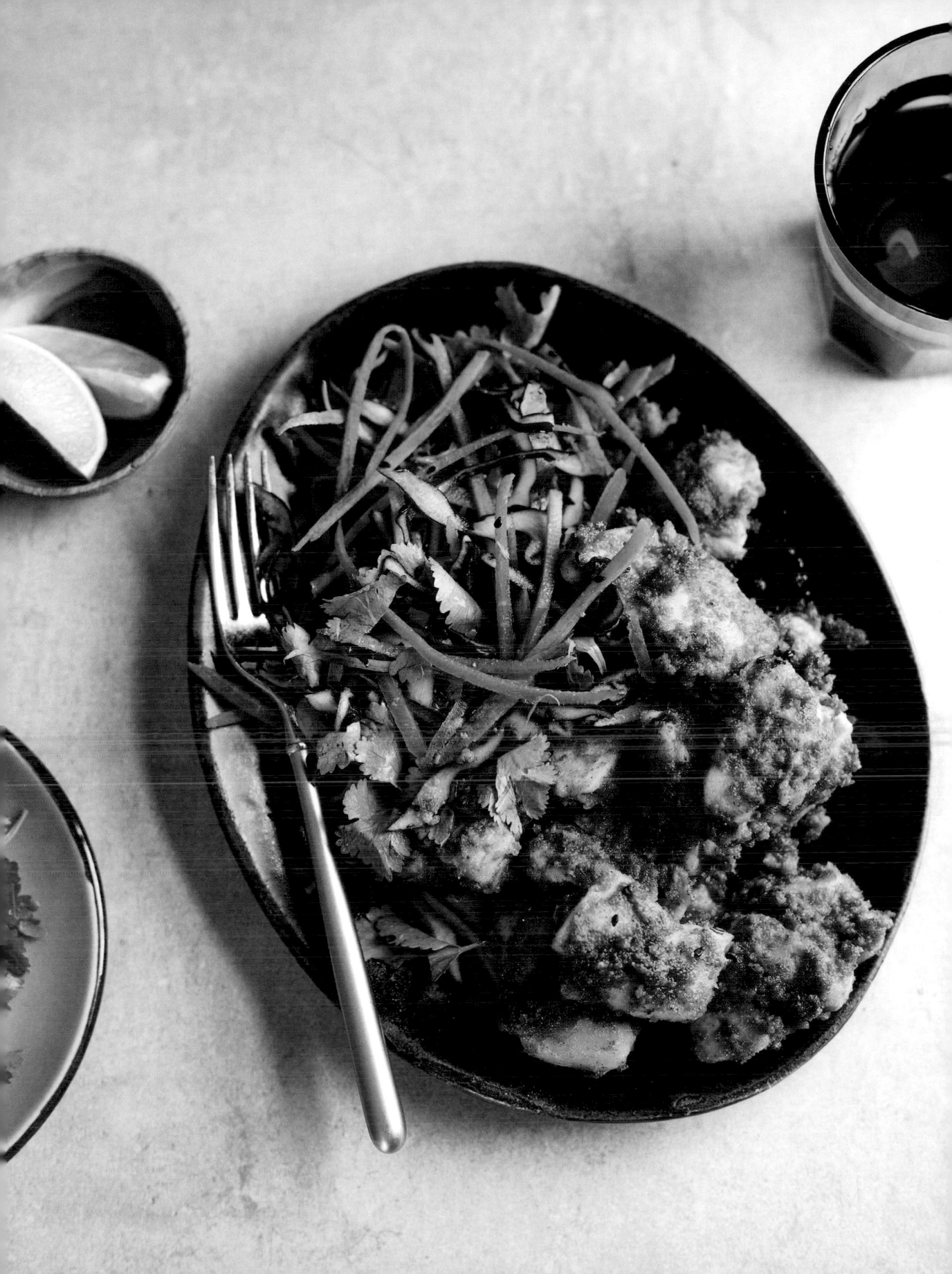

INGREDIENTS

100g radishes
2 tbsp salted roasted peanuts
handful of coriander
1 large carrot
1 lime
splash of fish sauce – optional
2 tbsp cornflour
big pinch of dried chilli flakes
salt and pepper
200g raw king prawns
2 tbsp coconut oil
sweet chilli sauce, to serve

SALT AND PEPPER PRAWNS WITH SWEET CHILLI

SERVES
ONE

1. Roughly chop the radishes, peanuts and coriander. Peel the carrot lengthways into long ribbons and put into a bowl. Scrape in the radishes, peanuts and most of the coriander. Cut the lime in half, squeeze the juice of one of the lime halves into the salad then splash in the fish sauce, if using. Mix everything together.

2. Stir the cornflour with the chilli flakes, a generous pinch of salt and a good whack of black pepper in a shallow bowl.

3. Using some kitchen roll, pat the prawns dry.

4. Melt the coconut oil in a wok or large frying pan over a high heat. Drop the prawns into the cornflour mix, toss so that each prawn becomes evenly coated, then carefully lower the prawns into the oil. Fry for 1½ minutes on each side. The raw grey colour of the prawns will turn pink, which shows you they are cooked.

5. Using a slotted spoon to get rid of any excess oil, pile the fried salt and pepper prawns onto a plate. Scatter over the remaining coriander. Serve with the carrot, radish and peanut salad, sweet chilli sauce and the remaining lime half for squeezing. Better than any takeaway.

REDUCED CARB

Veggie Swap

Swap the prawns for 140g firm tofu, cut into cubes and fried in the same way as the prawns.

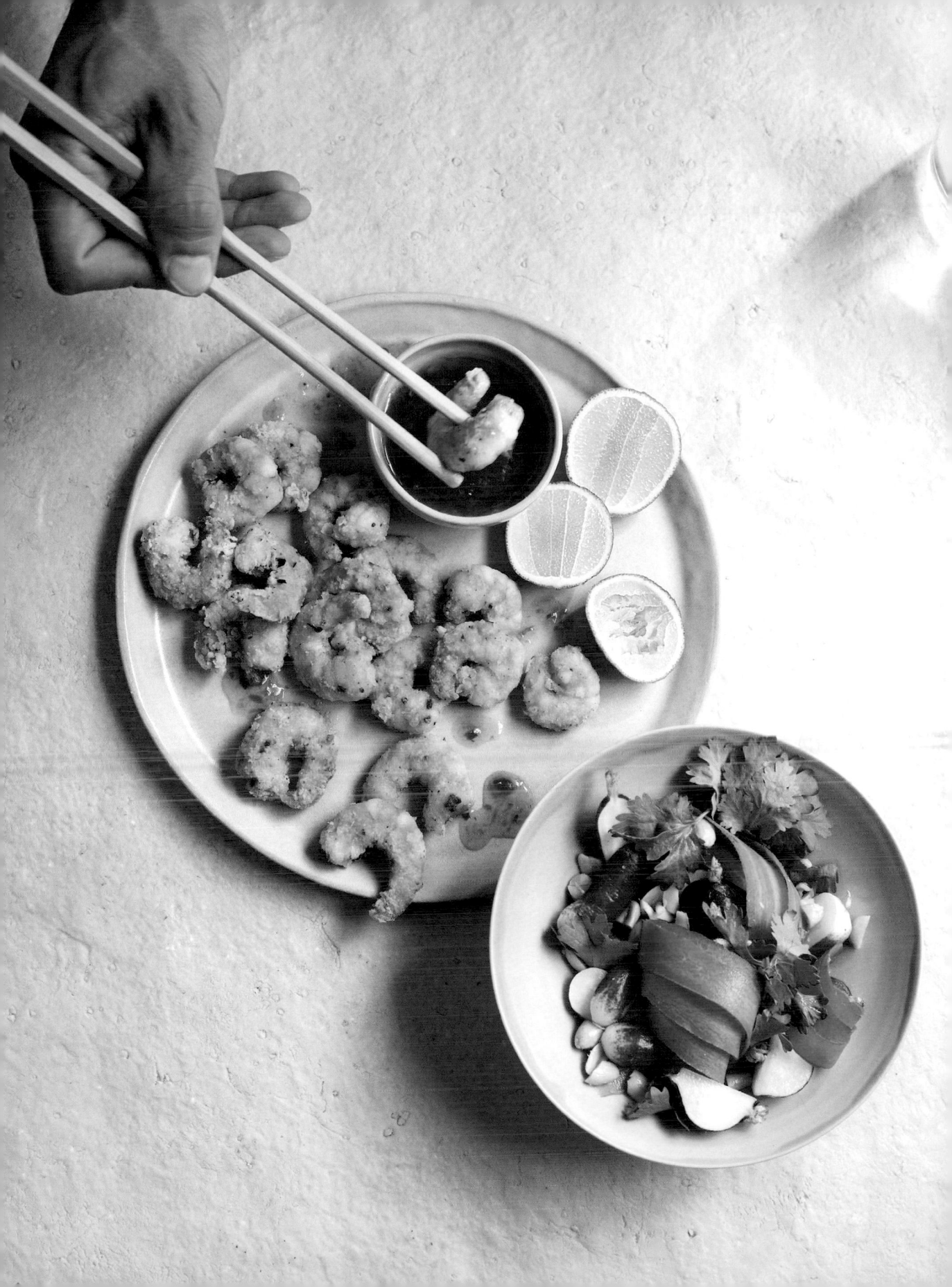

INGREDIENTS

1½ tbsp coconut oil
3 large handfuls of kale
big pinch of cayenne pepper
salt and pepper
220g reduced-fat beef mince,
   the freshest and best quality
   you can buy
2 sprigs of thyme
2 tsp Dijon mustard
1 small shallot, finely chopped
1 tbsp mayonnaise
½ tbsp ketchup

*** YOU COULD MAKE THE STEAK
HACHÉ (UP UNTIL STEP 3) THEN
KEEP RAW, COVERED IN THE
FRIDGE UNTIL READY TO COOK.
COOK THE KALE AND MAKE THE
SAUCE JUST BEFORE SERVING.**

STEAK HACHÉ

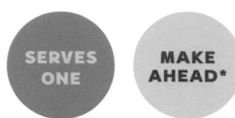

SERVES ONE   **MAKE AHEAD***

1. Preheat the oven to 220°C (fan 200°/gas mark 7). Dollop 1 tablespoon of coconut oil into a large roasting tray then place in the oven to melt.

2. Carefully bring the hot roasting tray out of the oven. Dump in the kale, season with a big pinch of cayenne, salt and pepper, then using tongs, separate the kale into a single layer. Roast in the oven for 8–10 minutes until crisp. Check after 5 minutes, removing any pieces of kale which are already crisp.

3. Meanwhile dump the beef mince into a bowl. Strip the thyme leaves off their sprigs into the bowl with the beef. Add 1½ teaspoons of mustard along with three-quarters of the chopped shallot and plenty of salt and pepper. Use your hands to combine all the flavourings, then shape the beef into a rough burger patty about the size of your hand. Put on a plate.

4. Melt the remaining coconut oil in a non-stick frying pan over a high heat. Lay the patty in the pan. Fry for 3 minutes on each side until nicely browned and mostly cooked through, then transfer the patty to a baking tray and put in the oven to finish cooking for 1–2 minutes. You want it crisp on the outside but juicy within – I like mine a little pink in the middle. Keep on cooking the patty if you like it more well done.

5. While the meat is in the oven, make your sauce. Mix the mayonnaise, ketchup, remaining mustard and shallot together in a small bowl.

6. Once you're happy with the burger patty, place onto a serving plate. Pile up the kale crisps and serve with the burger sauce. Dream food.

SEEDED CHICKEN SCHNITZEL SALAD

SERVES ONE

INGREDIENTS

1 x 200g skinless chicken
  breast fillet
salt and pepper
2 tbsp mixed seeds
1 tbsp mayonnaise
1 tbsp olive oil
2 large handfuls of kale
150g grilled vegetable
  antipasti selection
½ lemon

1. Place the chicken between two pieces of cling film or baking parchment on a chopping board. Using a rolling pin, meat mallet or any other blunt instrument, bash the chicken until it is about 1cm thick all over. Season with salt and pepper.

2. Spoon the mixed seeds onto a plate. Dollop the mayonnaise over the flattened chicken breast, using your fingers to make sure the whole fillet gets covered, then place the chicken fillet onto the seeds. Turn the chicken, patting the seeds into the flesh, until fully coated.

3. Heat the olive oil in a non-stick frying pan over a medium to high heat. Place the seeded chicken breast in the pan, cook for about 4 minutes on each side, carefully flipping halfway.

4. Meanwhile dump the kale leaves into a bowl. Tip in the grilled vegetables and squeeze over the lemon juice. Give the salad a good mix with your hands – massaging the kale leaves with the other ingredients will help the leaves soften slightly.

5. Come back to your chicken. Check it is cooked by slicing into a thicker part to make sure the meat is white all the way through with no raw pink bits left. Once you're happy, take the pan off the heat.

6. Pile the kale salad onto a plate and place the seeded chicken schnitzel on top.

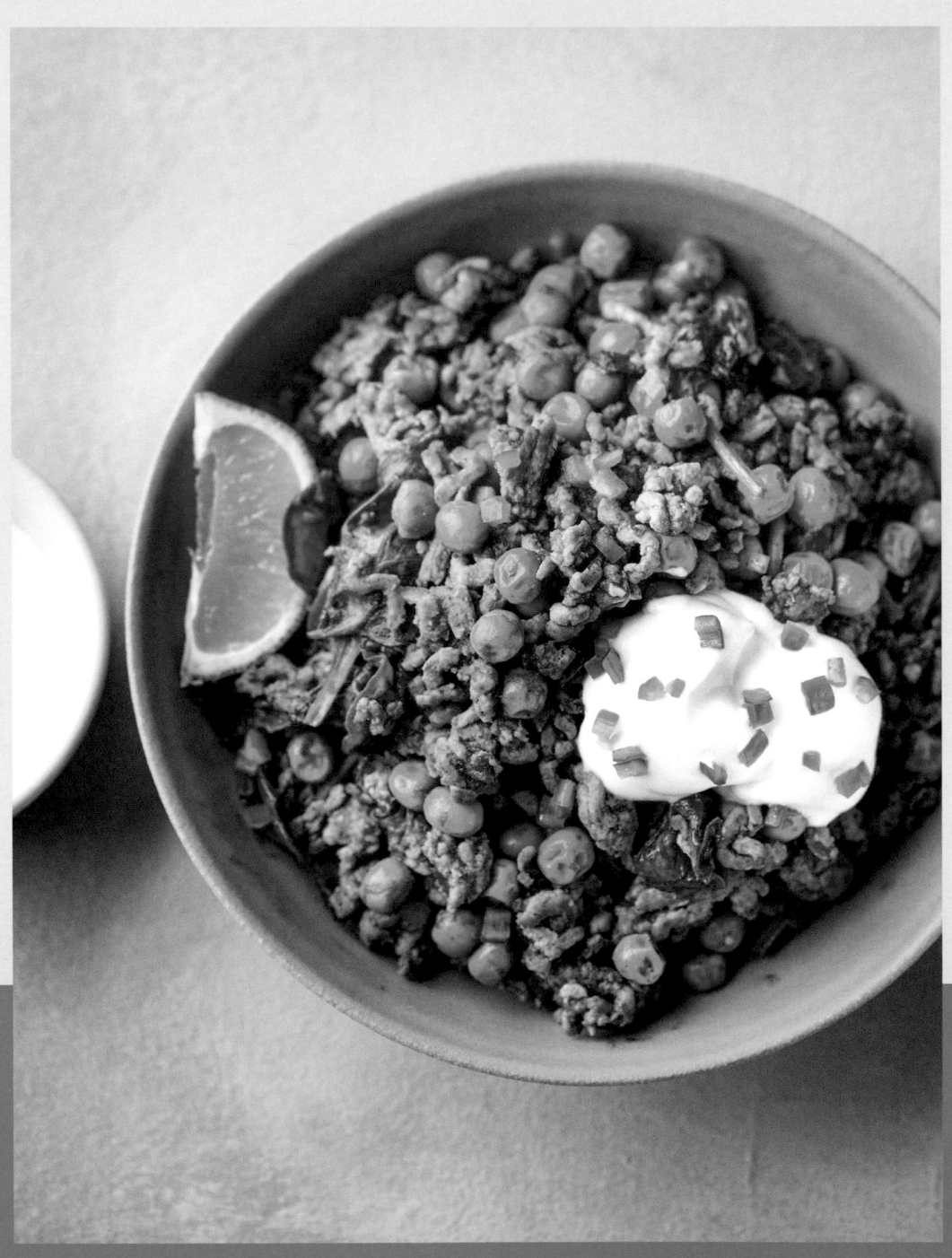

LAMB AND PEA KEEMA

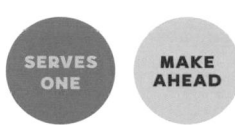

SERVES ONE   **MAKE AHEAD**

INGREDIENTS

½ tbsp coconut oil
220g reduced-fat lamb mince
2 tsp garam masala
½ tsp ground turmeric
salt and pepper
2 tsp garlic-ginger paste
2 tbsp tomato puree
2 large handfuls of spinach
150g frozen peas
juice of ½ lime
2 tbsp natural yoghurt
½ green chilli, finely sliced –
   remove the seeds if you don't
   like it hot

1. Melt the coconut oil in a saucepan over a high heat. Tip the lamb mince into the pan. Use the back of a wooden spoon to break the mince into small pieces.

2. Fry for around 5 minutes until the mince is no longer pink, then sprinkle in the garam masala and ground turmeric along with a good pinch of salt and pepper. Spoon in the garlic-ginger paste and tomato puree. Give everything a good mix and cook for 1 minute more.

3. Pour 200ml of water into the saucepan. Place a lid on top of the pan, reduce the heat to medium. Leave the keema to bubble away for around 5 minutes. Low-maintenance cooking.

4. Take the lid off the pan and crank up the heat. Drop in the spinach and peas. Cook for 1–2 minutes more until the spinach has wilted. Squeeze in the lime juice and season to taste.

5. Dish up the keema. Top with a dollop of yoghurt and the sliced green chilli.

REDUCED CARB

INGREDIENTS

1 avocado, de-stoned
½ small red onion
½ mango
½ red chilli
juice of ½ lime
salt and pepper
½ chorizo ring (around 110g)
1 egg
1 x 200g tin of sweetcorn,
    drained
2 tbsp self-raising flour
1 tbsp milk
½ tbsp coconut oil

*** SWEETCORN FRITTERS ONLY.
REHEAT IN A HOT OVEN FOR
5 MINUTES.**

SWEETCORN FRITTERS WITH CHORIZO AND MANGO AND AVOCADO SALSA

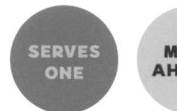

SERVES ONE

MAKE AHEAD*

1. Make the salsa. Scoop out the avocado, cut into cubes. Finely chop the red onion, mango and red chilli – remove the seeds if you don't like it hot. Scrape everything into a bowl. Squeeze in the lime juice and season with salt and pepper to taste.

2. Slice the chorizo.

3. Crack the egg into a large bowl. Mix in the drained sweetcorn, self-raising flour, milk and a big pinch of salt and pepper. Whisk together to form the fritter batter.

4. Heat two frying pans over a medium to high heat. Melt a dot of coconut oil in one of the pans, spoon the rest into the other. Into the pan with the dot of coconut oil, chuck in the chorizo. Fry, stirring occasionally, until crisp.

5. Meanwhile into the pan with the most coconut oil, spoon in the fritter mix to make four fritters, using the back of your spoon to flatten them slightly. Fry for 2 minutes on each side until golden, then transfer to a plate.

6. Spoon the chorizo along with its cooking oils over the sweetcorn fritters. Serve with the mango and avocado salsa.

REDUCED CARB

Veggie Swap

**Swap the fried chorizo
for 30g of feta crumbled
on top of the sweetcorn
fritters before eating.**

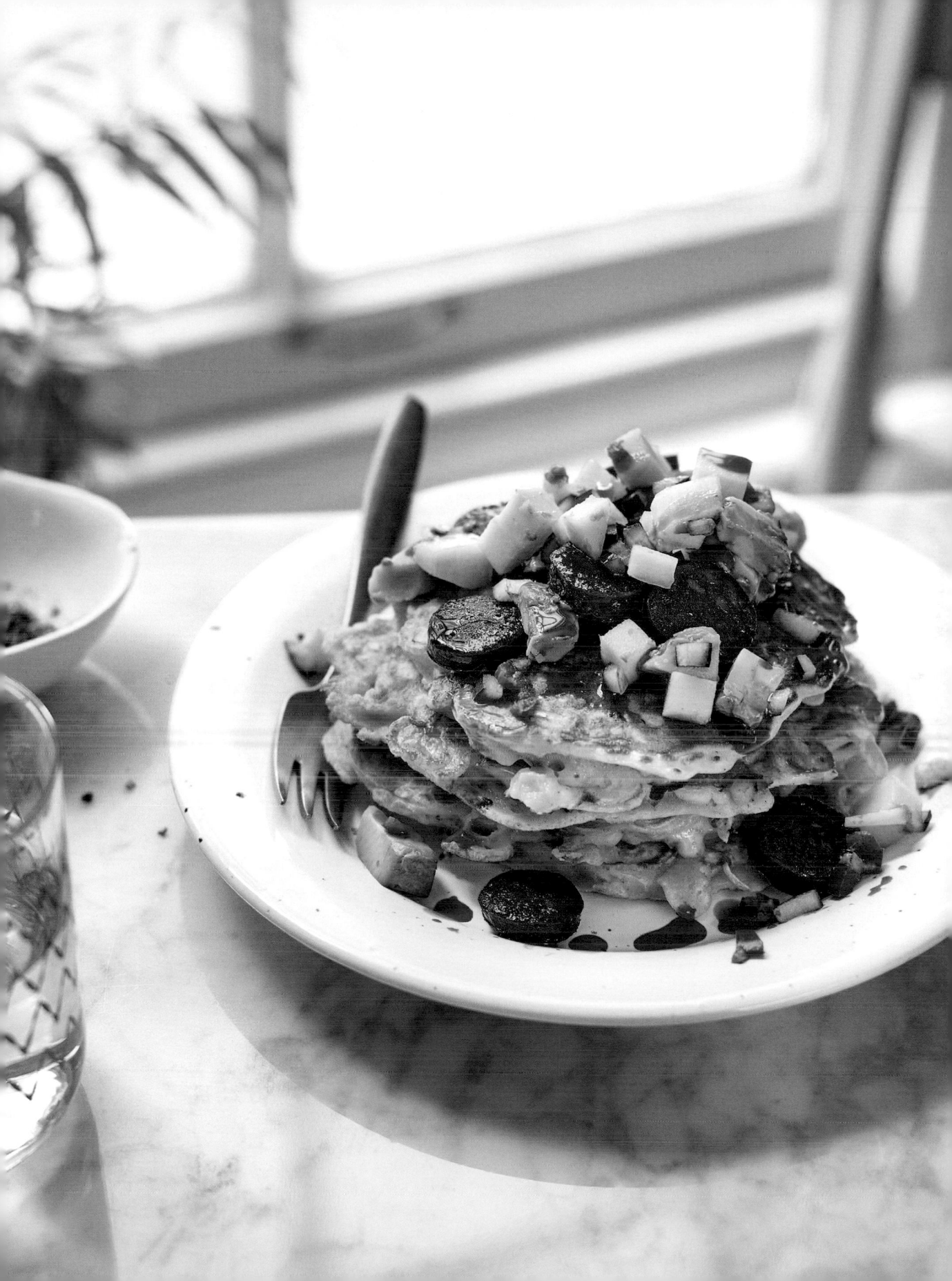

INGREDIENTS

1 tbsp olive oil

200g skinless, boneless
  chicken thighs, cut into
  large, bite-sized pieces

salt and pepper

1 fat clove garlic

8 pitted mixed olives

2 jarred roasted red
  peppers, drained

1 sprig of rosemary

glass of red wine

150g passata

big splash of balsamic vinegar

40g feta

*** ADD THE FETA JUST BEFORE
SERVING.**

CACCIATORE CHICKEN WITH MIXED OLIVES AND FETA

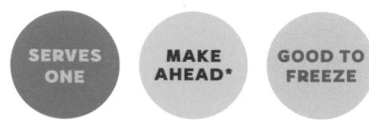

SERVES ONE · MAKE AHEAD* · GOOD TO FREEZE

1. Heat a frying pan over a high heat. Season the chicken thighs with salt and pepper. Add the oil to the hot pan, lay in the chicken pieces. Fry for 4 minutes, turning occasionally until nicely browned.

2. Meanwhile finely slice the garlic and roughly chop the olives and jarred red peppers.

3. Come back to the pan, lower the heat, chuck in the sliced garlic and rosemary sprig. Cook for 1 minute, then pour in the red wine. Bubble away for a couple of minutes, or until the wine has reduced by half, then pour in the passata and balsamic vinegar.

4. Scrape in the sliced olives and peppers, give everything a good mix then place a lid on the pan. Cook for about 6 minutes until the sauce has thickened slightly and the chicken is cooked through. Check by slicing into one of the larger pieces – the knife should cut through easily and the meat will have turned from pink to a whitish brown.

5. Pile the chicken cacciatore into a bowl, crumble over the feta to finish.

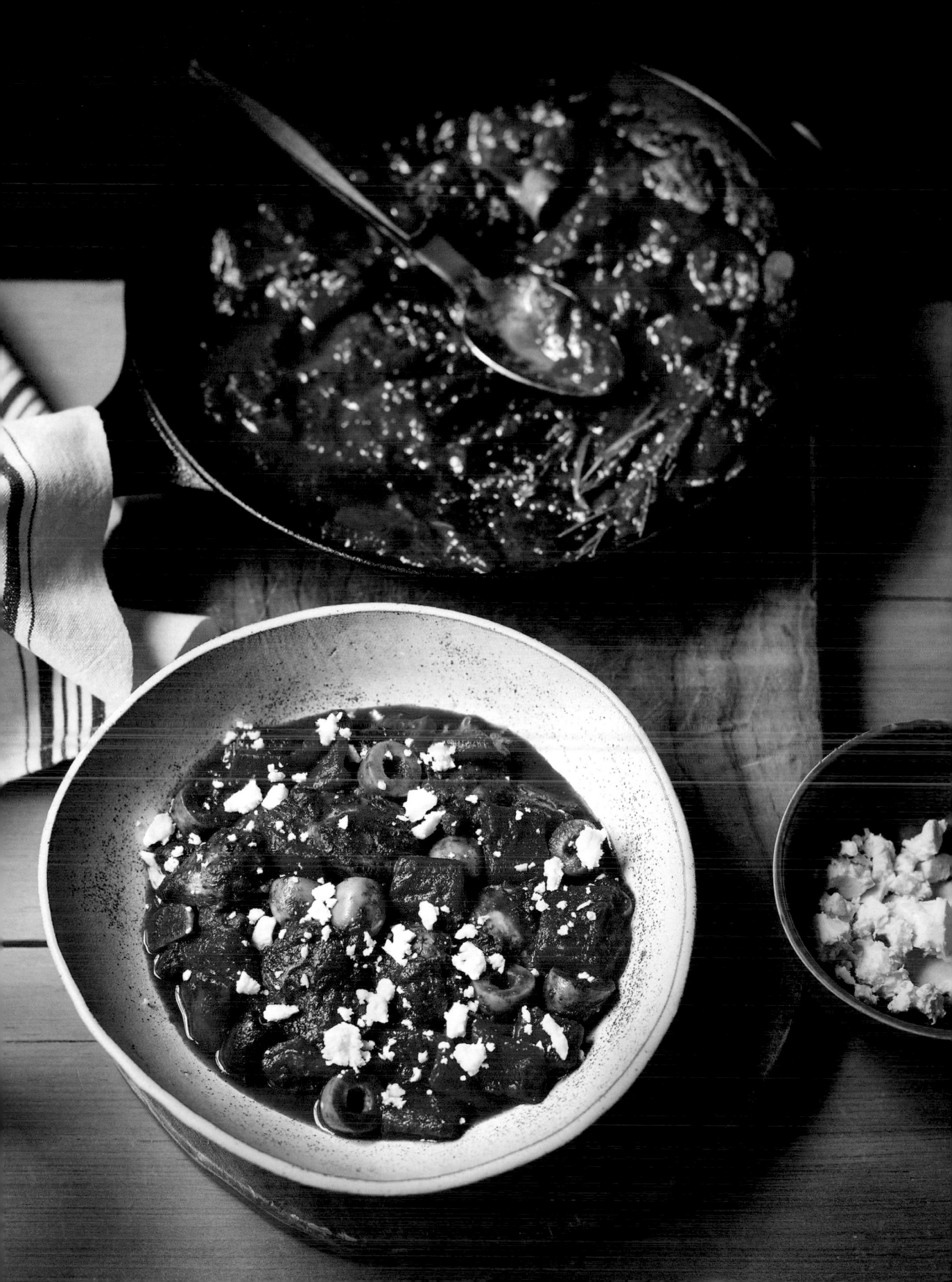

INGREDIENTS

1 medium courgette
100g green beans
1 jarred roasted red pepper,
  drained
1 clove garlic
6 cherry tomatoes
1 tbsp olive oil
1 tsp dried oregano
salt and pepper
2 tbsp almonds
80g halloumi (⅓ of a pack)
½ tbsp balsamic vinegar

*** YOU COULD DOUBLE THE
RECIPE FOR ANOTHER TIME AND
REHEAT IN THE MICROWAVE OR A
HOT OVEN.**

MEDITERRANEAN HALLOUMI TRAYBAKE

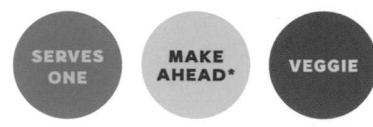

SERVES ONE   MAKE AHEAD*   VEGGIE

1. Preheat the grill to maximum.

2. Cut the courgette into diagonal slices. Trim the green beans, slice the roasted red pepper and garlic.

3. Dump everything onto a roasting tray. Chuck in the whole cherry tomatoes. Drizzle over the olive oil, sprinkle with the dried oregano, salt and pepper. Give everything a good mix, then spread into a roughly single layer and slide under the grill for 5 minutes.

4. While the vegetables are grilling, roughly chop the almonds and slice the halloumi.

5. After 5 minutes, flip the vegetables then place the halloumi onto the tray. Scatter over the almonds and drizzle everything with the balsamic vinegar. Slide back under the grill for 5 minutes until the veg is tender and the halloumi is golden.

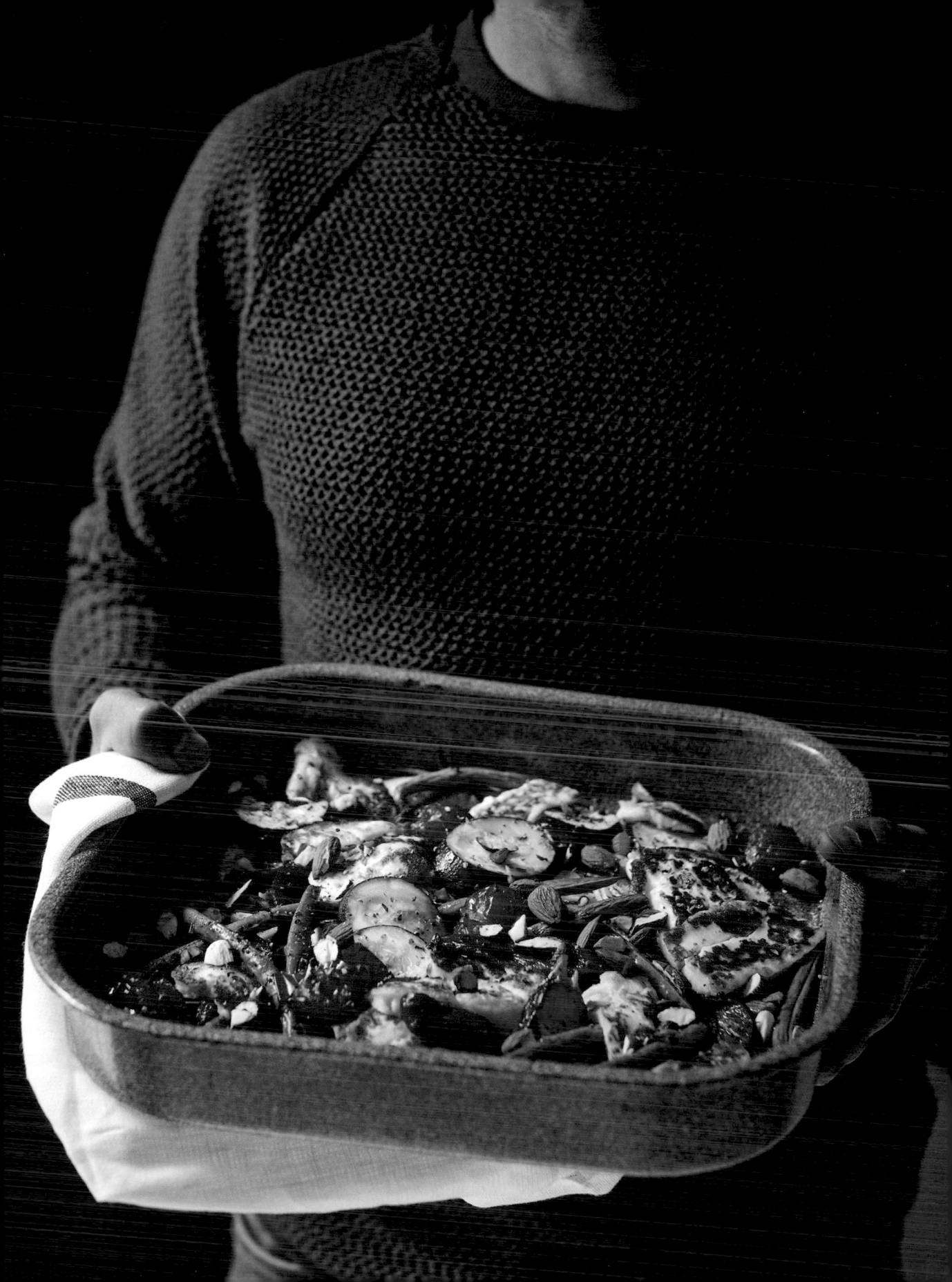

INGREDIENTS

2 x 110g sea bass fillets, skin on
2 tbsp olive oil
salt and pepper
1 large courgette
large handful of basil,
    leaves only
30g toasted pine nuts
juice of ½ lemon
½ red chilli, finely sliced – remove
    the seeds if you don't like it hot
small handful of mint, leaves
    picked

SEA BASS WITH PESTO AND CHARRED COURGETTE, CHILLI AND MINT

SERVES
ONE

1. Preheat your grill to maximum.

2. Lay the sea bass fillets, skin side up, on a baking tray lined with baking parchment. Drizzle over a little olive oil and season with salt and pepper. Slide the fish under the hot grill. Cook the fish without turning for 7 minutes, by which time the skin will have crisped up and blistered in places. Make sure the sea bass is cooked by checking that the flesh has turned from a raw pale colour to cooked bright white, then turn off the grill and leave the fillets to keep warm until you're ready to eat.

3. While the fish is cooking, slice the courgette into long strips around 1cm thick. Drizzle over 2 teaspoons of olive oil and season with salt and pepper. Heat a griddle pan over a high heat. Once the pan is searingly hot, carefully lay the courgette strips on. Griddle for 2 minutes on each side until they are charred and cooked through but not soggy. Move the charred courgette to a serving plate.

4. Make the pesto. Put the basil into a small food processor along with the toasted pine nuts, remaining 1 tablespoon olive oil and a squeeze of lemon juice. Pour in a splash of water and a good pinch of salt and pepper, then blitz to a smooth pesto. Add a little more water if you need it.

5. Scatter the chilli and mint leaves over the courgette and squeeze over some lemon juice. Lay the sea bass onto the plate and drizzle over the pesto, to serve.

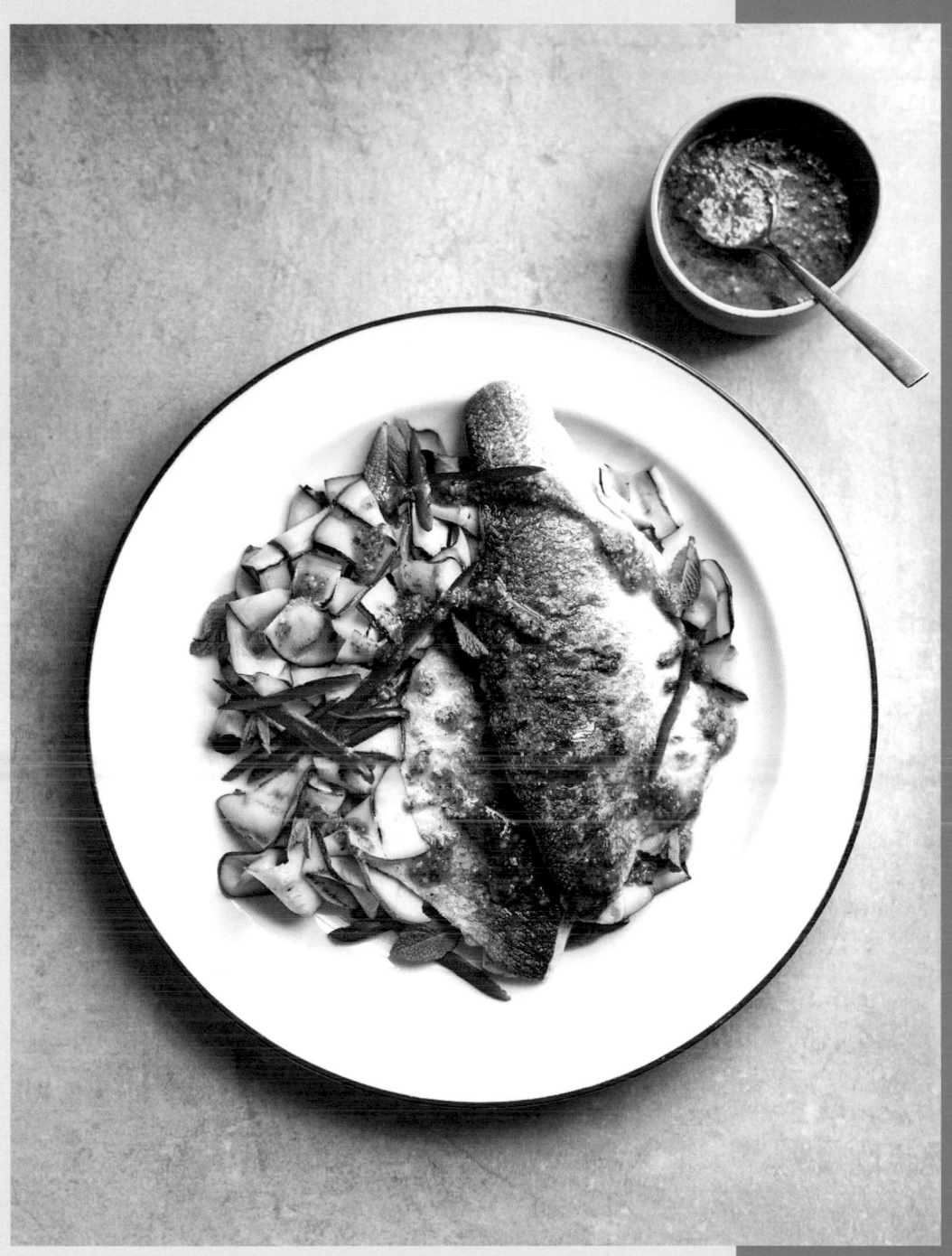

INGREDIENTS

½ chorizo ring (110g)

2 jarred roasted red peppers, drained

1 clove garlic

30g butter

1–2 tsp chipotle paste

200g chopped tomatoes

200g mixed beans, drained and rinsed

salt and pepper

2 large handfuls of kale

SMOKY CHORIZO MIXED BEAN STEW

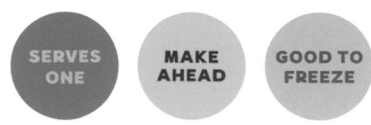

SERVES ONE   MAKE AHEAD   GOOD TO FREEZE

1. Slice the chorizo ring and the jarred red peppers, finely chop the garlic clove.

2. Melt the butter in a frying pan over a medium to high heat. Once bubbling, chuck in the chorizo. Fry for around 4 minutes, turning occasionally, until crisp.

3. Add the garlic and chipotle paste to the pan. Cook, stirring, for 1 minute then tip in the chopped tomatoes and mixed beans. Season with salt and pepper and leave to bubble away for 5 minutes.

4. Come back to the stew, drop the kale and sliced red peppers into the pan. Cook for a minute or two until the kale has wilted, then dish up the stew.

Veggie Swap

Swap the chorizo with 1 sliced red onion, fried for the same time as the chorizo would have been. Top with 4 slices of fried halloumi.

CORONATION CHICKEN SALAD

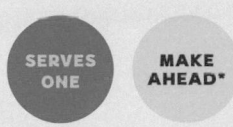

SERVES ONE   MAKE AHEAD*

INGREDIENTS

½ tbsp coconut oil

1 tbsp medium curry powder

1 x 200g skinless chicken breast, sliced into 1cm strips

2 tbsp Greek yoghurt

1 heaped tsp mango chutney

2 spring onions, finely sliced (green and white parts)

salt and pepper

2 handfuls of baby spinach leaves

1 tbsp pomegranate seeds

1 poppadum

* KEEP CORONATION CHICKEN SEPARATE FROM THE REST OF THE SALAD. MIX TOGETHER WHEN YOU'RE READY TO EAT.

1. Melt the coconut oil in a frying pan over a medium to high heat. Sprinkle in the curry powder, cook for 30 seconds, stirring the spices into the coconut oil, then tip in the sliced chicken. Fry for about 5 minutes or until the chicken is cooked through. Check by slicing into one of the larger pieces to make sure the meat is white all the way through, with no raw pink bits left.

2. Take the pan off the heat. Dollop in the yoghurt and mango chutney, and using a wooden spoon, stir into the chicken to create a creamy curried sauce. Dump in most of the spring onions and mix together. Season the coronation chicken with salt and pepper to taste.

3. Pile the spinach onto a plate. Top with the coronation chicken mixture. Scatter over the remaining spring onions and pomegranate seeds, then scrunch the poppadum with your hands into large shards over the salad.

Veggie Swap

Swap the chicken for ½ small head of cauliflower cut into smallish florets and cooked in the same way as the chicken breast.

REDUCED CARB

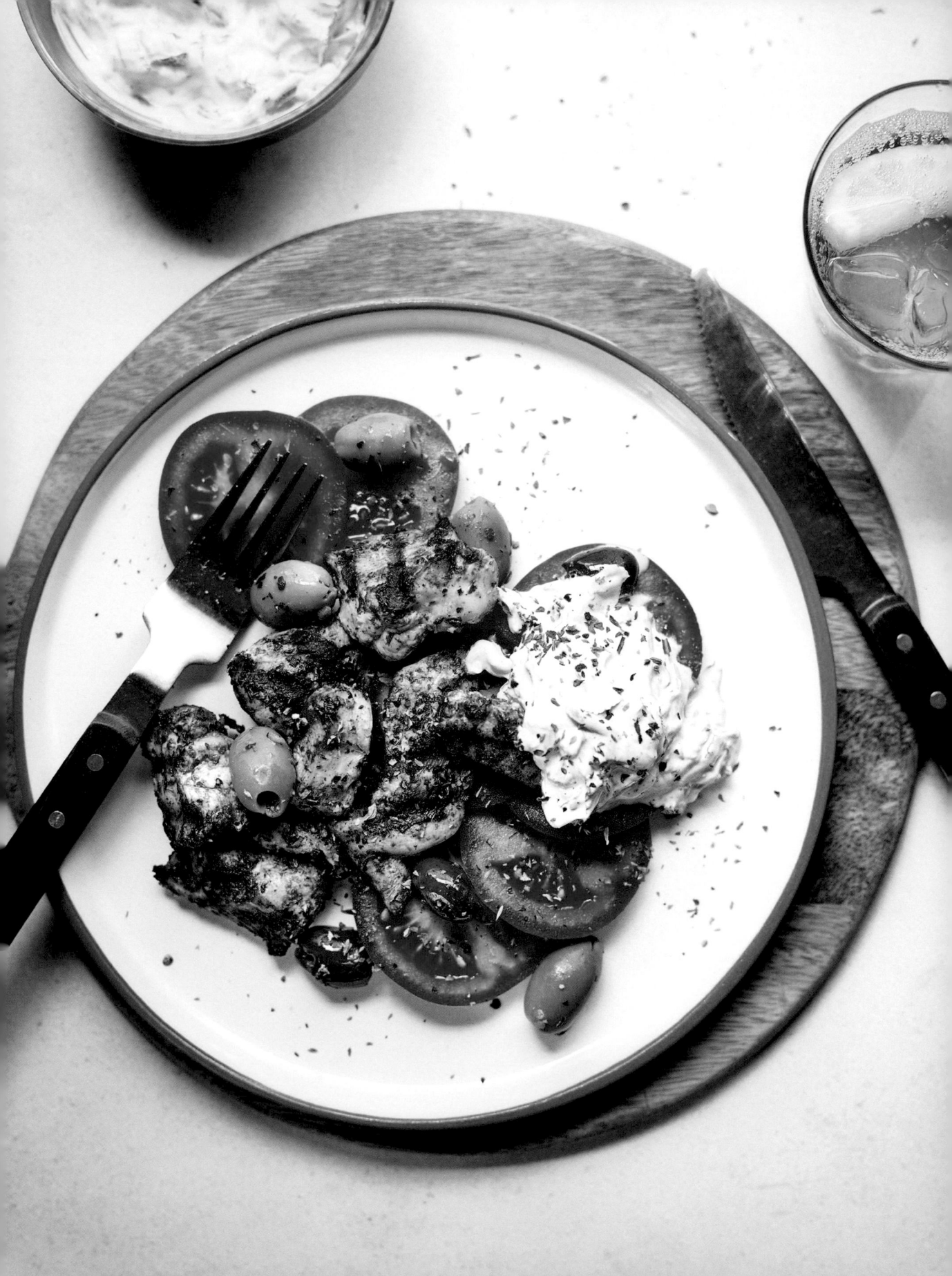

CHICKEN SOUVLAKI WITH TZATZIKI, SLICED TOMATO AND OLIVES

SERVES ONE

INGREDIENTS

1 x 200g skinless chicken
    breast fillet, cut into large,
    bite-sized pieces
½ tsp paprika
½ tsp dried oregano, plus a pinch
1 clove garlic
juice of ½ lemon
½ tbsp olive oil
salt and pepper
3 tbsp Greek yoghurt
½ cucumber
small handful of mint
1 large ripe tomato, sliced
8 pitted mixed olives

1. Tip the chicken breast pieces into a bowl. Sprinkle over the paprika and ½ teaspoon dried oregano. Using the fine side of a grater, grate half of the garlic into the bowl. Squeeze in the lemon juice, drizzle over the olive oil. Season with salt and pepper then mix the chicken with the herbs and spices.

2. Heat a griddle pan over the highest heat. Once the pan is searingly hot, lay the chicken pieces in. Cook for 4 minutes on each side, or until cooked through. Check by slicing into one of the larger pieces to make sure the meat is white all the way through, with no raw pink bits left.

3. Meanwhile make the tzatziki. Dollop the yoghurt into a small bowl. Grate the remaining garlic half into the yoghurt, then using the larger side of the grater, grate the cucumber. Squeeze out as much liquid as you can from the cucumber then drop it into the yoghurt. Finely chop the mint leaves, stir them into the yoghurt. Season the dip with salt and pepper.

4. Pile the chicken souvlaki onto a plate, place the sliced tomato and olives alongside, sprinkling over the remaining oregano. Serve with the tzatziki.

INGREDIENTS

½ fennel bulb
1 tbsp olive oil
salt and pepper
1 fat clove garlic
big pinch of dried chilli flakes
glass of white wine
1 x 227g tin of chopped tomatoes
handful of parsley
2 tbsp natural yoghurt
½ lemon
200g fish pie mix
2 tbsp toasted flaked almonds

*** SPOON OVER THE HERBY
YOGHURT AND ALMONDS
JUST BEFORE SERVING.**

TOMATO, FENNEL AND FISH STEW

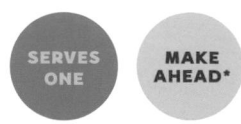

SERVES ONE   MAKE AHEAD*

1. Pick the green bits off the fennel – the 'fronds' – and save until later, then slice the fennel as finely as you can.

2. Heat a saucepan over a medium to high heat. Drizzle in the olive oil then dump the fennel into the pan along with some seasoning. Fry, stirring regularly for 3–4 minutes until the fennel is collapsed and beginning to caramelize.

3. Crush in the garlic clove and sprinkle in the chilli flakes. Cook for 1 minute more, then pour in the glass of white wine. Cook for 2 minutes, or until the wine has reduced by half, then tip in the chopped tomatoes. Crank up the heat. Bubble the sauce away for a few minutes while you make the herby yoghurt.

4. Put the parsley (stalks and all) into a small food processor. Blitz until finely chopped, then spoon in the yoghurt. Squeeze in a little lemon juice and blitz again to combine. Season to taste.

5. Come back to the tomato sauce. Lower the heat, drop in the fish pie mix. Place a lid on the pan and cook for 2–3 minutes more until the fish is cooked. Check by cutting into one of the thicker pieces to make sure the white fish has turned from raw, pale flesh to cooked bright white, and that the salmon flesh has turned matt pink in colour.

6. Take the pan off the heat. Season with salt, pepper and lemon juice to taste. Pile into a bowl, spoon over the herby yoghurt and top with the toasted flaked almonds.

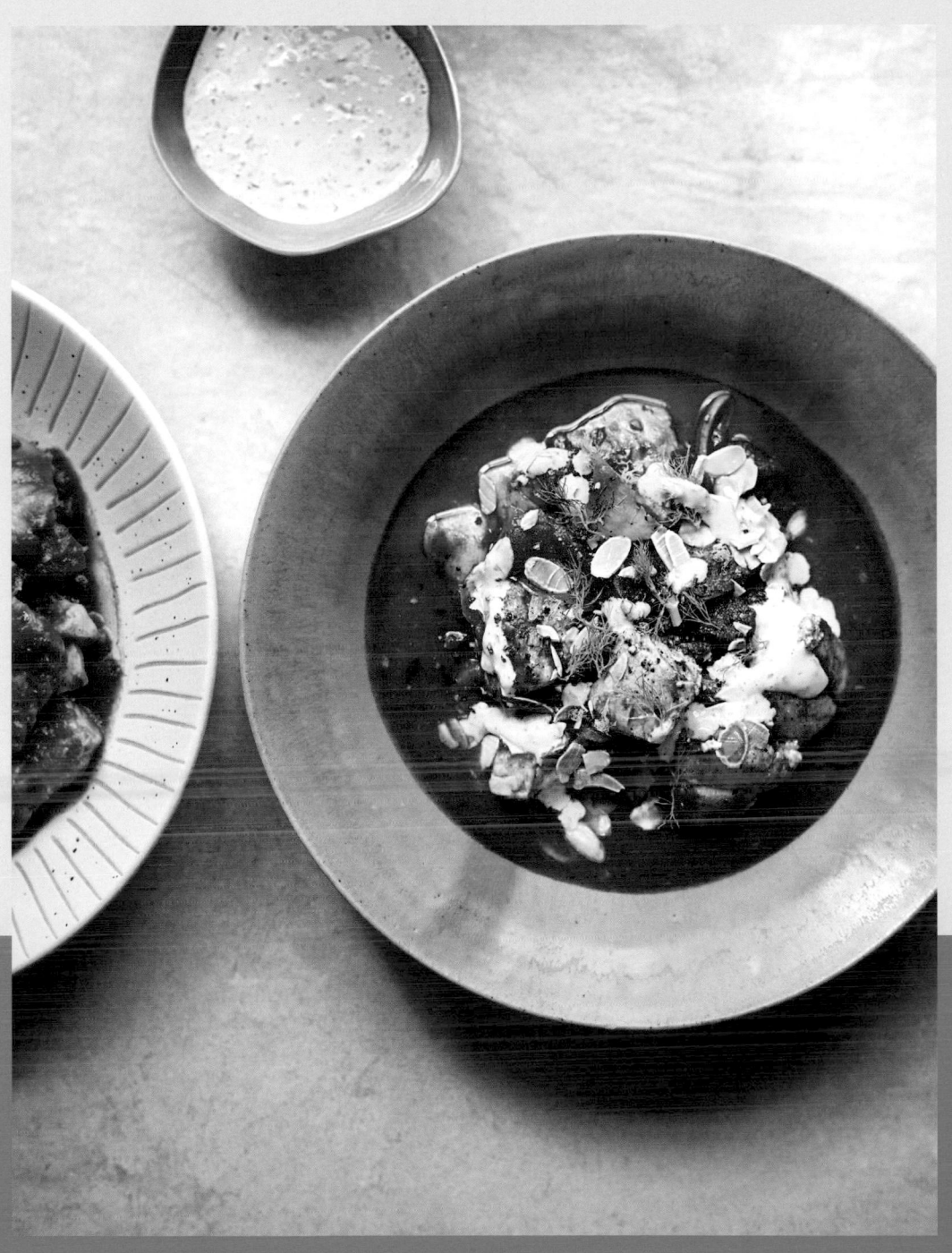

INGREDIENTS

2 pre-cooked beetroots
  (roughly 100g)
2 spring onions
handful of parsley
1 egg
50g ground almonds
50g feta
½ tsp ground coriander
zest and juice of ½ lemon
salt and pepper
2 tbsp olive oil
2 tsp pomegranate molasses
10 cherry tomatoes

* PATTIES ONLY.

BEETROOT AND FETA PATTIES WITH POMEGRANATE MOLASSES AND TOMATO SALAD

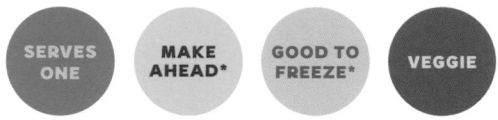

SERVES ONE · **MAKE AHEAD*** · **GOOD TO FREEZE*** · **VEGGIE**

1. Grate the beetroot then pat dry with some kitchen roll. Scrape into a bowl. Finely slice the spring onions (greens and all) and roughly chop the parsley. Drop half of the spring onions and parsley into the bowl with the grated beetroot.

2. Crack an egg into the bowl. Spoon in the ground almonds, crumble in the feta and sprinkle in the ground coriander and lemon zest with a generous pinch of salt and pepper. Mix together to form the patty mixture.

3. Heat a non-stick frying pan over a medium to high heat. Pour in half the olive oil. Using your hands shape the mixture into four patties straight into the pan. Fry for 3–4 minutes on each side until firm and golden.

4. Meanwhile whisk the pomegranate molasses and remaining olive oil together in a bowl. Season with lemon juice, salt and pepper to taste – you want the dressing to be quite tangy, it will mellow when everything else is added.

5. Add the remaining spring onions and parsley to the dressing. Halve the cherry tomatoes and chuck them in too, toss together.

6. Come back to the patties. Lay the patties onto a plate and pile the tomato salad next to them.

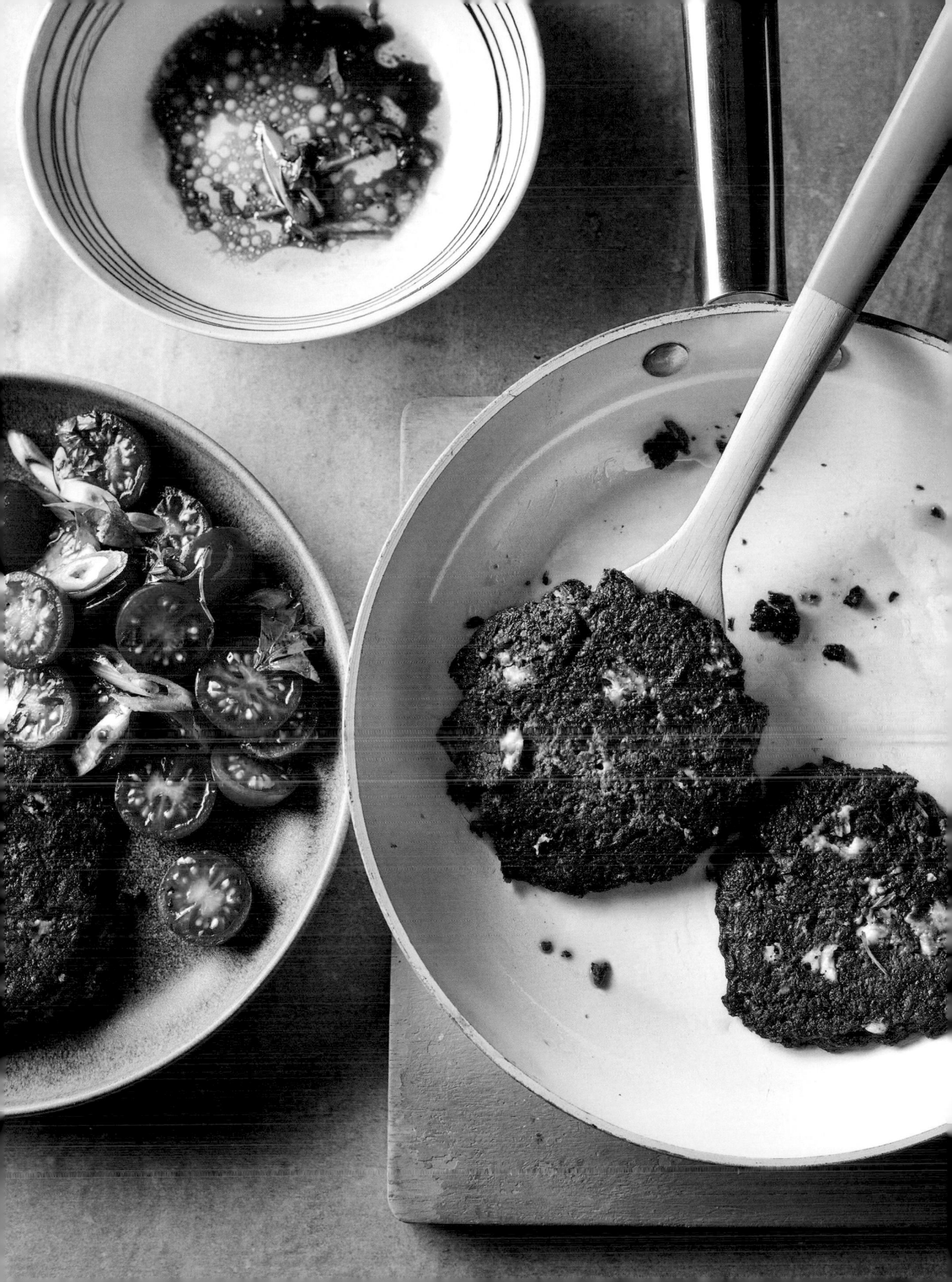

INGREDIENTS

1 lemongrass stalk, tender white part only, roughly chopped

1 clove garlic

1 small shallot, roughly chopped

knob of fresh ginger, peeled and roughly chopped

½ red chilli – remove the seeds if you don't like it hot

½ tsp each cumin and coriander seeds

½ tbsp coconut oil

200g skinless turkey breast fillets, sliced into 1cm strips

1 red pepper, sliced

200ml coconut milk

1 heaped tbsp peanut butter

1 tsp fish sauce

small handful of basil leaves

TURKEY AND RED PEPPER PANANG CURRY

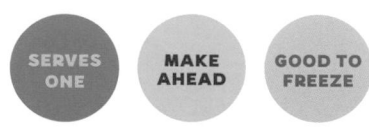

SERVES ONE   **MAKE AHEAD**   **GOOD TO FREEZE**

1. Put the first six ingredients into a small food processor with 1 tablespoon of water. Blitz to a smooth curry paste.

2. Melt the coconut oil in a wok or large frying pan over a medium to high heat. Spoon in the curry paste and cook, stirring almost constantly, for 1 minute, then chuck in the sliced turkey and red pepper.

3. Fry for around 2 minutes, then pour in the coconut milk. Dollop in the peanut butter. Give everything a good mix, then leave the curry to bubble away for 3 minutes or until the turkey is cooked. Check by slicing into one of the larger pieces to make sure the meat is white all the way through, with no raw pink bits left.

4. When you are happy that the turkey is cooked, take the curry off the heat, stir through the fish sauce and most of the basil leaves. Season to taste, then pile the curry into a bowl, scattering the remaining basil leaves on top.

Veggie Swap

Swap the turkey for 140g tofu, cut into cubes and dropped into the curry for the final 3-4 minutes of cooking time.

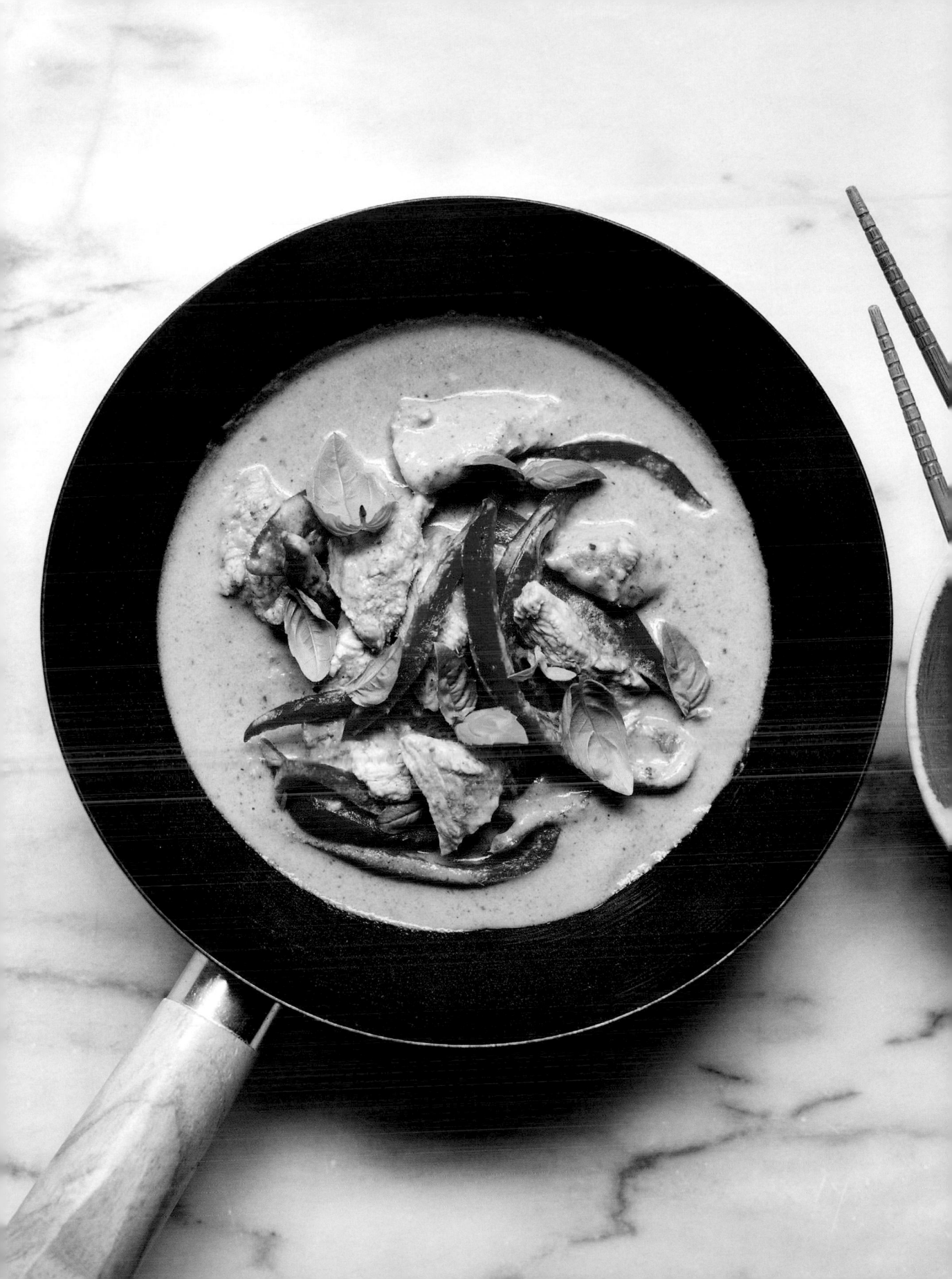

INGREDIENTS

200g passata
1 small garlic clove
½ tsp smoked paprika
splash of sherry or red wine
  vinegar
salt and pepper
large handful of chargrilled
  artichokes (from a pack
  or jarred)
1 tbsp capers
1 x 200g skinless boneless
  cod fillet
drizzle of olive oil
20g toasted pine nuts
green salad, to serve

TOMATO-BAKED COD WITH CAPERS AND PINE NUTS

SERVES
ONE

1. Preheat your oven to 220°C (fan 200°/gas mark 7).

2. Heat a small ovenproof dish over a medium heat. Pour in the passata, crush in the garlic clove, sprinkle in the smoked paprika, add a splash of sherry or red wine vinegar, a pinch of salt and pepper. Give the sauce a good stir. Drop in the chargrilled artichokes and capers, stir.

3. Make a space in the centre of the sauce. Season the cod with salt and pepper on both sides then place the cod into the sauce. Drizzle everything with a little olive oil. Roast in the oven for 10 minutes, or until the cod is cooked. Check by cutting into one of the thicker parts to make sure it has turned from raw, pale flesh to cooked bright white.

4. Carefully remove the dish from the oven, sprinkle over the toasted pine nuts and serve with a green salad.

Veggie Swap

Swap the cod for four big spoonfuls of ricotta dolloped into the sauce before baking for the same amount of time.

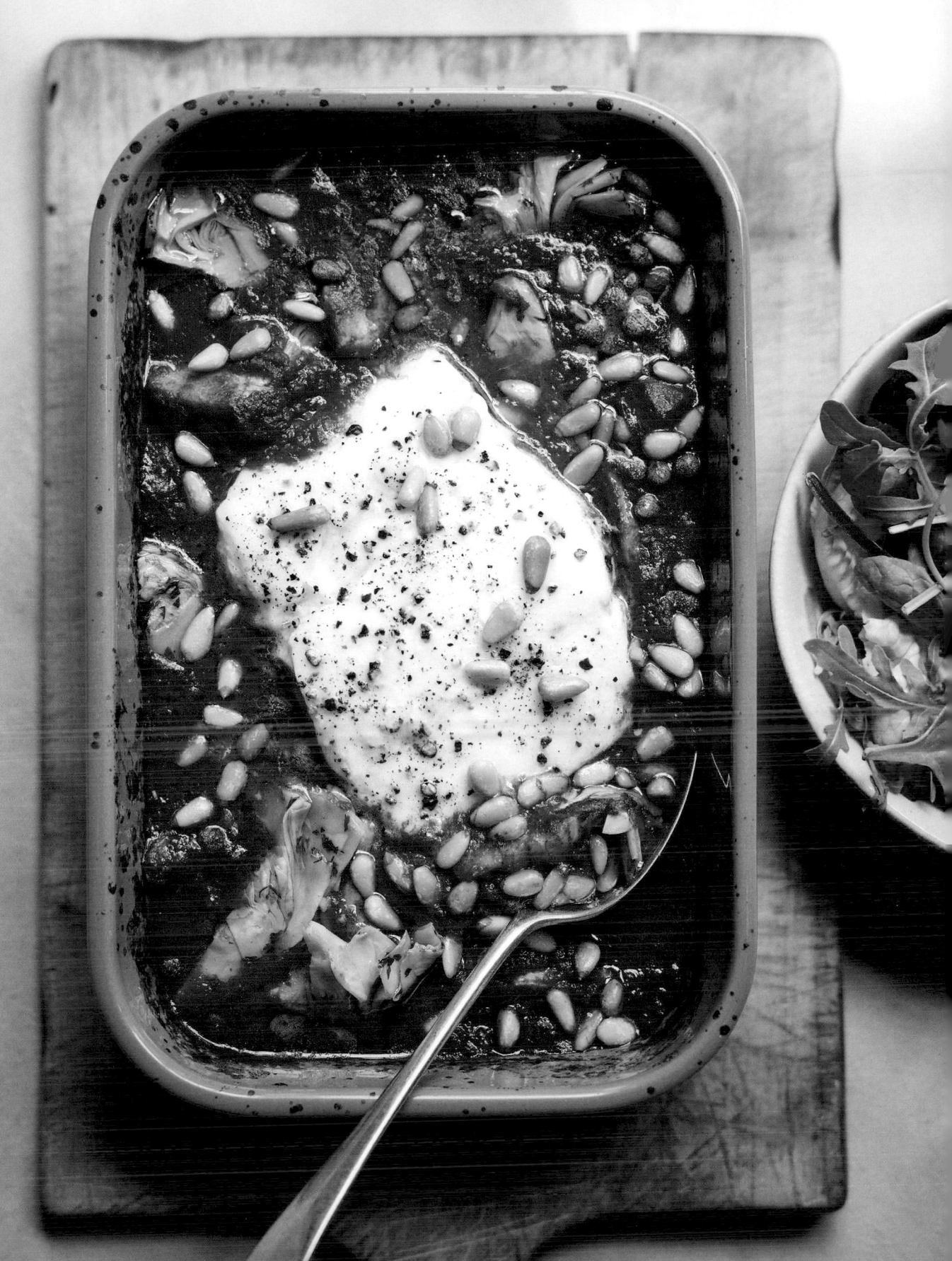

INGREDIENTS

½ large aubergine
1 tbsp olive oil
salt and pepper
6 slices of parma ham
2 tbsp sundried tomatoes
1 x 227g tin of chopped tomatoes
1 small clove garlic
pinch of dried chilli flakes
½ small ball of mozzarella
    (around 63g)
1 tbsp dried breadcrumbs
handful of basil leaves

PARMA HAM AND SUNDRIED TOMATO PARMIGIANA

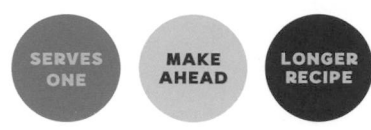

SERVES ONE   MAKE AHEAD   LONGER RECIPE

1. Preheat the grill to maximum.

2. Slice the aubergine into 2cm-thick rounds. Heat a frying pan over a high heat. Drizzle most of the olive oil over the aubergine rounds, rubbing the oil into the flesh. Season with salt and pepper. Lay the aubergine into the frying pan. Fry for 3 minutes on each side, until softened and golden brown. Transfer the aubergine to a plate and put the pan back on the heat.

3. Peel the parma ham slices straight out of their packaging into the hot frying pan. Fry for 1–2 minutes until the ham shrivels and crisps. Take the pan off the heat and leave to cool slightly.

4. Roughly chop the sundried tomatoes and scrape into a bowl. Tip in the chopped tomatoes, crush in the garlic clove, add a pinch of chilli flakes and some salt and pepper. Stir together.

5. Dollop a third of the sundried tomato sauce into the bottom of a small ovenproof dish. Layer in half the fried aubergine along with half the crispy parma ham, spoon over a third more sauce, then tear over half the mozzarella. Repeat with the remaining ingredients, finishing with the mozzarella. Scatter the breadcrumbs over the top and drizzle with the remaining oil. Slide under the grill and cook for 8 minutes until bubbling and golden brown.

6. Leave to cool for a couple of minutes and scatter over the basil leaves before tucking in.

Veggie Swap

Swap out the parma ham for 30g toasted pine nuts, layered into the parmigiana in the same way you would the ham.

REDUCED CARB

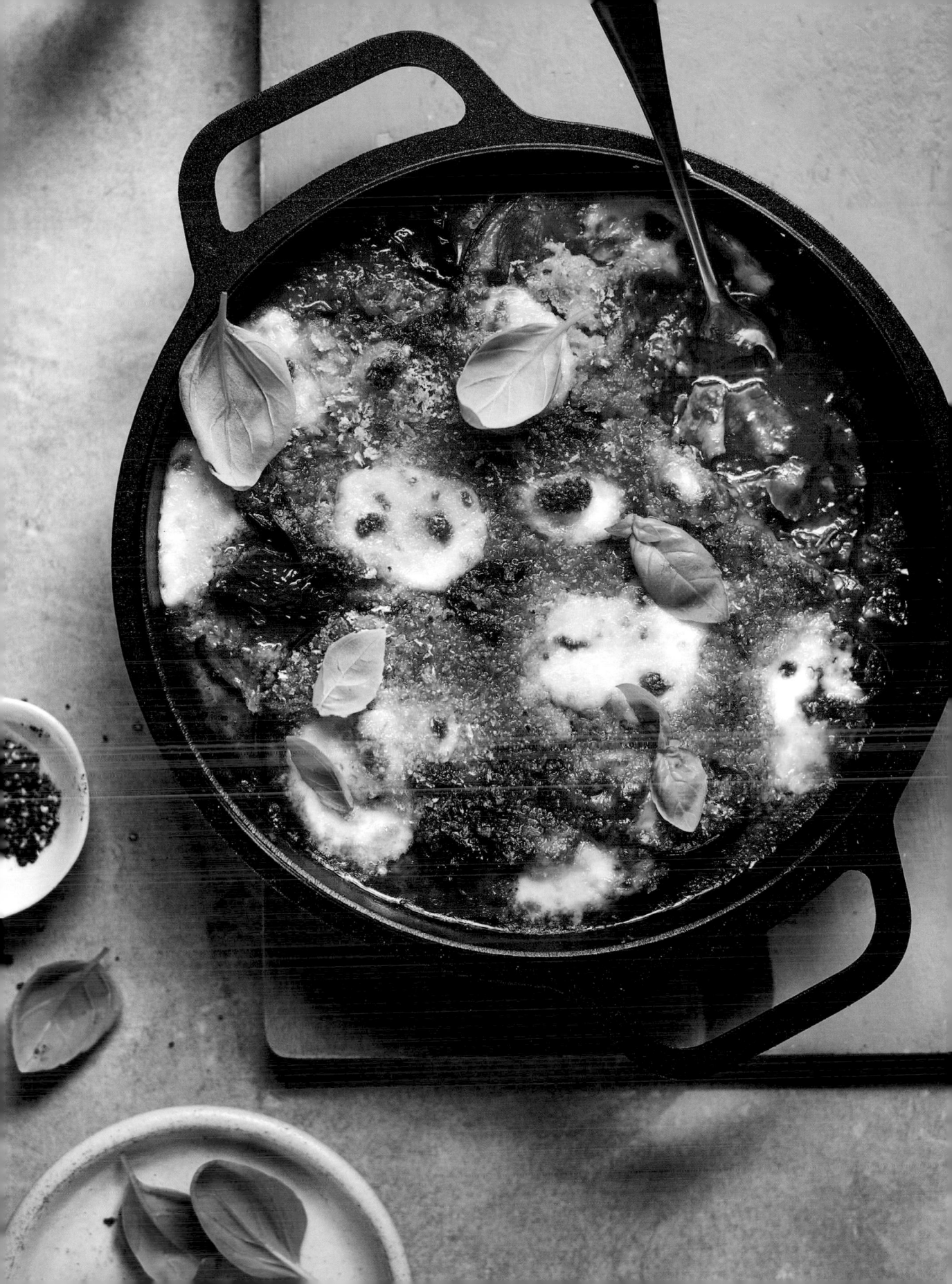

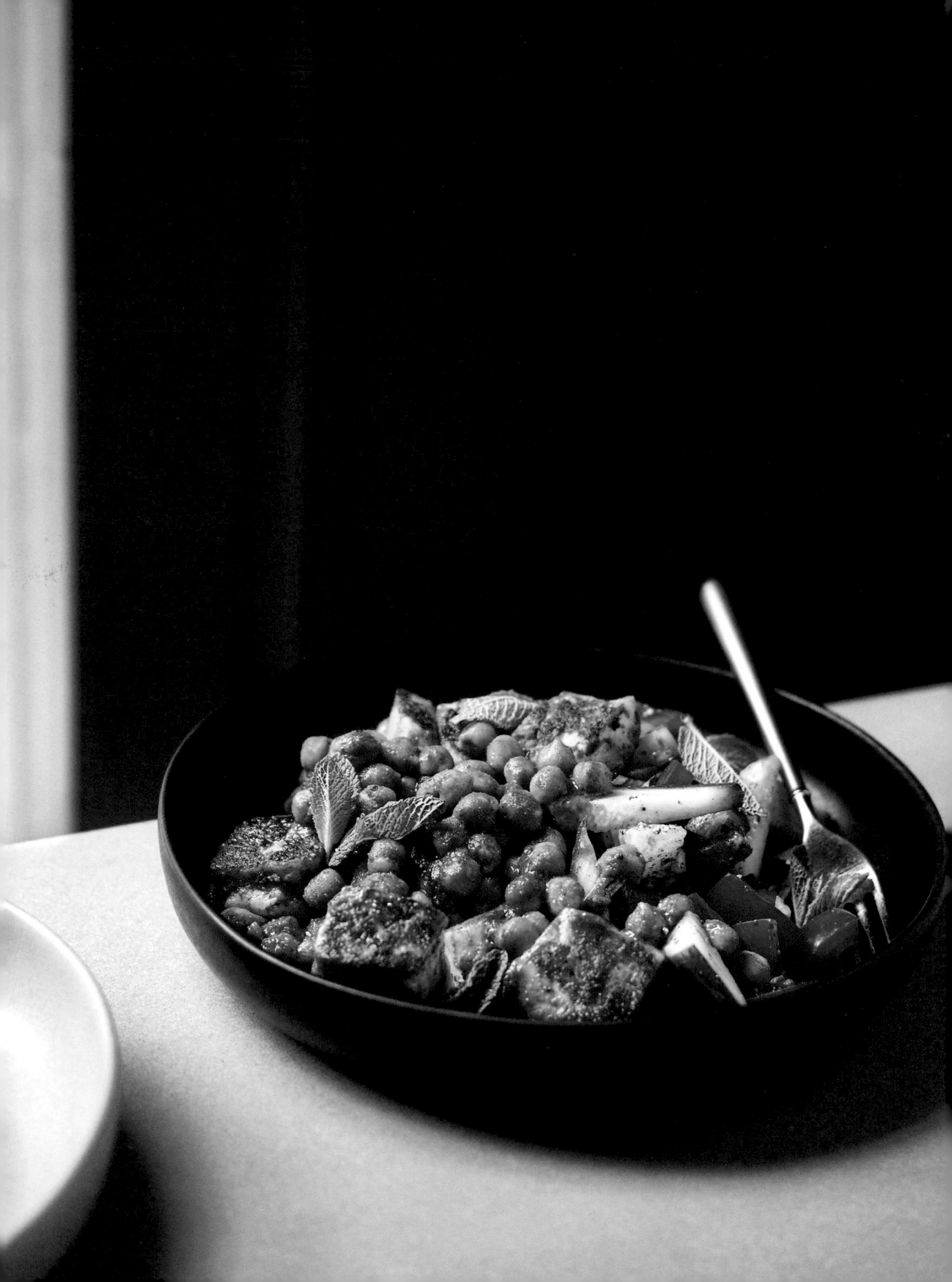

TIKKA MASALA, HALLOUMI AND CHICKPEA KACHUMBA

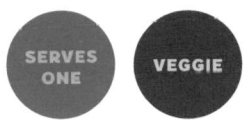

SERVES ONE   VEGGIE

INGREDIENTS

1 x 210g tin of chickpeas,
    drained and rinsed
½ small red onion
½ cucumber
1 large ripe tomato
pinch of cayenne pepper
salt and pepper
juice of ¼ lemon
80g halloumi (⅓ pack)
2 tsp coconut oil
1 tbsp tikka masala curry paste
handful of mint leaves

1. Drain the chickpeas in a sieve and rinse well. Leave in the sieve over a bowl to drain off any excess water.

2. Finely chop the red onion. Roughly chop the cucumber and tomato, scrape everything into a serving bowl. Sprinkle in a good pinch of cayenne, salt and pepper. Squeeze in the lemon juice, stir.

3. Cut the halloumi into large cubes. Ping the coconut oil in a large microwaveable bowl to melt. Stir in the tikka masala curry paste then drop in the cubed halloumi and rinsed chickpeas, toss to coat.

4. Heat a large non-stick frying pan over a high heat. Tip in the tikka masala halloumi and chickpeas. Fry, turning the halloumi with tongs as it browns on each side, for 5 minutes until golden and crisp.

5. Pile the halloumi and chickpeas on top of the kachumba salad. Finish with a scattering of mint leaves.

INGREDIENTS

150g chestnut mushrooms
1 tbsp coconut oil
salt and pepper
1 red pepper
½ onion
2 tomatoes
½ red chilli – remove the
   seeds if you don't like it hot
1 fat clove garlic
½ veggie stock cube
2 tbsp peanut butter
3 large handfuls of baby
   spinach leaves
squeeze of lemon juice
small handful of roasted
   salted peanuts

PEANUT BUTTER, MUSHROOM, SPINACH AND TOMATO STEW

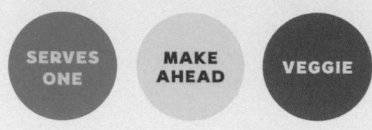

1. Roughly chop the mushrooms.

2. Melt the coconut oil in a large saucepan over a high heat. Chuck in the mushrooms, along with a pinch of salt. Fry for 5 minutes until golden and beginning to crisp.

3. While the mushrooms are frying, de-seed and core the red pepper. Roughly chop the onion and the tomatoes. Put them into a blender or small food processor along with the red chilli and garlic. Blitz to a paste.

4. Scrape the pepper and tomato paste into the saucepan with the mushrooms. Cook for 2 minutes, then pour in 150ml water. Crumble in the veggie stock cube.

5. Bring the stew to a boil. Once boiling, dollop in the peanut butter, mix well, then drop in the spinach. When wilted, season the stew with lemon juice, salt and pepper to taste and spoon into a bowl. Scatter over the peanuts to serve.

CREAMY COCONUT, CARROT AND SWEET POTATO SOUP WITH CHILLI PANEER CROUTONS

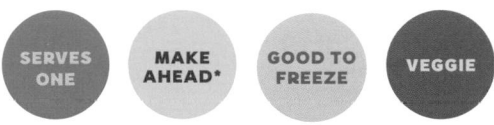

SERVES ONE MAKE AHEAD* GOOD TO FREEZE VEGGIE

INGREDIENTS

1 large carrot, peeled and cut into small chunks
1 small sweet potato, peeled and cut into small chunks
1 tbsp coconut oil
1 heaped tbsp korma curry paste
2 spring onions, finely sliced
200ml coconut milk
60g paneer (⅓ of a pack)
1 tsp cumin seeds
1 tsp hot chilli powder
juice of ½ lime
salt and pepper

* YOU COULD MAKE A BIG BATCH AND FREEZE THE REMAINING PORTIONS FOR ANOTHER TIME.

1. Put the carrot and sweet potato in a microwaveable bowl along with 2 tablespoons of water. Cover and zap on high for 5 minutes.

2. Meanwhile melt 2 teaspoons coconut oil in a saucepan over a medium heat. Dollop in the curry paste and most of the spring onions. Cook for 1 minute, stirring constantly, then pour in the coconut milk along with 100ml water. Leave to bubble away.

3. While the soup base is bubbling, cut the paneer into large cubes. Ping the remaining coconut oil in a small bowl in the microwave to melt. Spoon in the cumin seeds and chilli powder, add the paneer cubes and toss to coat.

4. Come back to the carrot and sweet potato. Carefully uncover, tip them along with their water into the soup saucepan. Cook for 5 minutes more while you fry the paneer.

5. Heat a non-stick frying pan over a medium heat. Tip in the spiced paneer and fry for 3–4 minutes, turning as each side becomes crisp and golden. Take the pan off the heat.

6. Come back to the soup. Take off the heat, squeeze in the lime juice and season with salt and pepper. Blitz with a soup blender or in a regular blender.

7. Pour into a bowl, top with the crispy paneer croutons. Scatter over the remaining sliced spring onion.

REDUCED CARB

SNACKS

INGREDIENTS

2 eggs
1 tbsp pumpkin seeds
1 tbsp tahini
juice of ½ lemon
salt and pepper
large handful of baby
   spinach leaves

***MAKE THE NIGHT BEFORE AND
KEEP IN THE FRIDGE.**

BOILED EGG PROTEIN POT WITH SPINACH AND TAHINI

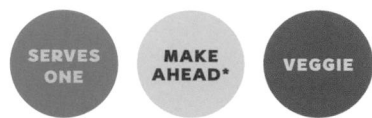

1. Bring a kettle of water to the boil.

2. Pour the boiling water into a saucepan over a medium heat, adjust the heat so the water is hissing rather than bubbling, then lower in your eggs. Cook for 6½–8 minutes, depending on whether you like soft- or hard-boiled.

3. Meanwhile toast the pumpkin seeds in a dry frying pan over a medium to high heat until they begin to pop. Take the pan off the heat and leave to cool. Mix the tahini with the lemon juice and a splash of water to create a creamy dressing. Season with salt and pepper to taste.

4. Carefully drain the cooked eggs in a sieve or colander, then rinse under cold running water until completely cool. Peel.

5. Dump your spinach into a bowl, or a pot to keep in the fridge for tomorrow. Pour in the tahini dressing. Place the cold, peeled eggs on top and scatter over the pumpkin seeds. Crack over some black pepper.

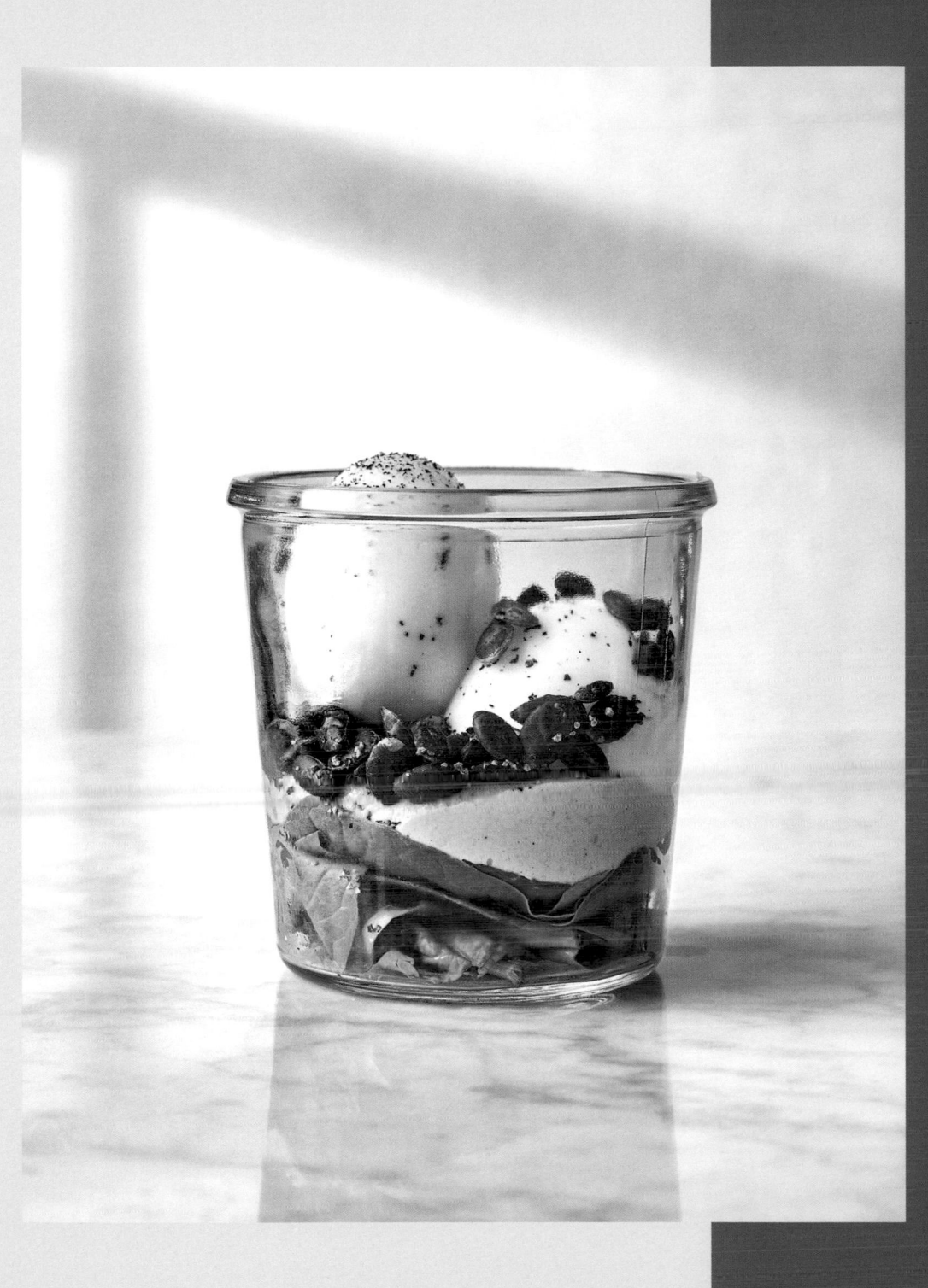

INGREDIENTS

500g turkey mince
4 sprigs of thyme
100g brie, cut into small cubes
salt and pepper
1 egg
plain flour, for dusting
1 sheet ready-rolled puff pastry
4 tbsp cranberry sauce
1 tbsp poppy or sesame seeds

*** FREEZE ONCE MADE, BEFORE
THEY GO INTO THE OVEN. BAKE
FROM FROZEN FOR AN EXTRA
10–15 MINUTES ON TOP OF THE
COOKING TIME UNTIL PIPING HOT
AND DEEP GOLDEN BROWN.**

TURKEY, BRIE AND CRANBERRY SAUSAGE ROLLS

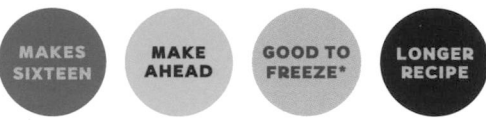

MAKES SIXTEEN   MAKE AHEAD   GOOD TO FREEZE*   LONGER RECIPE

1. Preheat the oven to 200°C (fan 180°/gas mark 6). Line a baking tray with baking parchment.

2. Dump the turkey mince into a bowl. Strip in the thyme leaves, discarding the stalks. Add the brie along with a generous pinch of salt and pepper. Mix everything together with a wooden spoon.

3. Crack the egg into a small bowl and whisk well with a fork until the white and yolk combine.

4. Lightly dust your work surface with flour. Unravel the sheet of puff pastry then, using a rolling pin, roll the pastry so that it becomes 1cm bigger on each side (see Tip).

5. Cut the pastry in half lengthways so that you have two long rectangles. Spread half the cranberry sauce across the middle of one of the rectangles, then form half the turkey mixture into a sausage shape over the top. Brush the borders with a little egg then roll the pastry over the filling to enclose. Using a fork, firmly press the edges of the pastry together. Repeat.

6. Using a sharp knife, cut the two long rolls into sixteen sausage rolls. Place the sausage rolls onto the lined baking tray. Brush the pastry with the remaining egg and sprinkle over the poppy or sesame seeds. Bake in the oven for 20–25 minutes until cooked through and deep golden brown.

Joe's Top Tip

If you don't have a rolling pin to thin out the pastry, don't worry. Rolling it thin just makes the sausage rolls a bit easier to form later on.

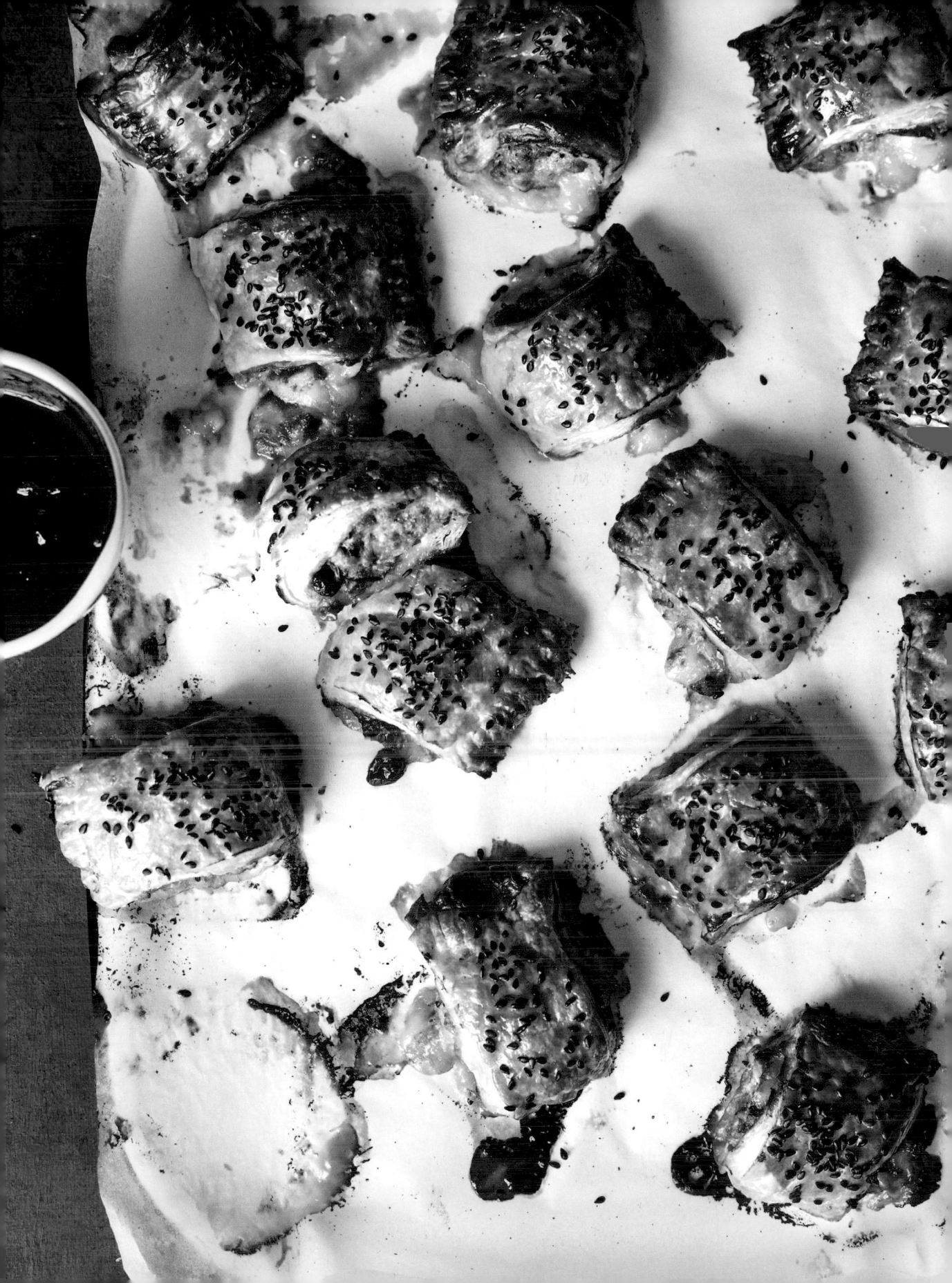

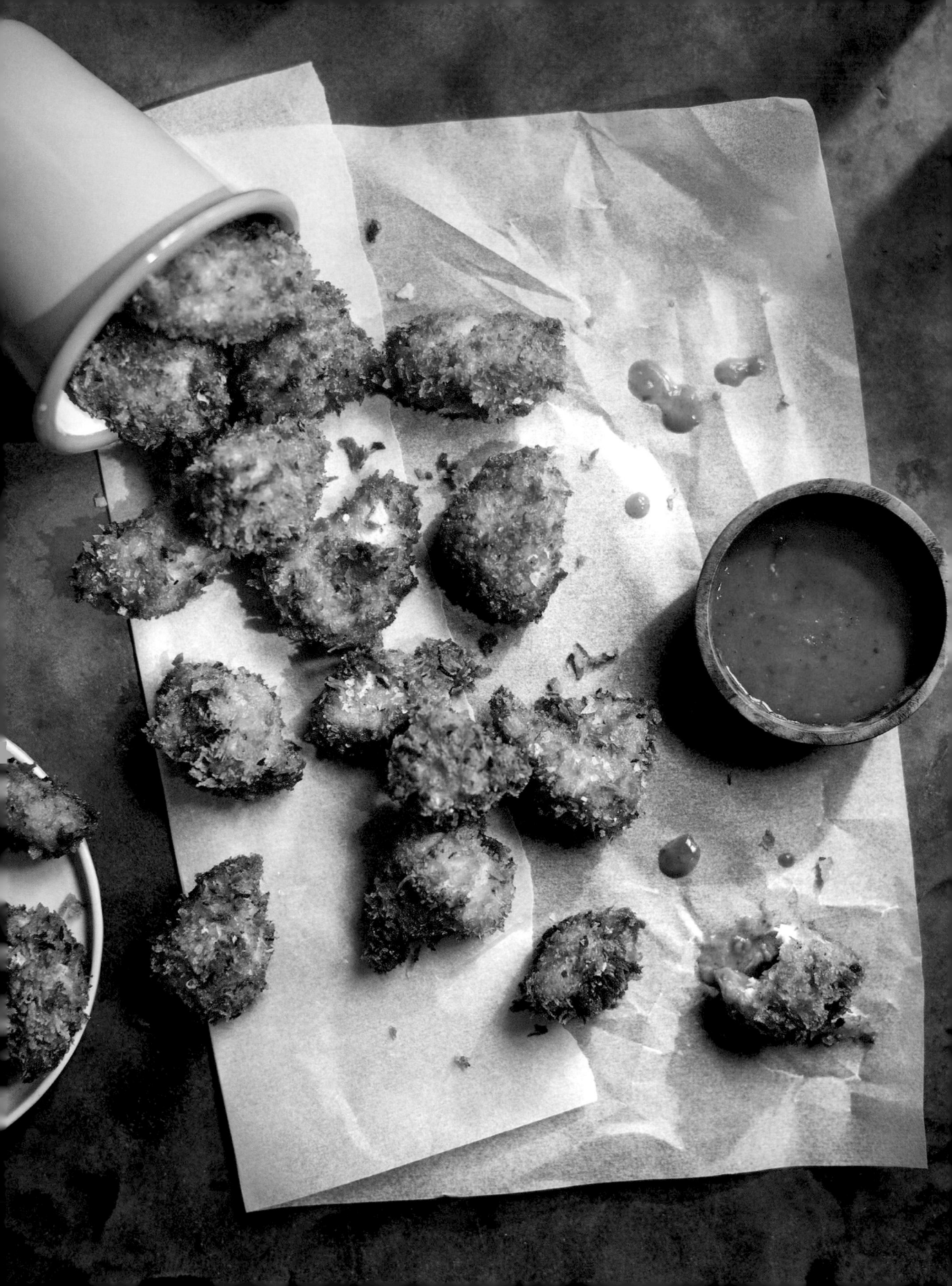

PERI PERI POPCORN CHICKEN

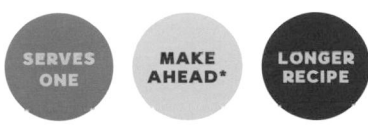

SERVES ONE **MAKE AHEAD*** **LONGER RECIPE**

INGREDIENTS

2 tbsp natural yoghurt
1 tbsp peri peri sauce, plus
   more to serve
50g dried breadcrumbs
1 x 200g skinless chicken
   breast fillet
salt and pepper
big pinch of smoked paprika

*** LEAVE TO COOL, THEN PUT
IN THE FRIDGE IN AN AIRTIGHT
CONTAINER FOR THE NEXT DAY.
KEEP SAUCE SEPARATE.**

1. Preheat the oven to 220°C (fan 200°/gas mark 7). Line a baking tray with baking parchment.

2. Spoon the yoghurt into a shallow bowl. Stir in the peri peri sauce. Measure the breadcrumbs into another shallow bowl.

3. Cut the chicken breast into popcorn-sized cubes. Season all over with a big pinch of salt, pepper and smoked paprika.

4. A few at a time, coat the chicken cubes in the peri peri sauce and then in the breadcrumbs, until completely coated. Lay out in a single layer on the lined baking tray. Roast in the oven for 12–14 minutes until cooked through and crisp. Check by slicing into one of the larger pieces to make sure the meat is white all the way through, with no raw pink bits left.

5. Gobble down with a little more peri peri sauce, for dipping.

SNACKS

139

INGREDIENTS

80g walnuts

2 jarred roasted red peppers,
    drained

½ tsp ground cumin

1 tbsp pomegranate molasses

½–1 tsp dried chilli flakes

2 tbsp olive oil

juice of ½ lemon

crudités of your choice, to serve
    – I love carrots and cucumber

*** THE DIP WILL KEEP IN THE
FRIDGE FOR UP TO 3 DAYS.**

WALNUT AND ROASTED RED PEPPER DIP

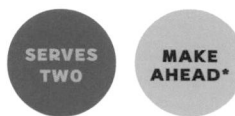

SERVES TWO

MAKE AHEAD*

1. Toast the walnuts in a dry frying pan over a medium heat until they smell nutty. Take the pan off the heat and leave to cool slightly.

2. Tip most of the walnuts into a small food processor. Add all the other ingredients and blitz until smooth. Season the dip with salt and pepper to taste.

3. Spoon into a bowl or container. Chop the remaining walnuts and scatter over the top. Serve with crudités, aka chopped raw vegetables, of your choice.

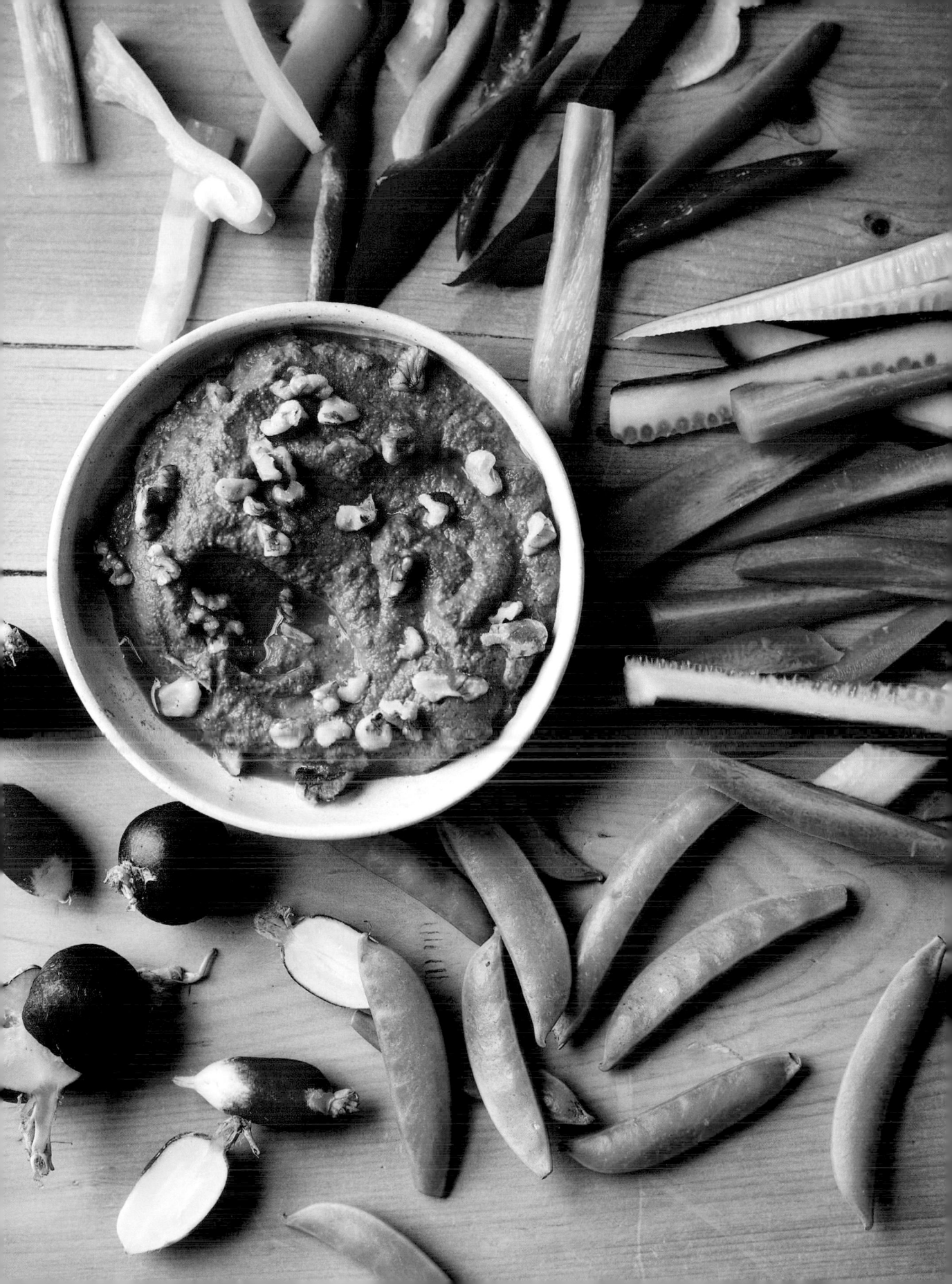

INGREDIENTS

100g almonds, very roughly
chopped
100g dark chocolate
1 tsp coconut oil
big pinch of sea salt – I like
the flaky stuff

DARK CHOCOLATE, ALMOND AND SEA SALT CLUSTERS

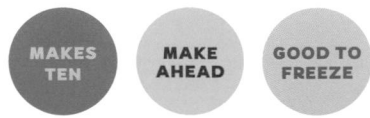

MAKES TEN

MAKE AHEAD

GOOD TO FREEZE

1. Line two small baking trays with baking parchment.

2. Toast the roughly chopped almonds in a dry frying pan over a medium heat until lightly golden.

3. Meanwhile break the chocolate into a microwaveable bowl, spoon in the coconut oil. Zap in the microwave in 30-second bursts, stirring in between, until the chocolate has all melted.

4. Tip the toasted almonds into the bowl of melted chocolate. Stir together so that all the almonds get coated in the melted chocolate, then dollop ten spoonfuls onto the lined baking trays. Sprinkle each with a generous pinch of sea salt and whack into the freezer for around 8 minutes, or until set.

5. Keep in an airtight container in the fridge for up to a week, for the ultimate cheeky snack.

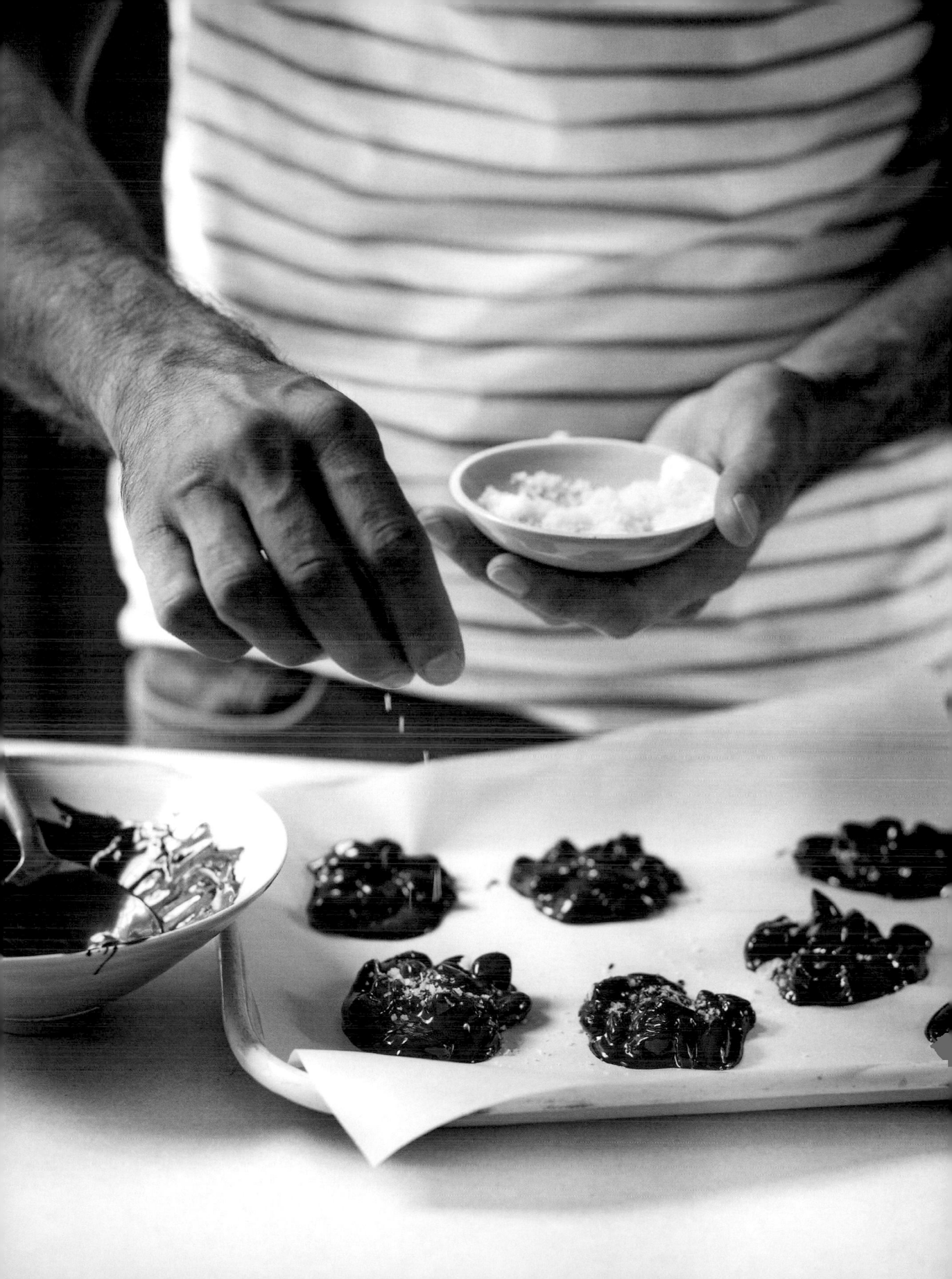

POST
WORKOUT

INGREDIENTS

1 tsp coconut oil
knob of fresh ginger, finely sliced
1 tsp coriander seeds
1 chicken stock cube
½ tsp five spice
1 x 200g skinless chicken breast
    fillet, cut into quarters
salt and pepper
½ red chilli
1 medium carrot
small handful of mint
200g pre-cooked rice noodles
1 tsp soy sauce
juice of ½ lime
splash of fish sauce

CHICKEN PHO

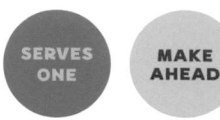

SERVES ONE

MAKE AHEAD

1. Bring a kettle of water to the boil.

2. Melt the coconut oil in a saucepan over a low heat. Add the sliced ginger and coriander seeds. Leave to gently toast.

3. Meanwhile put the chicken stock cube into a jug, measure in 400ml of boiling water and whisk with a fork to dissolve.

4. Come back to the pan, turn up the heat to medium and sprinkle in the five spice. Cook, stirring, for 30 seconds then pour in the chicken stock.

5. Season the chicken breast pieces with salt and pepper then carefully drop them into the saucepan. Place a lid on the pan and cook for 8 minutes.

6. While the chicken is cooking, finely slice the red chilli – remove the seeds if you don't like it hot. Peel the carrot into long ribbons and pick the mint leaves.

7. After 8 minutes the chicken should be cooked. Check by slicing into one of the pieces to make sure the meat is white all the way through, with no raw pink bits left. Once you're happy, using a slotted spoon lift the chicken onto a plate.

8. Drop the carrot ribbons and rice noodles into the broth. Shred the cooked chicken with two forks then put it back into the pan, season with soy sauce, lime juice and fish sauce to taste.

9. Serve up into a bowl, discarding the ginger slices and coriander seeds. Scatter over the mint leaves and sliced red chilli to finish.

Veggie Swap

Swap the chicken breast for 140g firm tofu, cut into cubes, dropped into the pho with the carrot and rice noodles.

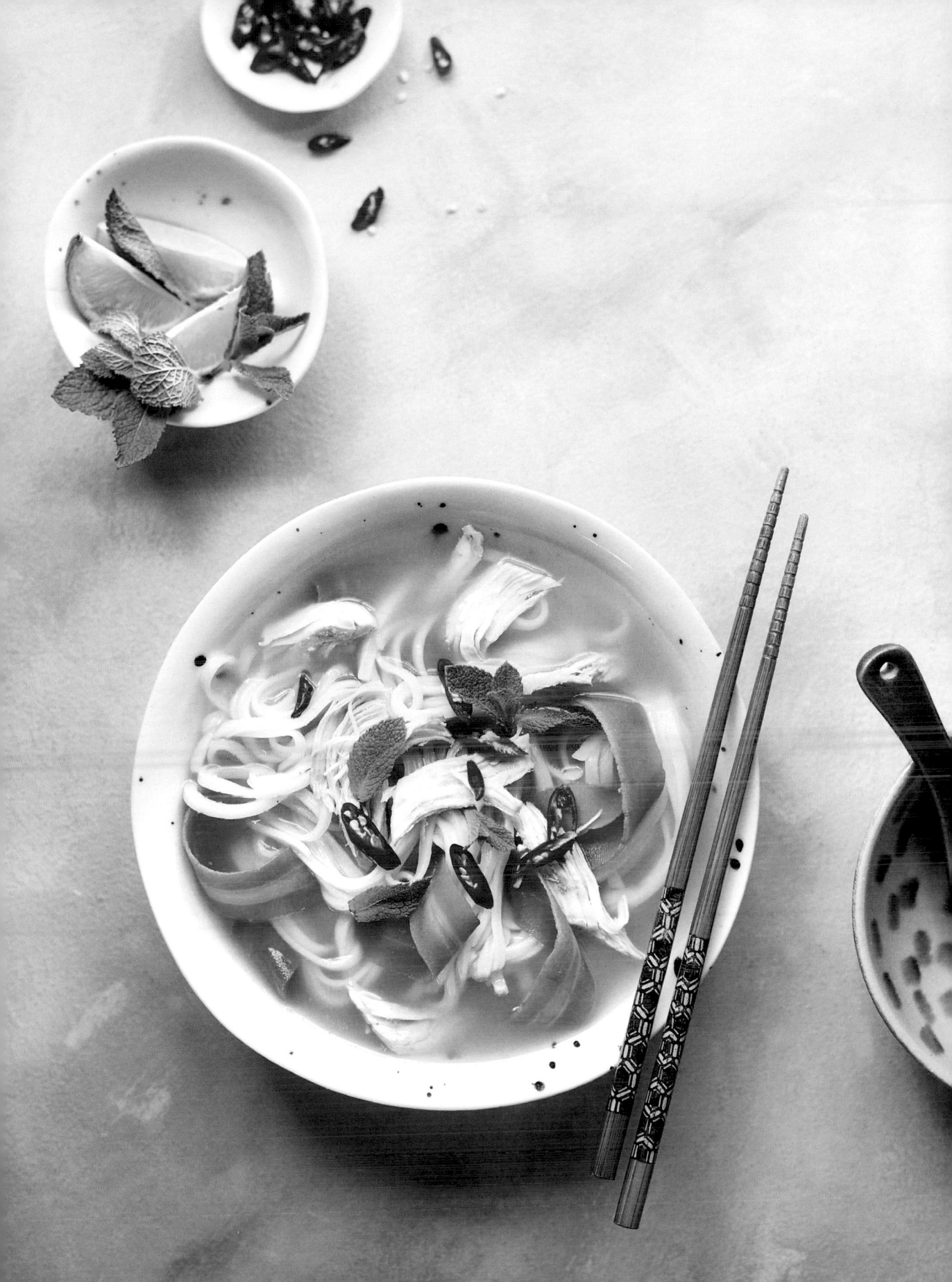

INGREDIENTS

2 tbsp coconut oil

800g beef braising steak, cut
into medium chunks

salt and pepper

6 shallots, halved

4 medium carrots, cut into
large chunks

4 celery sticks, cut into
large chunks

4 cloves garlic, chopped

3 bay leaves

2 tbsp self-raising flour,
plus 120g

330ml bottle of ale

1 x 400g tin of plum tomatoes

60g cold butter, cut into cubes

handful of chives

2 tbsp creamed horseradish
mash, to serve – optional

*** YOU COULD FREEZE THE STEW
FOR A LATER DATE AT THE END OF
STEP 4. WHEN READY TO SERVE,
DEFROST AND CONTINUE WITH
THE RECIPE.**

BEEF COBBLER WITH CHIVE AND HORSERADISH DUMPLINGS

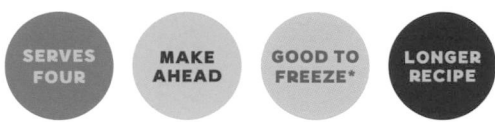

SERVES FOUR · MAKE AHEAD · GOOD TO FREEZE* · LONGER RECIPE

1. Preheat the oven to 180°C (fan 160°/gas mark 4).

2. Melt the coconut oil in a large shallow casserole pot or heavy-bottomed saucepan over a medium to high heat. Season the steak all over with salt and pepper. Fry the steak in two batches until browned, then tip all of the meat back into the pan.

3. Chuck in the shallots, carrots, celery, garlic and bay leaves. Sprinkle over 2 tablespoons of self-raising flour, give everything a good mix. Cook for 1–2 minutes, then tip in the ale, 400ml water and the tin of plum tomatoes. Use the back of your wooden spoon to break up the tomatoes. Season everything with a generous pinch of salt and pepper, bring the stew to a boil.

4. Once boiling, place a lid on the pan and shove in the oven. Cook for 2 hours, until the meat is pretty much falling apart. Check by trying to shred a piece with two forks.

5. Meanwhile make the dumplings. Tip the remaining 120g of self-raising flour into a bowl. Dump in the cold butter, then use your fingers to rub the butter into the flour until it resembles sand. Using scissors, snip in the chives, spoon in the creamed horseradish and season with salt and pepper. Pour in 2–4 tablespoons of water and mix together with a wooden spoon to create a thick dough. Add a little more water if you need it. Keep the dough, covered, in the fridge to rest.

6. When the meat in the stew is nearly tender, flour your hands then roll the dumpling dough into twelve small balls.

7. Crank up the oven to 200°C (fan 180°/gas mark 6). Place the dumplings on top of the stew, and return to the oven for 20 minutes, uncovered, until the dumplings are puffed up and golden. I like to eat this with mash – proper comfort food.

Joe's Top Tip

Flavours in this stew improve after a day or so, making this a great recipe to make ahead and reheat in a hot oven.

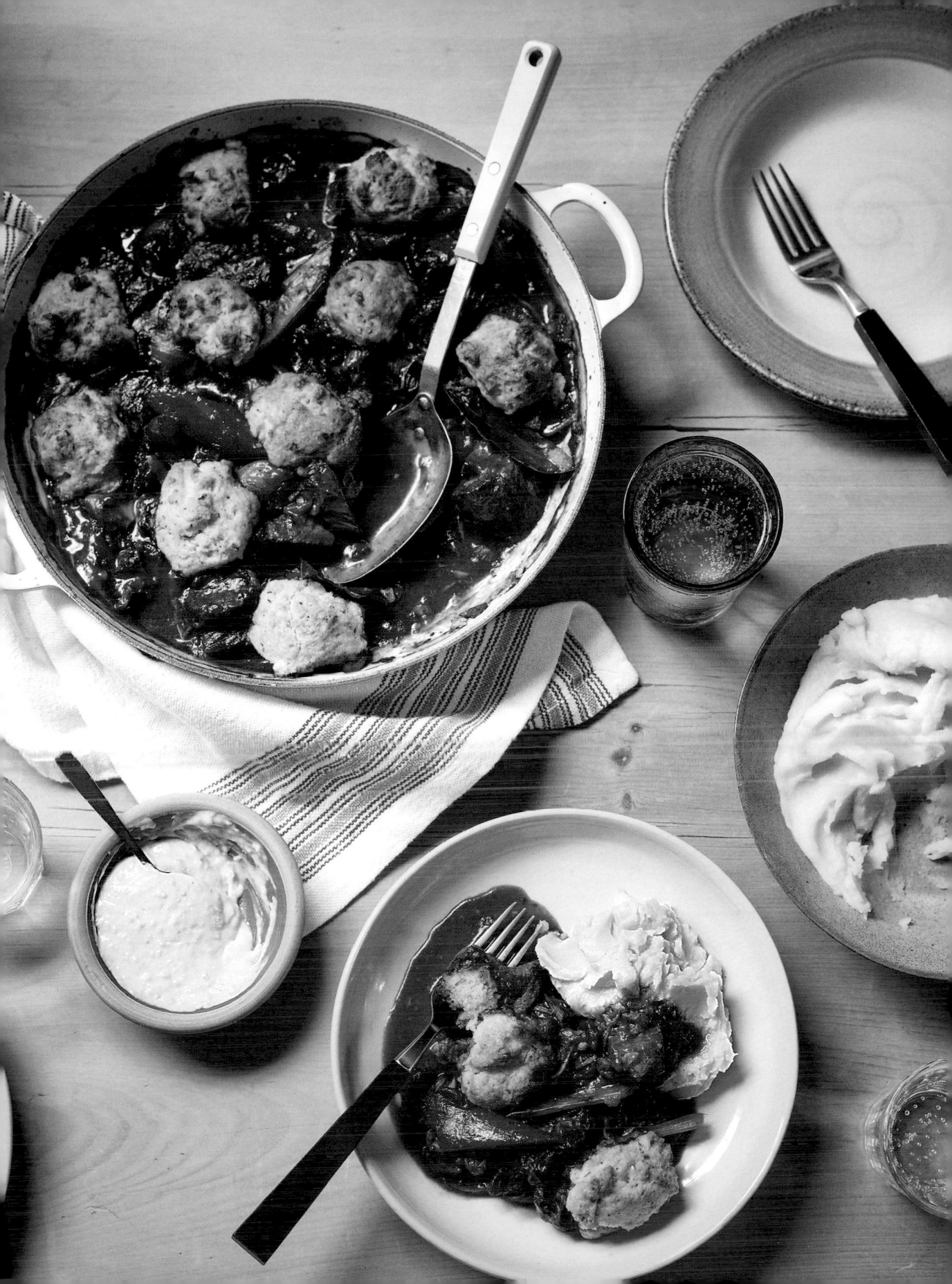

INGREDIENTS

50g walnuts
3 large handfuls of kale
1 small clove garlic
zest and juice of ½ lemon
2 tbsp olive oil
15g vegetarian hard cheese
    or parmesan (if not veggie),
    grated
salt and pepper
250g fresh gnocchi

KALE AND WALNUT PESTO GNOCCHI

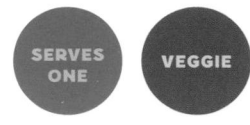

SERVES ONE **VEGGIE**

1. Bring a kettle of water to the boil.

2. Toast the walnuts in a dry frying pan over a medium heat until they smell nutty. Leave to cool.

3. Pour the boiling water into a saucepan over a medium heat. Salt the water, drop in the kale. Once wilted, lift the kale out of the water using a slotted spoon. Keep the pan of water on the heat. Tip the kale into a bowl of cold water. Once cool, drain and squeeze out as much water as possible.

4. Roughly chop the walnuts. Put the kale into a small food processor along with most of the walnuts, garlic, lemon zest and juice, olive oil and most of the grated cheese. Blitz to a textured pesto. Season to taste.

5. Come back to the pan of boiling water. Drop in the gnocchi and cook according to packet instructions. Drain, saving a mugful of cooking water, then tip the gnocchi back into the pan and spoon in the pesto. Mix together, adding a splash of the cooking water to loosen the pesto, until everything is heated through.

6. Pile the gnocchi into a bowl, scatter over the remaining walnuts then gobble down.

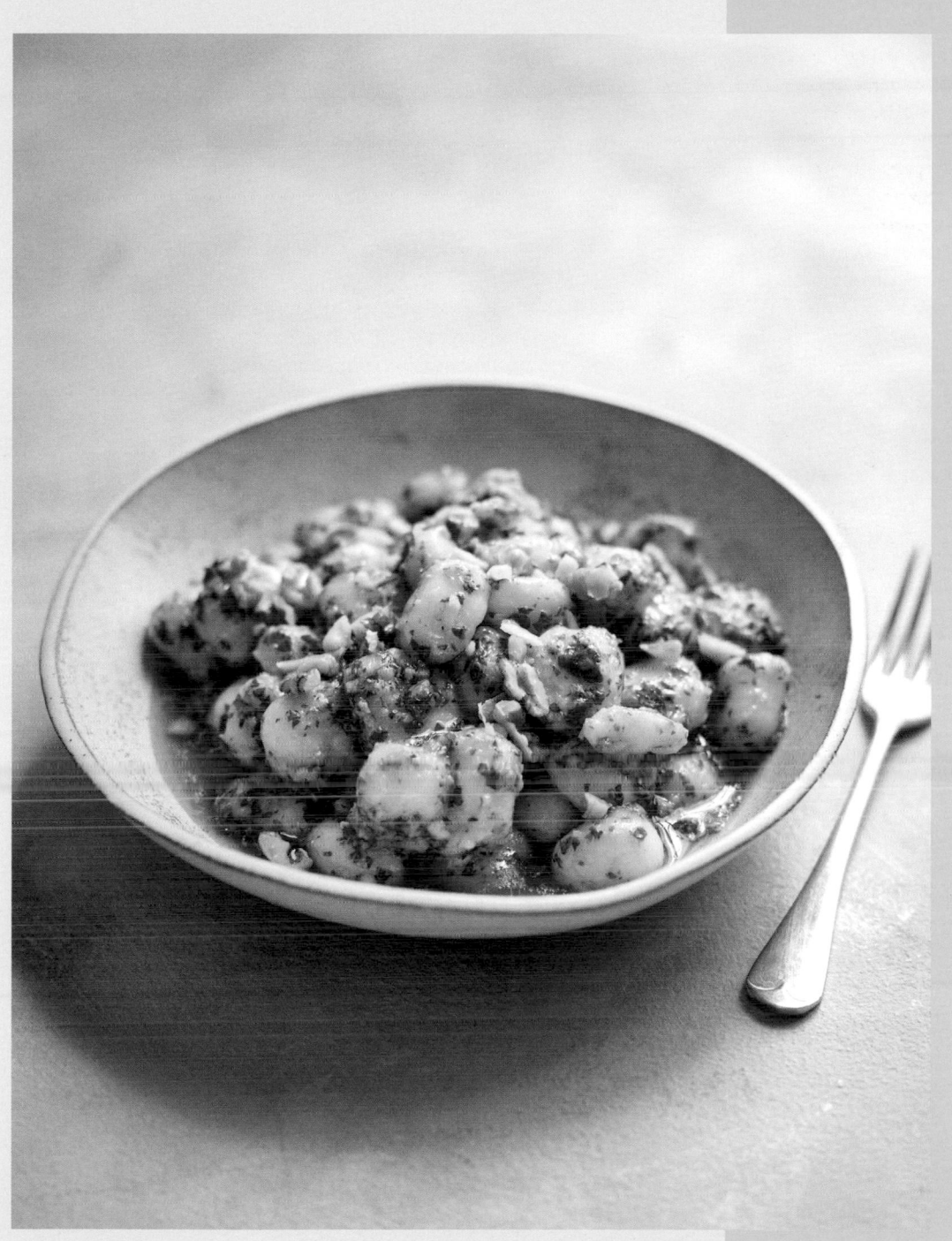

LANCASHIRE HOTPOT

INGREDIENTS

good drizzle of olive oil

400g lamb neck, cut into medium chunks

salt and pepper

50g butter

2 onions, sliced

1 chicken stock cube

1 tbsp plain flour

2 bay leaves

a few sprigs of thyme

big splash of Worcestershire sauce

2 large potatoes, peeled and cut into 1cm slices

buttery peas, to serve

* FREEZE COOKED HOTPOT.

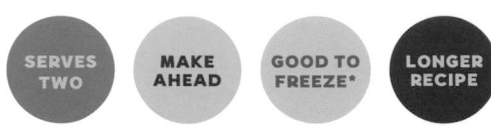

SERVES TWO

MAKE AHEAD

GOOD TO FREEZE*

LONGER RECIPE

1. Preheat the oven to 180°C (fan 160°/gas mark 4).

2. Heat a small casserole pot or heavy-bottomed saucepan over a medium to high heat. Pour in the olive oil, season the lamb all over with salt and pepper. Fry the lamb until browned all over, then remove with tongs onto a plate.

3. Reduce the heat to medium and melt half the butter into the pan. When bubbling, chuck in the sliced onions, along with a pinch of salt. Cook for 10 minutes, stirring occasionally until soft.

4. Meanwhile bring a kettle of water to the boil. Put the chicken stock cube into a jug, measure in 250ml boiling water and whisk with a fork to dissolve.

5. Come back to the onions, tip the lamb back into the pan. Sprinkle over the plain flour, give everything a good mix then pour in the chicken stock. Add the bay leaves, thyme and a decent splash of Worcestershire sauce. Stir, take the pan off the heat.

6. Lay the potato slices on top of the lamb casserole, overlapping each one a little bit. Season the potatoes with salt and pepper and dot over the remaining butter.

7. Place a lid on the pan and cook for 1½ hours. Remove the lid, crank up the heat to 200°C (fan 180°/gas mark 6) and cook for a further 30 minutes, until a cutlery knife can easily cut through the potatoes and they are nicely golden. Serve with buttery peas.

Joe's Top Tip

I like to use Maris Piper potatoes because they soak up the sauce and get crispy. Double win!

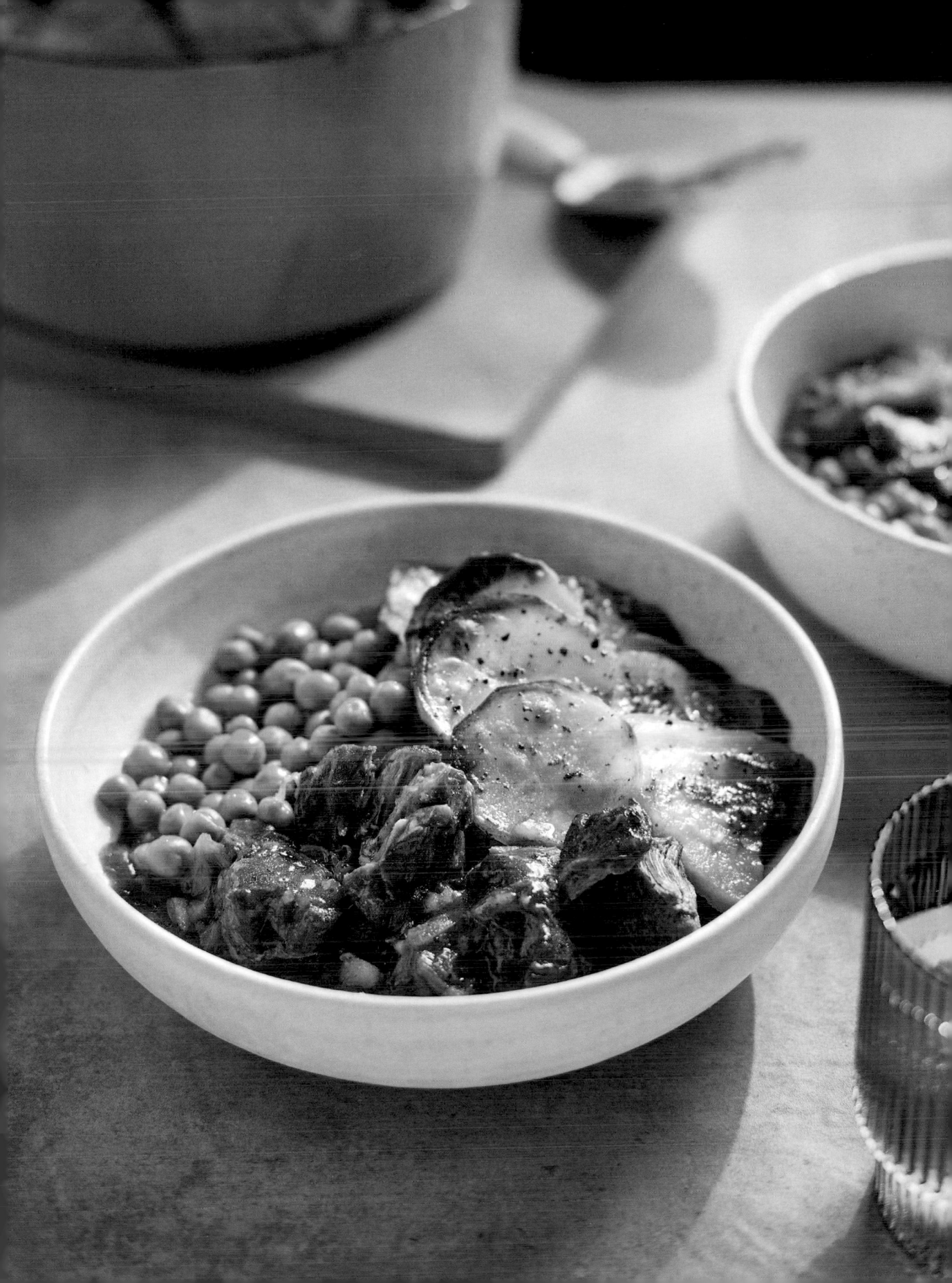

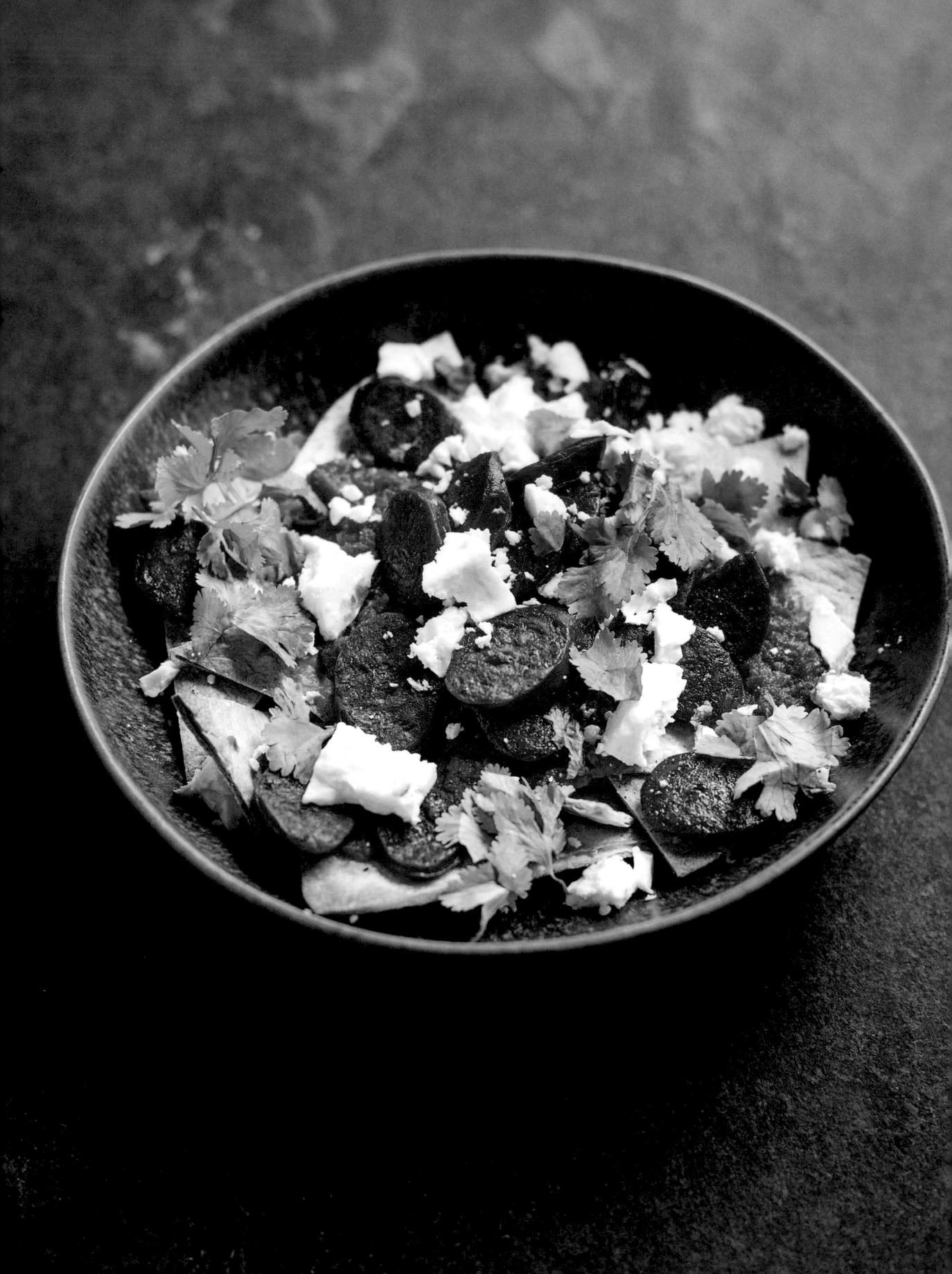

CHORIZO CHILAQUILES

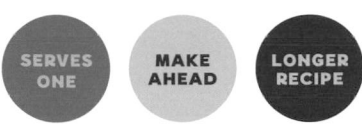

SERVES ONE · MAKE AHEAD · LONGER RECIPE

INGREDIENTS

3 flour tortillas
1 tbsp olive oil, plus a drizzle
salt and pepper
¼ chorizo ring (110g)
2 ripe medium tomatoes
½ red onion
½ jalapeño
30g feta
small handful of coriander

1. Preheat the oven to 220°C (fan 200°/gas mark 7).

2. Using kitchen scissors, cut each tortilla into eight triangles, the same size as tortilla chips. Dump them onto a large baking tray. Toss with 1 tablespoon of oil and a generous pinch of salt and pepper. Spread out into a single layer, then bake for 8–10 minutes, flipping halfway through. Homemade nachos done.

3. Meanwhile slice the chorizo. Heat a non-stick frying pan over a medium to high heat. Drizzle in a little oil, chuck in the chorizo and fry, stirring occasionally, for 5 minutes until crisp.

4. While the chorizo is frying, roughly chop the tomatoes, red onion and jalapeño – remove the seeds if you don't like it hot. Put everything into a small food processor, blitz to a sauce.

5. Come back to the chorizo. Using a slotted spoon, remove from the pan onto a plate. Pour the tomato sauce into the frying pan with the chorizo oils. Crank up the heat and bubble away for 2–3 minutes until no longer watery. Season to taste.

6. Pile the homemade nachos into a bowl. Pour over the warm tomato sauce. Top with the fried chorizo, then crumble over the feta and tear over some coriander. Epic.

Veggie Swap

Swap the chorizo for 2 eggs, fried to your liking, placed on top of the chilaquiles.

POST WORKOUT

INGREDIENTS

1 fat clove garlic
½ lemon
salt and pepper
100g spaghetti
1 tbsp olive oil
6 turkey meatballs (200g)
200g passata
2 tsp harissa
handful of basil leaves

* SAUCE ONLY.

TURKEY MEATBALLS AND HARISSA SPAGHETTI

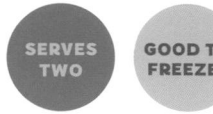

SERVES TWO   GOOD TO FREEZE*

1. Bring a kettle of water to the boil.

2. Meanwhile finely chop the garlic and zest the lemon.

3. Pour the boiling water into a saucepan over a medium heat. Salt the water, drop in the spaghetti. Cook for 1 minute less than packet instructions.

4. While the pasta is cooking, heat a non-stick frying pan over a high heat. Pour in the olive oil, lay in the meatballs. Fry for 4 minutes, turning regularly until evenly browned. Scrape in the chopped garlic, cook for 30 seconds then add the passata and harissa. Season with salt and pepper, then leave to bubble away for 5 minutes until the sauce has thickened and the meatballs are cooked through. Check by slicing into one to make sure the meat is white all the way through, with no raw pink bits left.

5. Drain the spaghetti into a colander, saving half a mugful of pasta water. Drop the spaghetti into the frying pan with the meatballs and sauce. Add the lemon zest, a squeeze of lemon juice, a splash of pasta water, half the basil leaves and a generous crack of black pepper. Mix to combine.

6. Serve up the spaghetti and meatballs. Scatter over the remaining basil leaves, then dive in.

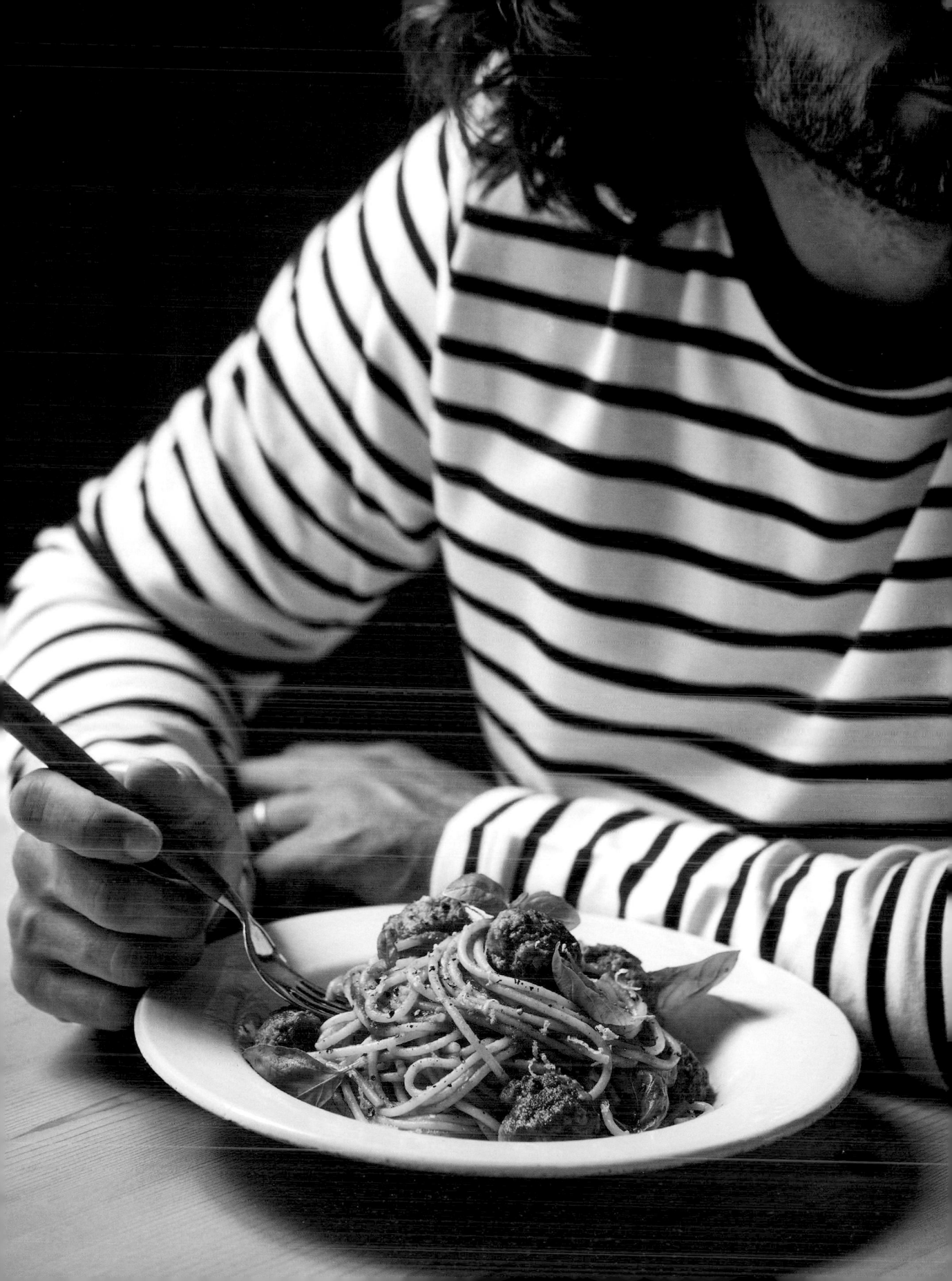

INGREDIENTS

2 large potatoes
salt and pepper
2 tbsp olive oil
big pinch of smoked paprika
2 x gammon steaks
    (around 180g each)
1 tbsp wholegrain mustard
drizzle of honey
2 eggs
condiments of your choice
    to serve

* CHIPS ONLY. REHEAT IN A HOT OVEN TO CRISP UP.

JOE'S MUSTARDY HAM, EGG AND CHIPS

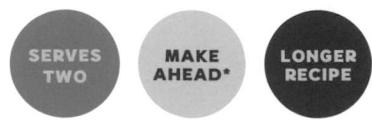

SERVES TWO   MAKE AHEAD*   LONGER RECIPE

1. Preheat the oven to 220°C (fan 200°/gas mark 7). Bring a kettle of water to the boil.

2. Cut the potatoes into chunky chips, leaving the skin on.

3. Pour the boiling water into a saucepan over a medium to high heat. Salt the water, drop in the chips and cook for 3 minutes. Drain into a colander and shake off any excess water. Leave the chips to steam for a few minutes, then tip onto a baking tray.

4. Drizzle over 1 tablespoon of olive oil, season well with a generous pinch of salt, pepper and smoked paprika. Toss together with tongs, then spread the chips out into a single layer. Roast for 25–30 minutes until golden brown and crisp, flipping the chips halfway.

5. Once the chips have 15 minutes of cooking time left, heat a large non-stick frying pan over a medium heat. Pour in ½ tablespoon of oil then place the gammon steaks in the pan. Fry for 5 minutes on each side, then transfer to a baking tray lined with tin foil.

6. Spoon the wholegrain mustard over the gammon steaks and drizzle over the honey. Slide into the bottom of the oven while you fry the eggs.

7. Put the same pan back onto the heat (no need to wash it first – extra flavour). Pour in the remaining oil, then crack in the eggs and fry to your liking.

8. Dish up the chips between two plates. Lay a honey and mustard ham alongside, with a fried egg. Serve with condiments of your choice – I like ketchup. Dream food!

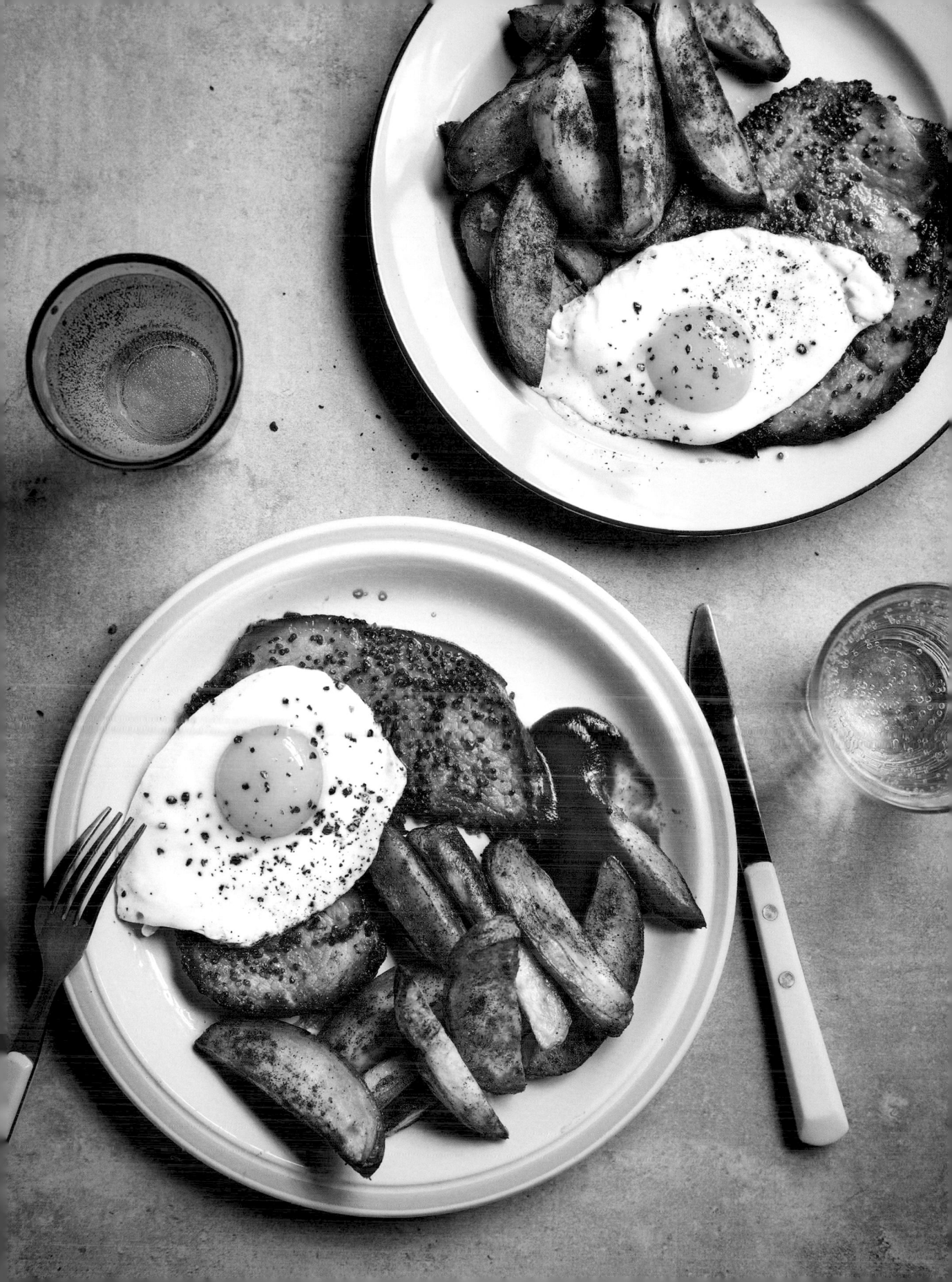

INGREDIENTS

1 large sweet potato
½ lime
1 clove garlic
2 spring onions (green and
    white parts)
small handful of coriander
    (stalks and all)
1 red pepper
20g butter
salt and pepper
2 tsp Cajun seasoning
180g raw king prawns

CAJUN-STYLE PRAWNS WITH LIME SWEET POTATO MASH

SERVES
ONE

1. Cut the sweet potato into medium chunks, leaving the skin on. Put in a microwaveable bowl with the lime half and 1 tablespoon of water. Cover and zap on high for 10 minutes until completely soft.

2. Meanwhile, finely slice the garlic, spring onions, coriander stalks and red pepper. Keep some of the sliced spring onion to one side.

3. Melt the butter in a frying pan over a medium heat. Scrape in the veggies along with a pinch of salt and pepper. Cook, stirring almost constantly, for 4 minutes until the peppers are soft, then sprinkle over the Cajun seasoning and chuck in the prawns. Cook for 2–3 minutes. The raw grey colour of the prawns will turn pink, which shows you they are cooked.

4. Turn down the heat to low to keep the prawns warm, and come back to your sweet potato. Carefully uncover and, using a fork, squeeze out the juice from the lime. Season with salt and pepper, roughly mash.

5. Pile the mash into a bowl. Spoon over the Cajun prawn mix, finish with a scattering of coriander leaves and the remaining spring onion.

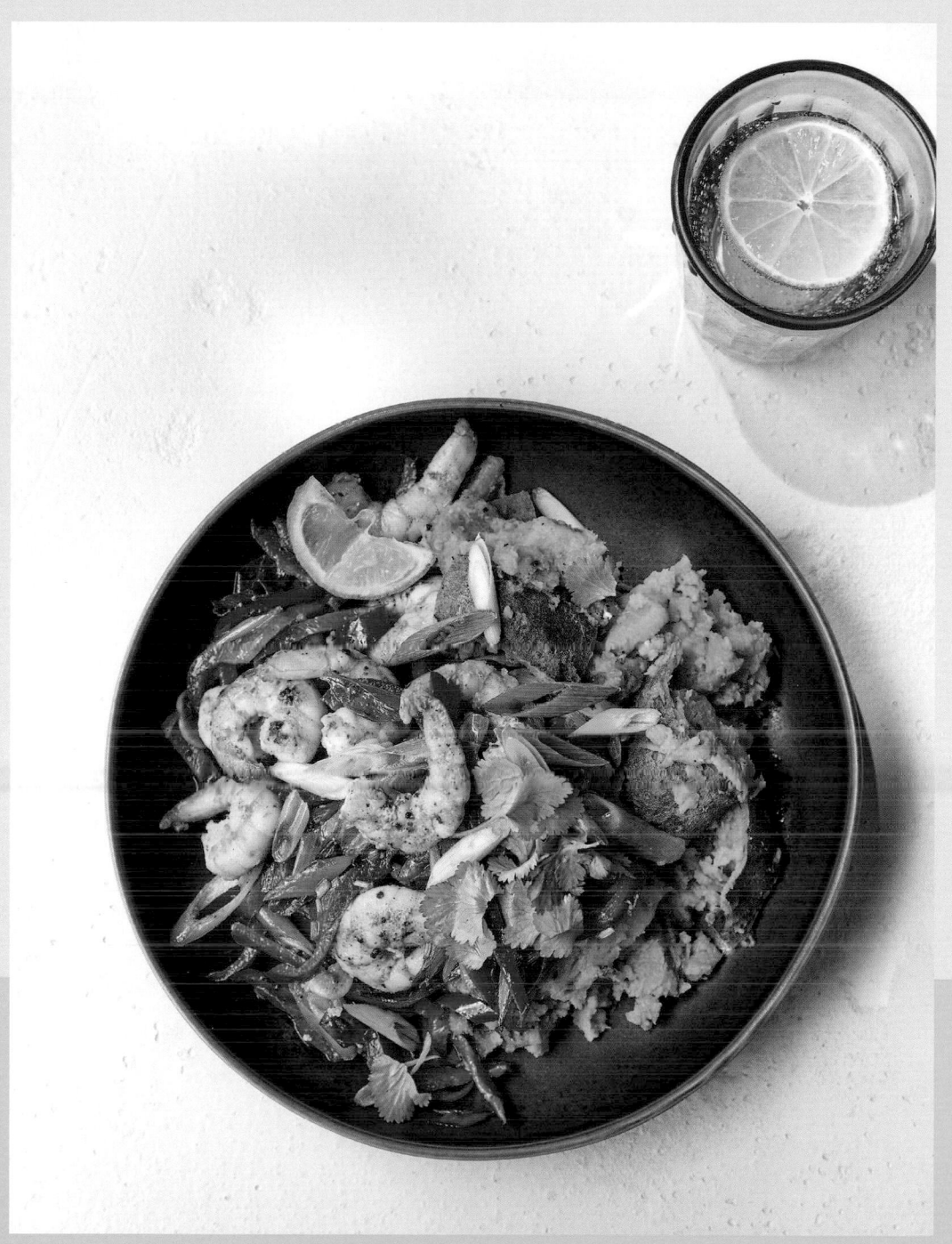

INGREDIENTS

2 tbsp butter

½ chorizo ring (110g), sliced

2 x 150g skinless chicken breast fillets, sliced into 1cm strips

1 large red onion, sliced

2 mixed peppers – I like orange and red – sliced

2 fat cloves garlic, finely chopped

2 tsp smoked paprika

2 tsp dried oregano

1 x 400g tin of cherry tomatoes

salt and pepper

splash of sherry or red wine vinegar

½ pack filo pastry (6 sheets)

2 tbsp flaked almonds

rocket salad, to serve

CHICKEN AND CHORIZO FILO PIE

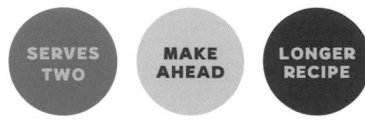

SERVES TWO   MAKE AHEAD   LONGER RECIPE

1. Preheat the oven to 220°C (fan 200°/gas mark 7).

2. Melt half the butter in an ovenproof frying pan over a high heat. Once bubbling, chuck in the sliced chorizo, chicken, onion and peppers. Fry, stirring regularly, for around 5 minutes until the chicken is mostly cooked through and the onion and peppers have collapsed and softened.

3. Add the garlic, smoked paprika and oregano to the pan. Give everything a good mix, cook for 1 minute then tip in the tin of cherry tomatoes. Bring the pie mixture to a boil, season with salt, pepper and a splash of sherry or red wine vinegar. Take the pan off the heat.

4. Melt the remaining butter in the microwave. Lay the pastry sheets out. Brush each one with the melted butter. Take a sheet of filo and roughly crumple it in your hand.

5. Place the crumpled sheet on top of the frying pan, then repeat with the remaining filo sheets until the chorizo and chicken pie mixture is completely covered.

6. Whack the pie in the oven for 10 minutes, then sprinkle the flaked almonds over the top. Return to the oven for 5–10 minutes until the pastry is deep golden brown and crisp.

7. Leave to rest for a few minutes before serving – no one likes a burnt mouth. Serve with a rocket salad.

Veggie Swap

Swap the chicken and chorizo for 60g feta, crumbled into large pieces and 1 x 400g tin of drained and rinsed chickpeas, both added to the pie mix at the same time as the tin of cherry tomatoes.

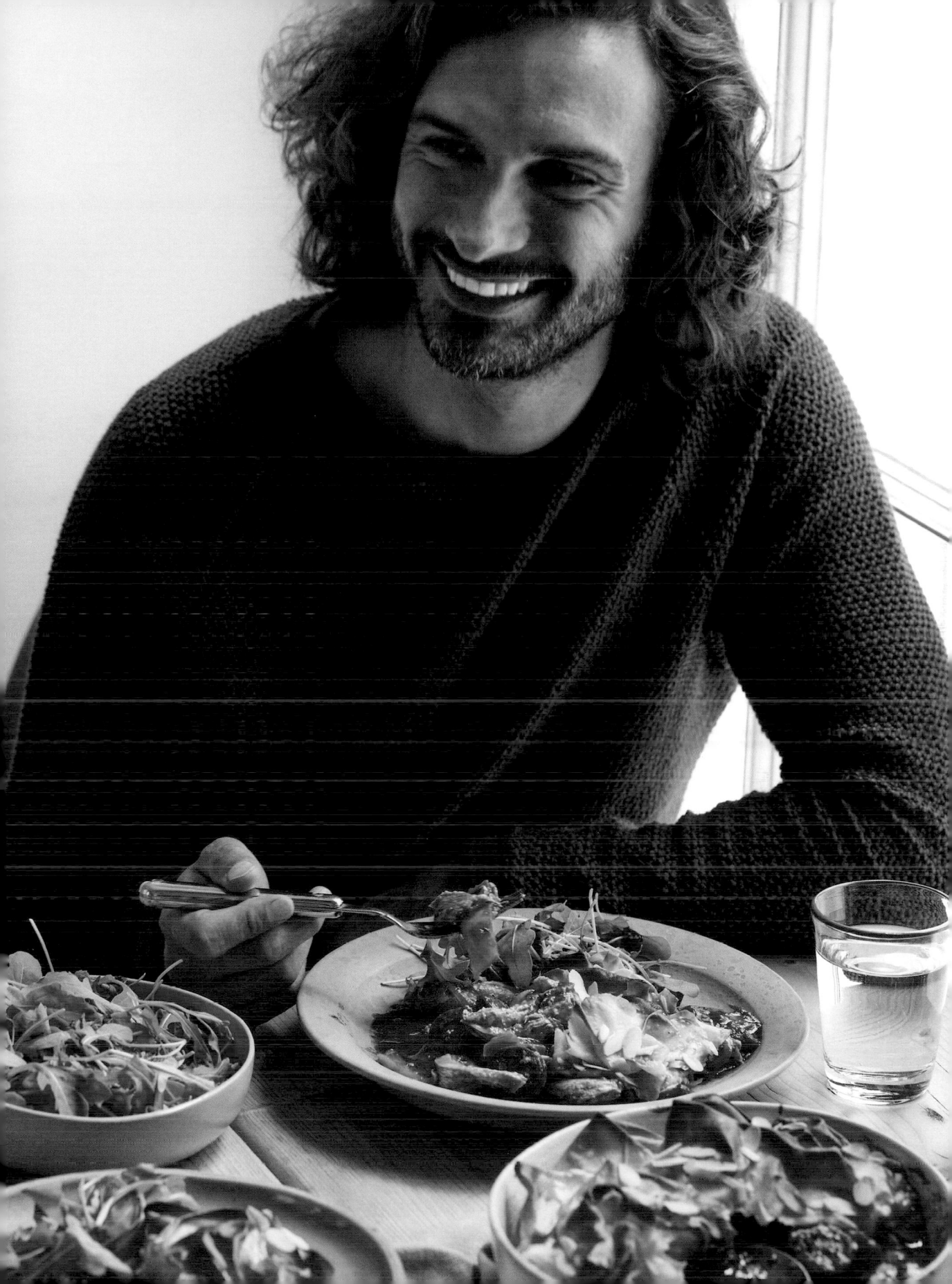

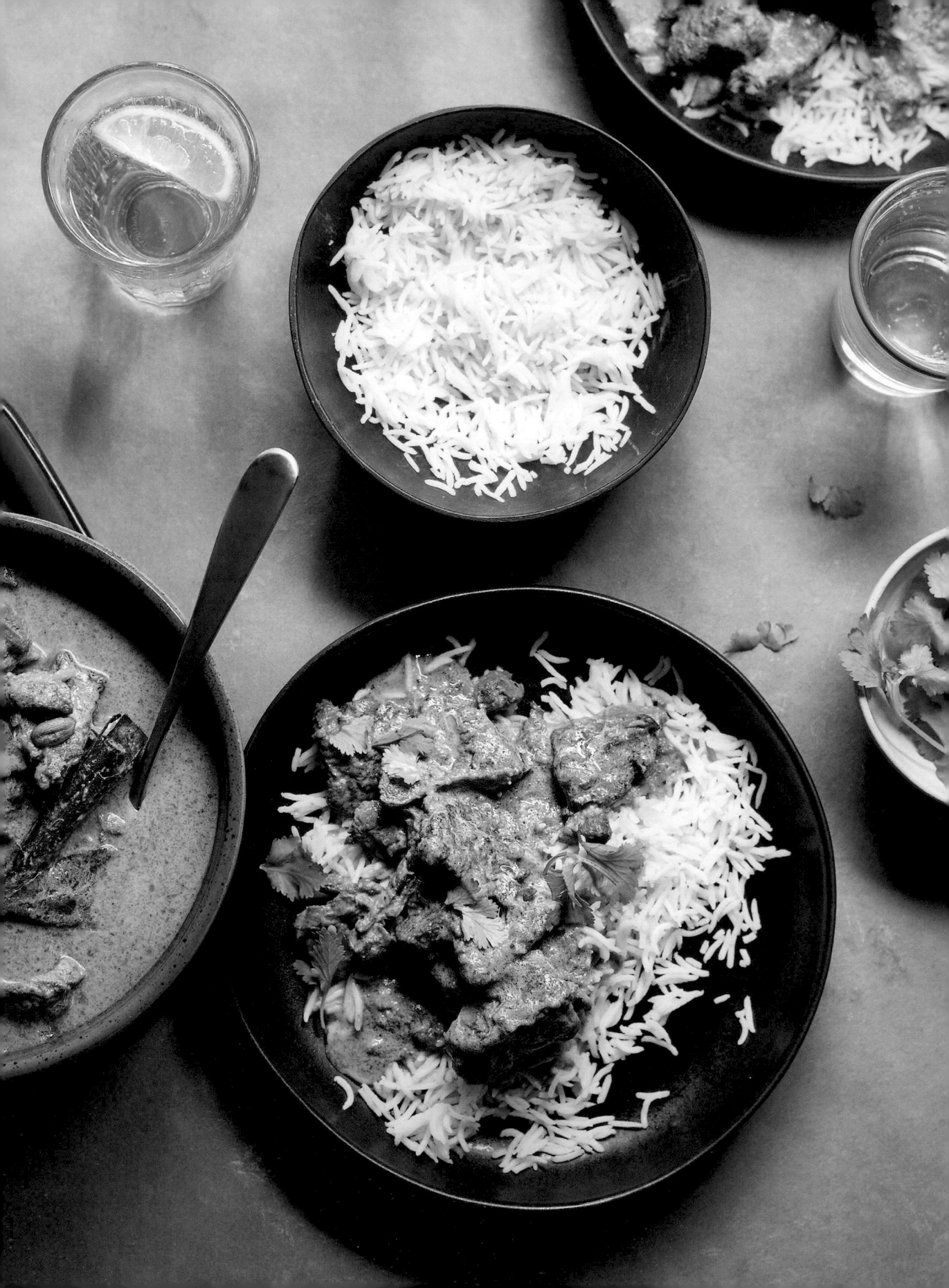

LAMB ROGAN JOSH

 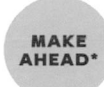 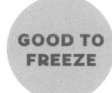 

SERVES FOUR · MAKE AHEAD* · GOOD TO FREEZE · LONGER RECIPE

1. Preheat the oven to 150°C (fan 130°/gas mark 2).

2. Put the ginger and garlic into a small food processor with 2 tablespoons water. Blitz to a paste.

3. Melt the coconut oil in a large casserole pot or heavy-bottomed saucepan over a medium to high heat. Season the lamb pieces all over with salt and pepper. Once the oil is melted, fry the lamb in two batches until browned, remove with tongs onto a plate.

4. Add the cinnamon stick, cardamom pods and bay leaves into the melted oil, cook, stirring for 30 seconds until the bay leaves begin to change colour, then chuck in the onions. Fry for 5 minutes then tip in the ginger and garlic paste. Cook, stirring for a minute or so until all the water has evaporated, sprinkle in the ground cumin, coriander and chilli powder. Give everything a good mix, then tip the lamb back into the pan.

5. While stirring, add the yoghurt, one spoonful at a time – this is important because if you add all the yoghurt at once it can split. After each spoonful of yoghurt, mix well and cook for around 30 seconds before adding the next spoonful – this is the hardest bit of the recipe, I promise.

6. Once all the yoghurt has been added, pour in 400ml water. Sprinkle in a good pinch of salt and pepper, mix everything together. Place a lid on the pan, whack in the oven for 1½ hours or until the meat is tender. Check by trying to shred a piece with two forks.

7. Once you are happy with the meat, stir through the garam masala and season to taste. Serve the lamb rogan josh with rice and roughly chopped fresh coriander. Dream food.

INGREDIENTS

large knob of fresh ginger, roughly chopped
4 fat cloves garlic
1½ tbsp coconut oil
800g boneless lamb shoulder, cut into medium chunks
salt and pepper
1 cinnamon stick
8 cardamom pods
4 bay leaves
2 onions, chopped
2 tsp ground cumin
2 tsp ground coriander
1 tbsp chilli powder
6 tbsp low-fat natural yoghurt
2 tsp garam masala
rice and fresh coriander, to serve

* KEEPS FOR UP TO 2 DAYS COVERED IN THE FRIDGE.

Joe's Top Tip

Don't be put off by the list of ingredients – most of them are dried spices you will use again. Trust me, once you've made this once, you'll be wanting to cook it again and again.

> "
>
> I used to stand back and let my husband lift heavy things for me. Now I can say 'it's OK, I can do it, I'm Joe Wicks strong'. I feel more independent and ready to face the world.
>
> "
>
> **VALERIE, 59**

66

My health is unrecognizable! I have more energy and look forward to physical challenges now. The best bit for me is that I can now keep up and play with my boys. It brings us so much joy and has created so many happy family moments that we can all play and explore together. Amazing!

99

CHARLOTTE, 32

INGREDIENTS

knob of butter
1 onion, finely chopped
150g smoked cubed pancetta
1 chicken stock cube
2 fat cloves garlic, finely
    chopped
160g arborio risotto rice
glass of white wine
1 egg and 2 egg yolks
30g parmesan, finely grated
black pepper

CARBONARA RISOTTO

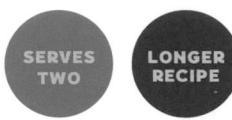

SERVES TWO

LONGER RECIPE

1. Bring a kettle of water to the boil.

2. Meanwhile melt the butter in a large frying pan over a medium heat. When bubbling, chuck in the chopped onion and pancetta. Cook, stirring occasionally, for 8–10 minutes until the onion is completely soft and the pancetta crisp.

3. Put the chicken stock cube into a jug, measure in 700ml boiling water and whisk with a fork to dissolve.

4. Scrape the garlic into the pan with the onion and pancetta. Cook, stirring, for 1 minute then tip in the rice. Give everything a good mix, let the rice toast in the frying pan for a minute or so then pour in the white wine. Using a wooden spoon, scrape your pan to get all of the tasty bits off the bottom. Once the wine has evaporated, pour in 650ml chicken stock.

5. Bubble the risotto away, stirring occasionally so it doesn't stick to the bottom of the pan, until most of the stock has been absorbed by the rice. This usually takes 20 minutes. Keep tasting the rice after 15 minutes – you want it to be creamy with a little bite, but not crunchy.

6. Once the rice is nearly cooked, crack the egg into the jug with the remaining cooled chicken stock and add the egg yolks. Add the finely grated parmesan and a decent crack of black pepper. Whisk together with a fork.

7. When you are happy with the risotto, turn down the heat to low and pour in the egg mixture. Stir for a minute or so until all the cheese has melted into the risotto and the rice is coated in a shiny rich sauce.

8. Dish up the carbonara risotto, crack over some more black pepper and, if you're feeling cheeky, grate over a little more parmesan.

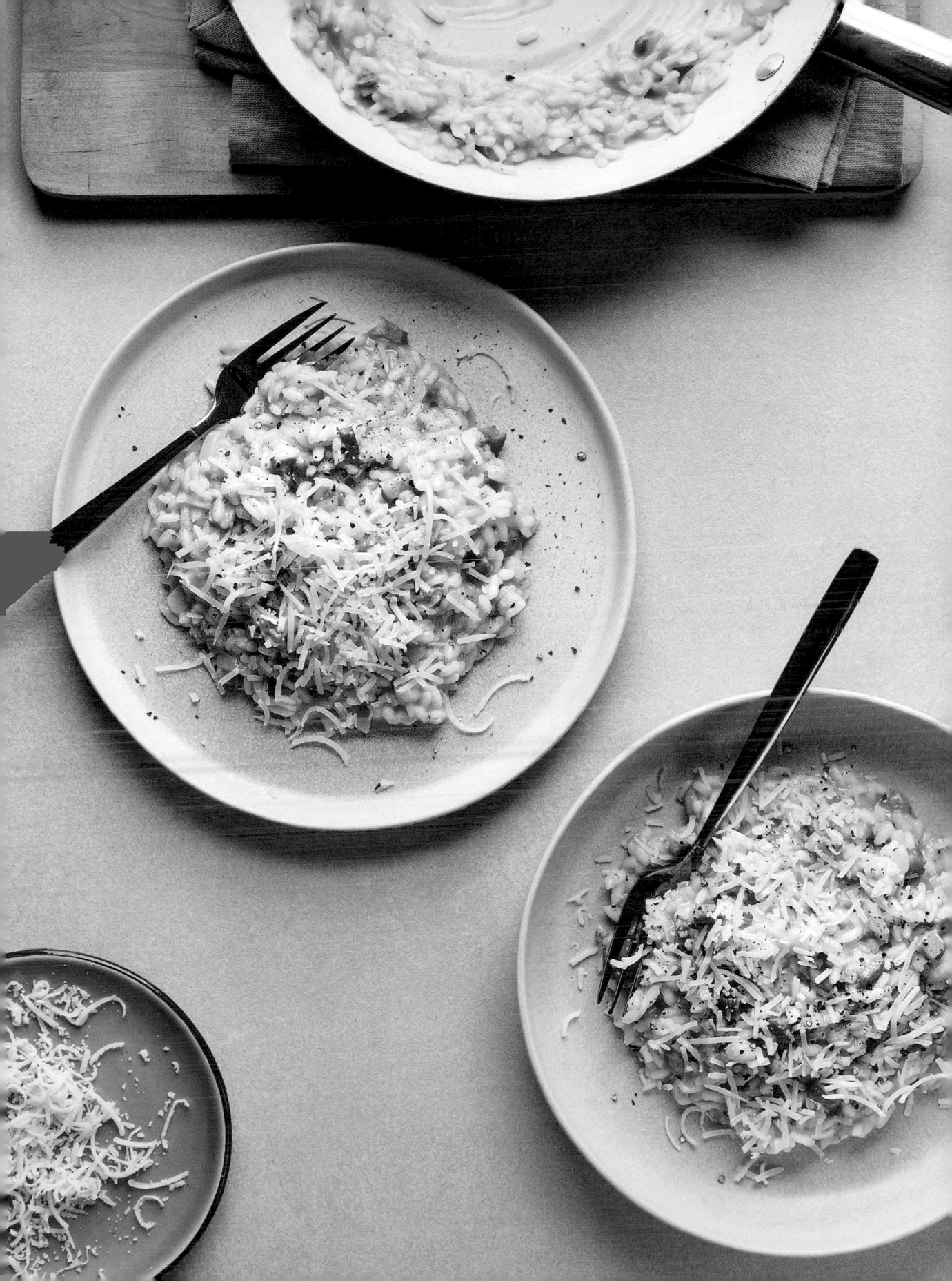

INGREDIENTS

2 large red onions
2 large sweet potatoes
3 fat cloves garlic
2 tbsp coconut oil
salt and pepper
1 tbsp ground cumin
2 tsp dried oregano
1 tbsp chipotle paste, plus a
    little extra to serve
2 x 400g tins of chopped
    tomatoes
2 x 400g tins of black beans,
    drained and rinsed
150g quinoa
1½ limes
4 spoonfuls of low-fat natural
    yoghurt of your choice,
    to serve
handful of coriander leaves

*** YOU COULD FREEZE THIS IN
INDIVIDUAL PORTIONS FOR QUICK
MEALS ANOTHER TIME.**

BLACK BEAN, QUINOA AND SWEET POTATO CHILLI

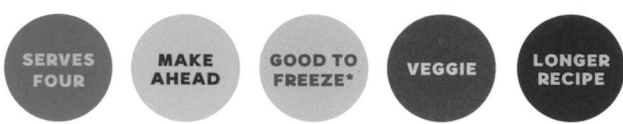

SERVES FOUR   MAKE AHEAD   GOOD TO FREEZE*   VEGGIE   LONGER RECIPE

1. Chop 1½ red onions, finely slice the remaining half. Scrape the sliced half into a bowl to be used later.

2. Peel the sweet potatoes and cut into small chunks, finely chop the garlic.

3. Melt the coconut oil in a large saucepan over a medium to high heat. Chuck in the chopped onions along with a pinch of salt. Cook, stirring regularly, for 5–6 minutes until soft. Scrape in the garlic. Cook, stirring, for 1 minute more then sprinkle in the ground cumin and oregano. Give everything a good mix, then dump in the sweet potato chunks. Spoon in the chipotle paste, stir.

4. Tip in the chopped tomatoes, black beans and quinoa. Fill both of the cans from the chopped tomatoes with water and pour that in, too. Bring the chilli to a boil, season well with salt and pepper then lower the heat to medium. Leave to bubble away for 35 minutes, or until the sweet potato is soft, quinoa cooked and chilli thick.

5. Meanwhile, squeeze half a lime over the sliced red onion, sprinkle with salt and black pepper. Use your hands to scrunch the onion with the lime juice – this will encourage it to soften. Leave to lightly pickle.

6. Once you are happy with the chilli, serve up into bowls. Top each with a dollop of yoghurt and if you like, for some extra heat, swirl through a little more chipotle paste. Scatter over the quick-pickled red onions and tear over some coriander leaves. Serve with the remaining lime, cut into wedges, for squeezing.

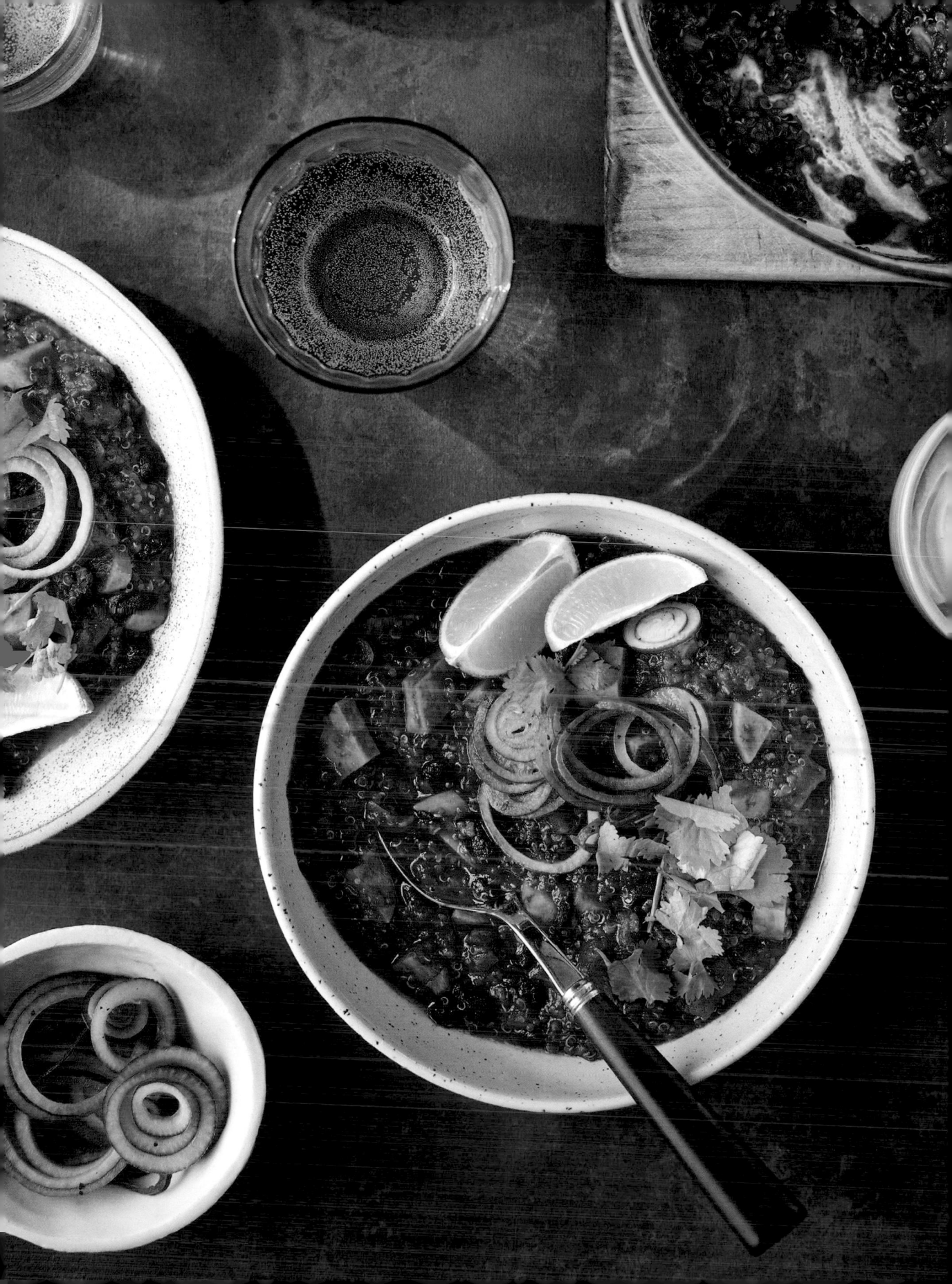

INGREDIENTS

1 part-baked baguette
¼ cucumber
4 radishes
splash of rice wine vinegar
salt
small handful of salted roasted
    peanuts
small handful of coriander
3 portobello mushrooms
1 tbsp sesame oil
1–2 tsp hot sauce – I like Sriracha
1 tbsp low-fat natural yoghurt
1 tbsp soy sauce

SOY MUSHROOM BANH MI

 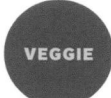

SERVES ONE   VEGGIE

1. Preheat the oven to 220°C (fan 200°/gas mark 7).

2. Put the baguette on a baking tray, sprinkle over a little water. Whack in the oven for 10–12 minutes until cooked through and golden.

3. Meanwhile peel the cucumber into long ribbons and finely slice the radishes. Scrape into a bowl, splash in some rice wine vinegar, sprinkle in a pinch of salt. Toss together. Roughly chop the peanuts and coriander.

4. Cut the portobello mushrooms into thick slices. Heat a large non-stick frying pan over the highest heat. Pour in the sesame oil then carefully lay the mushroom slices in the pan so that they all have enough space to fry evenly. Cook for 2 minutes on each side.

5. Meanwhile mix the hot sauce with the yoghurt in a small bowl.

6. After the mushrooms have been frying for 4 minutes, pour the soy sauce into the pan. Bubble away for 30 seconds, then take the pan off the heat.

7. Assemble your banh mi. Cut open the baguette. Spread in the hot sauce yoghurt, stuff with the soy mushrooms and cucumber salad. Scatter over the peanuts and coriander before gobbling down.

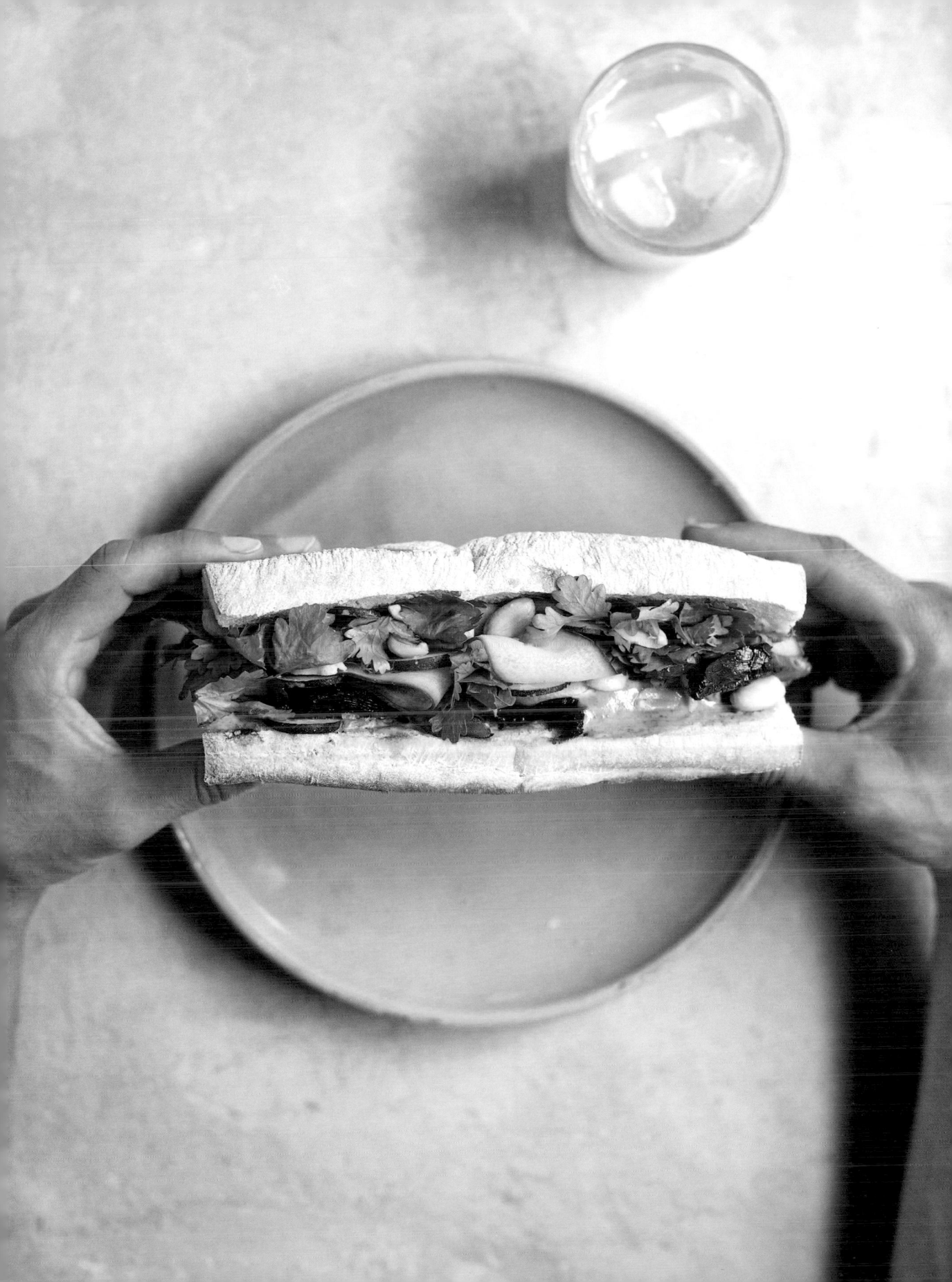

INGREDIENTS

1 medium sweet potato,
    skin left on, cut into eight
    wedges
1 x 200g skinless chicken
    breast fillet
1 tbsp tandoori curry paste
salt and pepper
1 tbsp coconut oil
1 brioche bun, cut in half
¼ cucumber
1½ tbsp low-fat Greek yoghurt
big pinch of garam masala
2 leaves of iceberg lettuce
squeeze of lemon juice
1 tbsp crispy onions – optional

TANDOORI CHICKEN BURGER WITH CUCUMBER RAITA

SERVES
ONE

1. Put the sweet potato wedges into a microwaveable bowl with 2 tablespoons of water, cover and zap on high for 6 minutes.

2. Meanwhile place the chicken between two pieces of cling film or baking parchment on a chopping board. Using a rolling pin, meat mallet or any other blunt instrument, bash the chicken until it is about 1cm thick all over. Spoon the tandoori curry paste over the chicken breast, rubbing it into the flesh, and season with salt and pepper.

3. Melt 1 teaspoon of coconut oil in a non-stick frying pan over a medium to high heat. Once melted, lay the chicken in the pan, cook for around 4 minutes on each side.

4. While the chicken is cooking, melt the remaining coconut oil in a separate frying pan over a medium to high heat. Carefully uncover the sweet potato wedges, tip out their water and place the wedges into the hot pan. Season. Fry for 3–4 minutes, turning halfway, until crisp. Once nearly cooked, move the wedges to one side of the frying pan and toast the burger bun, cut side down, in the other.

5. Make the raita. Grate the cucumber, squeeze out as much liquid as you can, dump into a small bowl. Add the Greek yoghurt, garam masala, salt and pepper, stir together. Slice the lettuce and squeeze over some lemon juice.

6. Come back to the chicken, which by now will be cooked through. Check by slicing into a thicker part to make sure the meat is white all the way through with no raw pink bits left. Cut the chicken in half.

7. Assemble your burger. Spread half the cucumber raita onto the base of the bun. Place the lettuce on top, followed by the tandoori chicken, remaining raita and crispy onions, if you like. Serve with the sweet potato wedges.

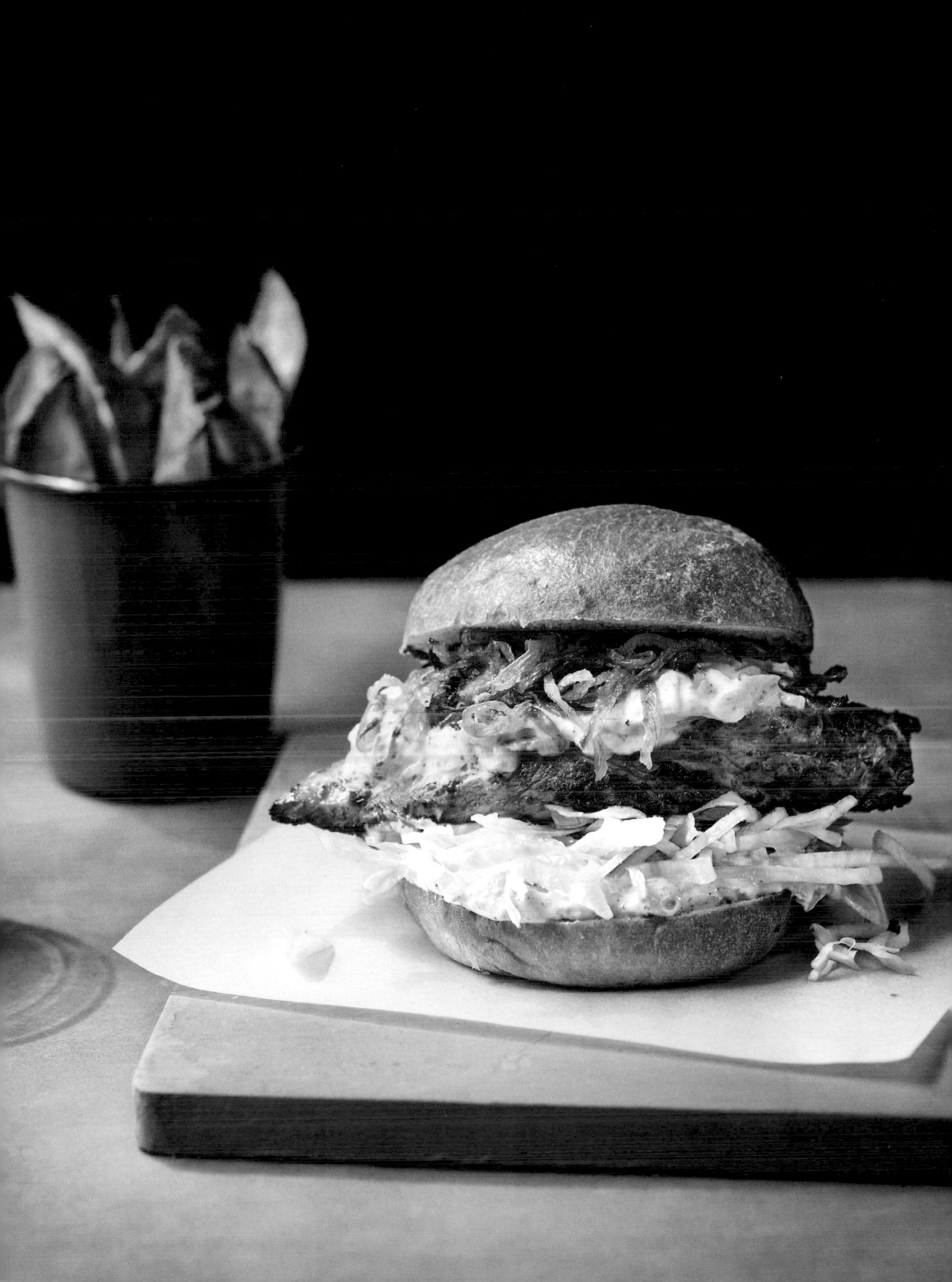

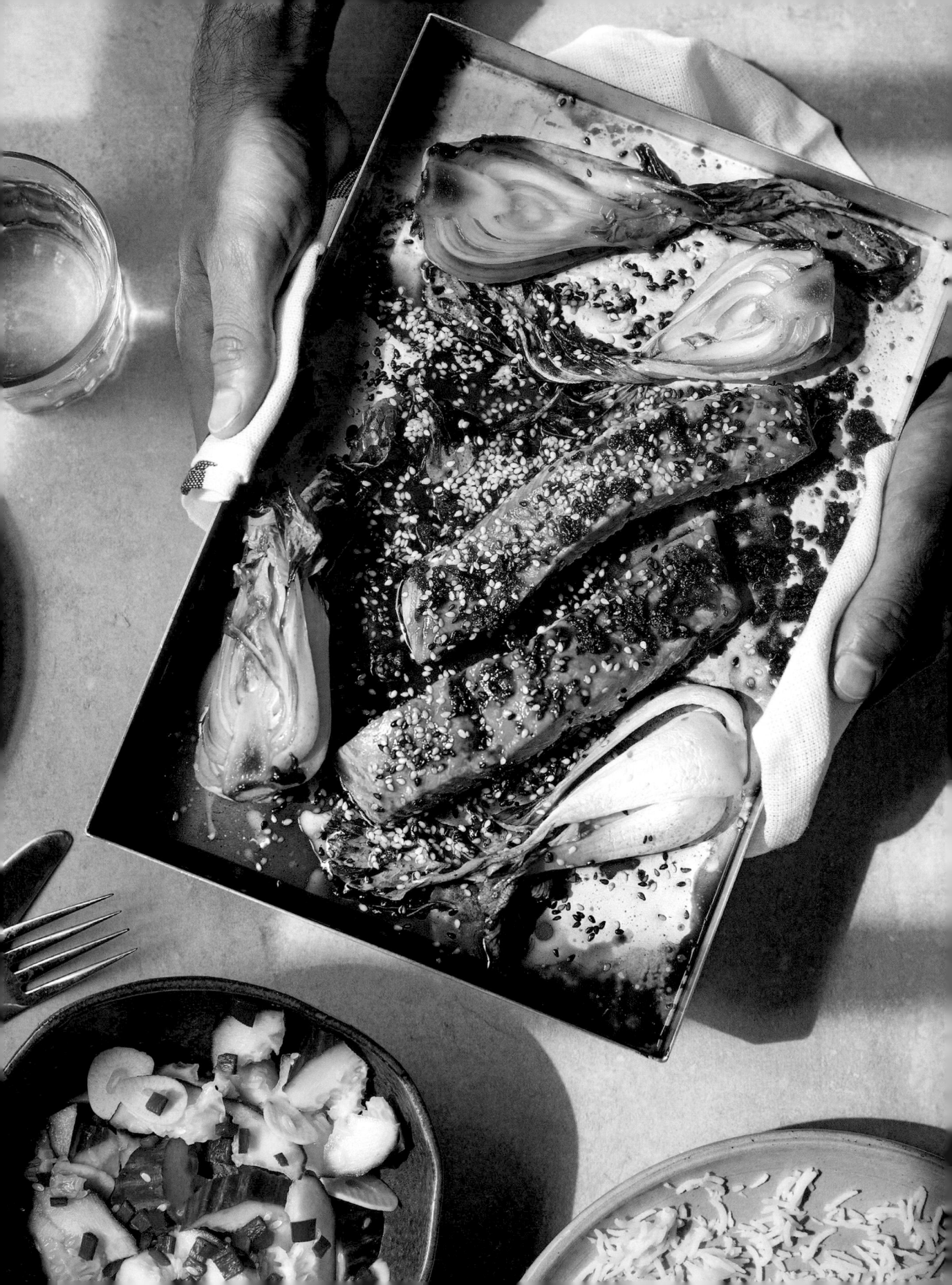

VIETNAMESE STICKY SALMON WITH COCONUT RICE

SERVES ONE

½ small cucumber
salt
1 x 200g skinless boneless
    salmon fillet
1 small clove garlic
½ red chilli
1 pak choi
1 tbsp fish sauce
1 tbsp soft brown sugar
½ tbsp soy sauce
1 tbsp sesame seeds
250g pre-cooked coconut rice
2 tsp rice wine vinegar

1. Preheat the grill to maximum.

2. Using a rolling pin or any other blunt instrument, bash the cucumber until it starts to split, then cut into rough diagonal pieces. Put into a sieve over a bowl and season with a pinch of salt. Leave for a few minutes for the water to drain off.

3. Cut the salmon fillet in half. Lay on a baking tray, slide under the grill for 5 minutes.

4. Meanwhile finely chop the garlic and red chilli – remove the seeds if you don't like it hot. Cut the pak choi in half lengthways. Mix together the fish sauce, soft brown sugar and soy sauce in a small bowl, stirring until the sugar has dissolved.

5. Come back to the salmon. Lay the pak choi, cut side down, on the baking tray, then drizzle the sauce over the salmon. Scatter over the sesame seeds and slide back under the grill for 3 minutes.

6. While the salmon and pak choi are grilling, ping the coconut rice in the microwave according to packet instructions. Drain away any water from the bowl underneath the cucumber, then tip the cucumber into the bowl. Stir in the finely chopped garlic, chilli and rice wine vinegar.

7. By now the salmon should be cooked – you can check this by slicing into the thickest part of one of the pieces to make sure the flesh has turned matt pink in colour.

8. Pile the coconut rice into a bowl, lay the sticky salmon and pak choi on top. Drizzle over the cooking juices and serve with the smacked cucumber.

INGREDIENTS

6–8 new potatoes (200g)
1 tbsp coconut oil
1 small onion, finely chopped
salt and pepper
2 tsp garlic-ginger paste
1 tsp cumin seeds
1 tsp coriander seeds
½ tbsp medium curry powder
150g frozen peas
80g halloumi (⅓ pack), cut into
    four slices
mango chutney, to serve –
    optional

BOMBAY POTATO HASH WITH HALLOUMI

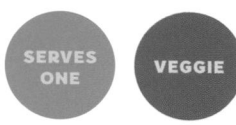

SERVES ONE

VEGGIE

1. Quarter the new potatoes, leaving the skin on. Put in a microwaveable bowl with 2 tablespoons of water, cover and zap on high for 5 minutes.

2. Meanwhile melt the coconut oil in a large non-stick frying pan over a medium to high heat. Chuck in the onion, along with a pinch of salt. Cook, stirring regularly, for 3 minutes until nearly soft. Spoon in the garlic-ginger paste. Cook for 30 seconds more, then sprinkle in the cumin seeds, coriander seeds and curry powder. Mix everything together.

3. Come back to the potatoes, carefully uncover then tip the potatoes along with their water into the frying pan. Crank up the heat. Fry for 2 minutes, then dump in the frozen peas. Season with salt and pepper, stir then move everything to one half of the pan.

4. Add the halloumi slices to the other half of the frying pan, fry for 1–2 minutes on each side until crisp.

5. Dish up the potato hash into a bowl, top with the halloumi slices and serve with mango chutney if you like.

Joe's Top Tip

If you are extra hungry,
add a fried egg.

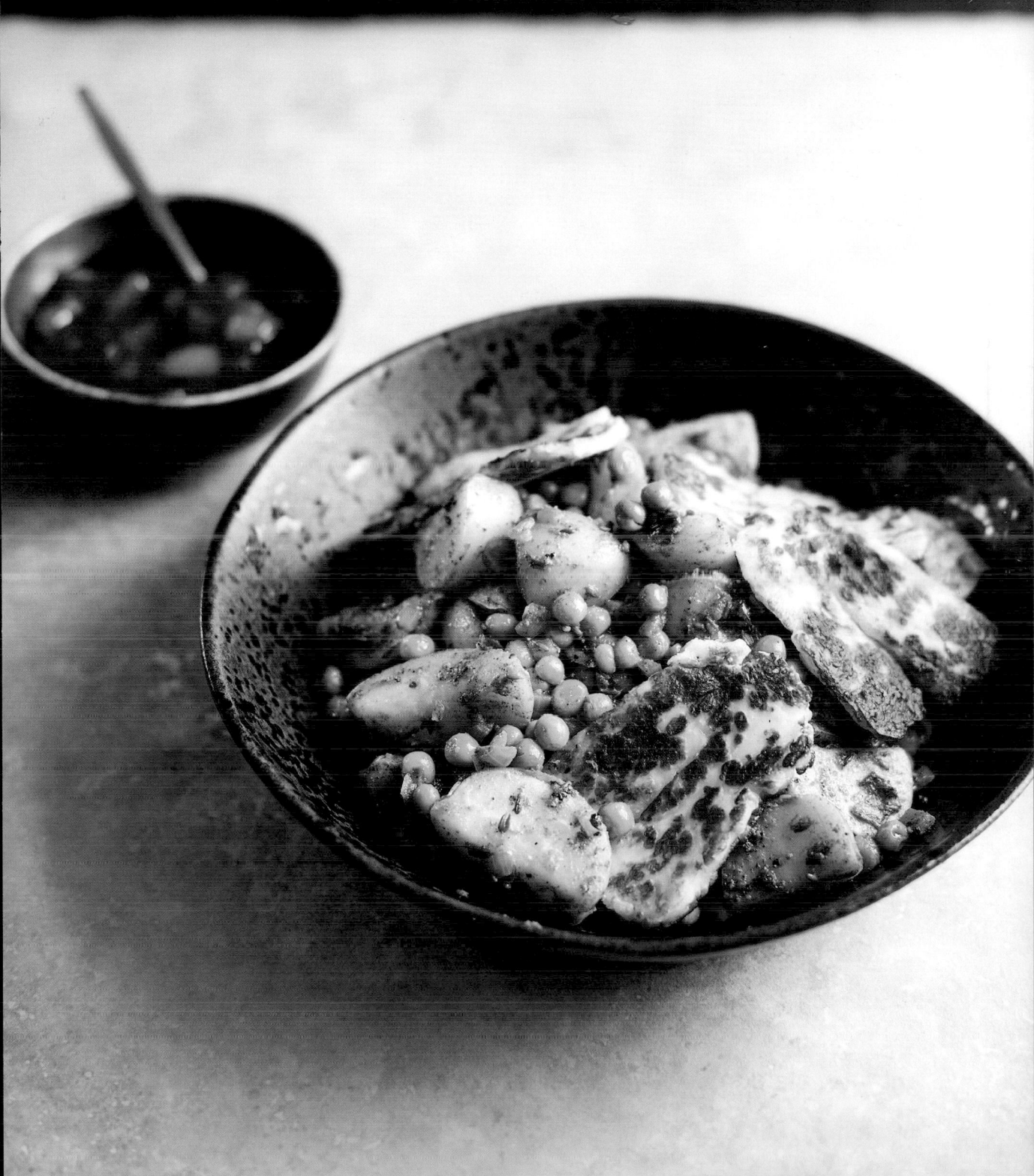

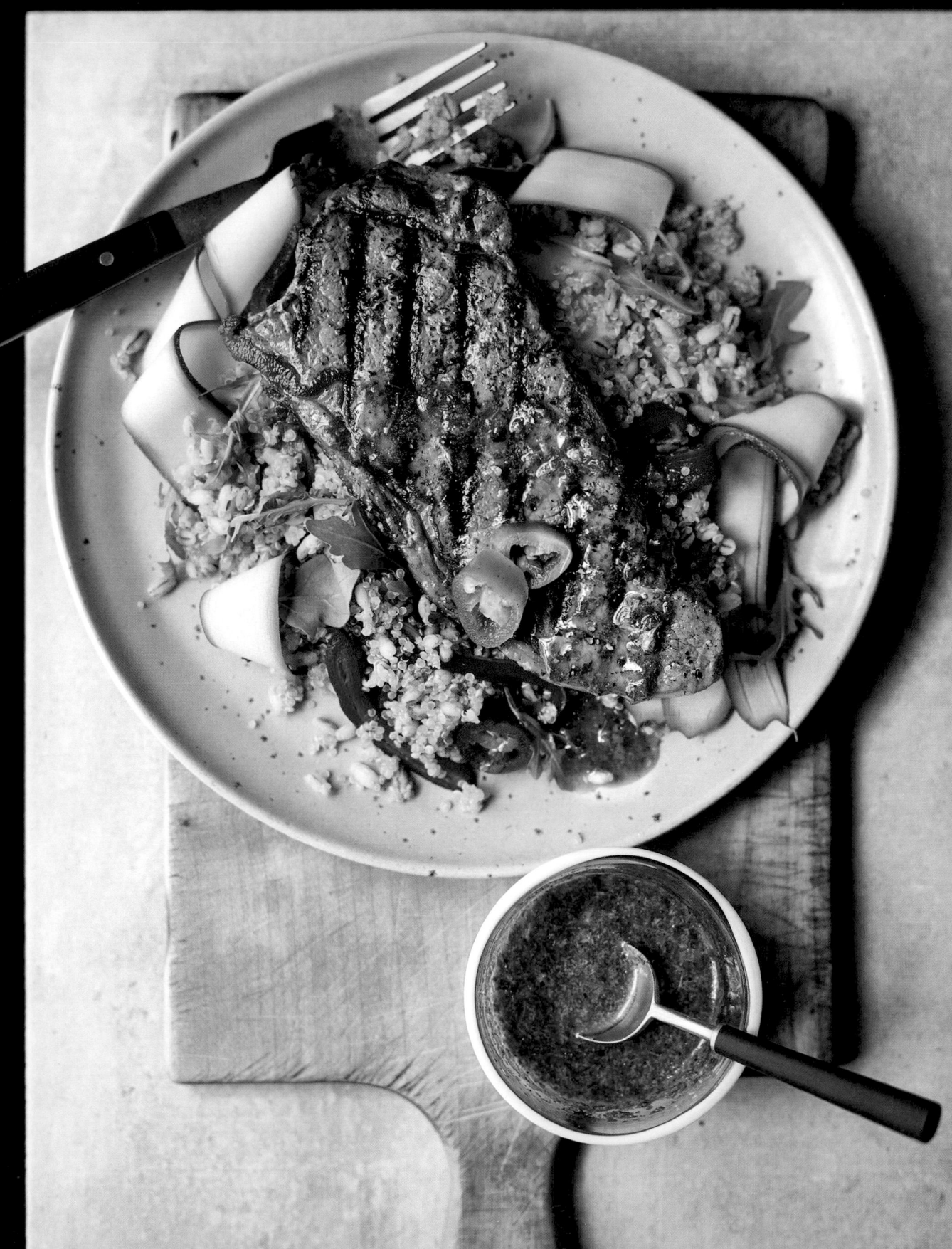

CHIMICHURRI STEAK WITH MIXED GRAINS

SERVES ONE

small handful of parsley
small handful of coriander
1 small clove garlic
2 pickled jalapeños and 1 tbsp
   pickling juice, plus a few extra to
   serve – optional
1 tbsp olive oil
salt and pepper
1 x 225g sirloin steak, trimmed
   of visible fat
200g pre-cooked mixed grains
½ medium courgette
1 jarred roasted red pepper,
   drained
large handful of rocket
squeeze of lemon juice

1. Make the chimichurri. Put the parsley and coriander (stalks and all) into a small food processor with the garlic, pickled jalapeños, 1 tablespoon of pickling juice and most of the olive oil. Blitz to a smooth green sauce. Add a little water if you need it. Season to taste with salt and black pepper – you want it to be nice and tangy.

2. Heat a griddle pan over the highest heat. Drizzle the steak with the remaining oil, rubbing it into the flesh, and season all over with salt and pepper. When searingly hot, carefully lay the steak into the pan. Cook according to preference – I like my steaks medium rare, so 2½ minutes on each side, turning regularly – then leave to rest, covered, until you're ready to eat.

3. While the steak is cooking, ping the mixed grains in the microwave according to packet instructions. Peel the courgette into long ribbons. Slice the red pepper. Mix the warmed grains, courgette and pepper together in a serving bowl, along with the rocket. Season with salt, pepper and lemon juice, to taste.

4. Thinly slice the steak on a diagonal, then pile on top of the mixed grains. Drizzle over the chimichurri. If you like it spicy, scatter over a couple more pickled jalapeños.

Veggie Swap

Swap the steak for 30g
toasted chopped hazelnuts
and 30g feta, crumbled and
stirred into the mixed grains
along with the chimichurri.

INGREDIENTS

½ fennel bulb
salt and pepper
100g rigatoni
1 tbsp olive oil
2 fat sausages (200g)
1 tsp fennel seeds
½–1 tsp dried chilli flakes
10 cherry tomatoes
big splash of balsamic vinegar
2 tsp capers

SAUSAGE, FENNEL AND CHILLI RIGATONI

SERVES ONE

1. Bring a kettle of water to the boil.

2. Meanwhile pick the green bits off the fennel – the 'fronds' – and save until later. Finely slice the fennel bulb.

3. Pour the boiling water into a saucepan over a medium heat. Salt the water, drop in the rigatoni. Cook for 1 minute less than packet instructions.

4. While the pasta is cooking, heat a frying pan over a medium to high heat. Add the olive oil then squeeze the sausages from their skins straight into the frying pan. Chuck in the sliced fennel along with a good pinch of salt and pepper. Fry, stirring occasionally, for 5 minutes until the sausage has browned and fennel has collapsed.

5. Sprinkle the fennel seeds and chilli flakes into the pan. Cook for 30 seconds more, then chuck in the cherry tomatoes. Spoon in a little pasta water and leave to bubble away for a few minutes until the tomatoes have burst, then stir through the balsamic vinegar and capers. Keep warm.

6. Drain the rigatoni into a colander then tip into the pan with the sauce. Give everything a good mix, season to taste and serve up in a bowl. Finish with a scattering of fennel fronds.

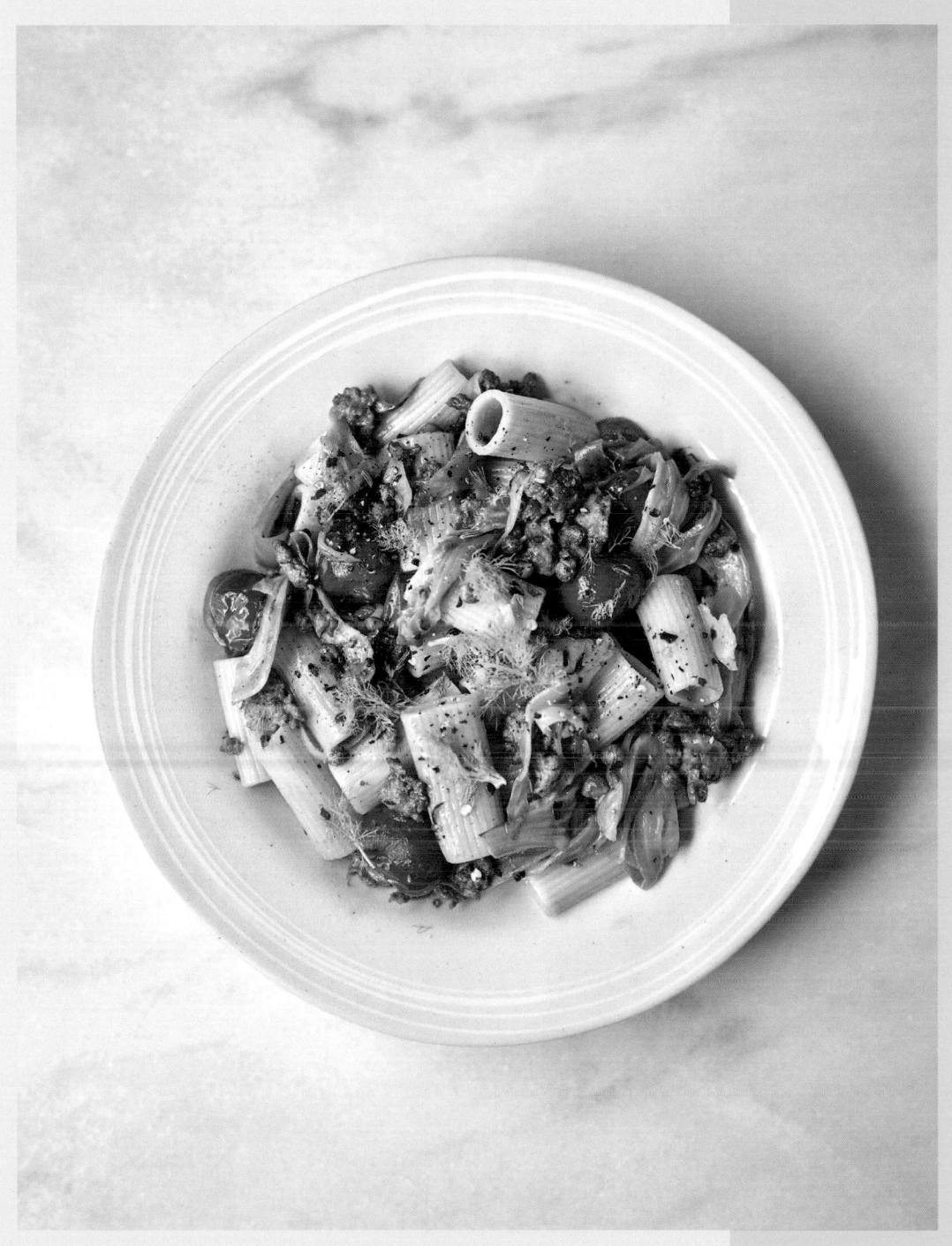

INGREDIENTS

1 fat clove garlic
½ red chilli
100g little trees (tenderstem broccoli)
salt and pepper
100g penne
2 tbsp pumpkin seeds
3–4 anchovies in olive oil
juice of 1 lemon
drizzle of olive oil
grated pecorino or parmesan, to serve – optional

BROCCOLI AND ANCHOVY PENNE WITH TOASTED PUMPKIN SEEDS

SERVES ONE

1. Bring a kettle of water to the boil.

2. Meanwhile finely slice the garlic clove and red chilli – remove the seeds if you don't like it hot. Cut the broccoli into finger-length pieces, slicing any of the bigger stalks in half lengthways.

3. Pour the boiling water into a saucepan over a medium heat. Salt the water, drop in the penne. Cook for 1 minute less than packet instructions.

4. While the pasta is cooking, toast the pumpkin seeds in a dry frying pan over a medium heat until they begin to pop. Tip the seeds into a bowl and put the pan back onto the heat.

5. Add the anchovies to the pan, along with 1 tablespoon of their oil. Scrape in the sliced garlic and chilli. Cook, stirring, until the anchovies have 'melted' into the oil then chuck in the broccoli. Squeeze in half the lemon juice, along with 2 tablespoons of water. Cook for 4–5 minutes, until all the liquid has evaporated and the broccoli is tender and vivid green. Keep warm.

6. Drain the penne into a colander, saving half a mugful of pasta water. Tip the pasta into the pan with the broccoli, stir and splash in a little pasta water, enough to make the penne shiny. Drizzle in a little olive oil and season with lemon juice and a good grind of black pepper, to taste.

7. Pile the penne into a bowl, scatter over the pumpkin seeds and serve with some grated pecorino or parmesan, if you like.

MOROCCAN-SPICED CARROT, POMEGRANATE AND HAZELNUT WILD RICE

INGREDIENTS

3 medium carrots, roughly sliced
1 tbsp olive oil
½ tbsp ras el hanout
salt and pepper
30g hazelnuts
juice of ½ lemon
1 tsp harissa
250g pre-cooked wild rice
2 tbsp pomegranate seeds
handful of mint leaves
30g feta

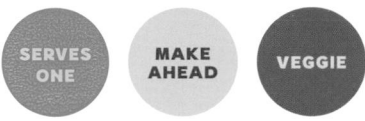

SERVES ONE   MAKE AHEAD   VEGGIE

1. Preheat the oven to 220°C (fan 200°/gas mark 7).

2. Put the carrots in a microwaveable bowl with 1 tablespoon of water, cover and zap on high for 3 minutes.

3. Tip the carrots onto a roasting tray, drizzle over half the olive oil, sprinkle over the ras el hanout, salt and pepper. Mix the carrots with the oil and spices, then spread them out into a single layer. Roast in the oven for 11 minutes.

4. While the carrots are roasting, toast the hazelnuts in a dry frying pan over a medium heat until they smell nutty, then leave to cool. Mix the lemon juice, harissa and remaining olive oil together in a serving bowl with a pinch of salt and pepper, to make the dressing.

5. Ping the wild rice in the microwave according to packet instructions, then tip the rice into the dressing. Roughly chop the hazelnuts and scrape most of them into the rice. Add the pomegranate seeds and most of the mint leaves, give everything a good mix.

6. Tip the cooked carrots into the wild rice salad. Mix, then crumble over the feta and scatter over the remaining hazelnuts and mint leaves to finish.

INGREDIENTS

100g firm tofu

1 pak choi, halved

1 vegetable stock cube

2 tsp chilli oil, plus a drizzle to
serve – optional

2 tsp garlic-ginger paste

100g dried egg noodles

100g mange tout

2 tbsp tahini

2 tsp soy sauce

splash of rice wine vinegar

2 tsp toasted sesame seeds

SESAME TAHINI RAMEN

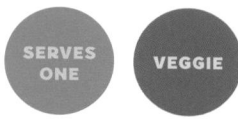

1. Bring a kettle of water to the boil.

2. Meanwhile, using a fork, break the tofu into small scrambled-egg sized pieces in a bowl. Cut the pak choi halves into quarters.

3. Put the vegetable stock cube into a jug. Measure in 500ml of boiling water and whisk with a fork to dissolve. Pour the stock into a saucepan over a medium heat.

4. Heat a non-stick frying pan over a high heat. Pour in the chilli oil, spoon in the garlic-ginger paste, cook, stirring for 30 seconds, then tip in the tofu. Fry, stirring occasionally for 5 minutes until the tofu is crisp.

5. Come back to the pan of stock. Drop in the noodles and pak choi. Cook for 3 minutes then add the mange tout. Spoon in the tahini, 1 teaspoon soy sauce and a splash of rice wine vinegar. Stir to incorporate the tahini into the stock, making a creamy broth. Take the pan off the heat.

6. Add the remaining soy sauce and sesame seeds to the fried tofu, stir. Dish up the tahini ramen, spoon over the crispy sesame tofu and drizzle with a little more chilli oil, if you like.

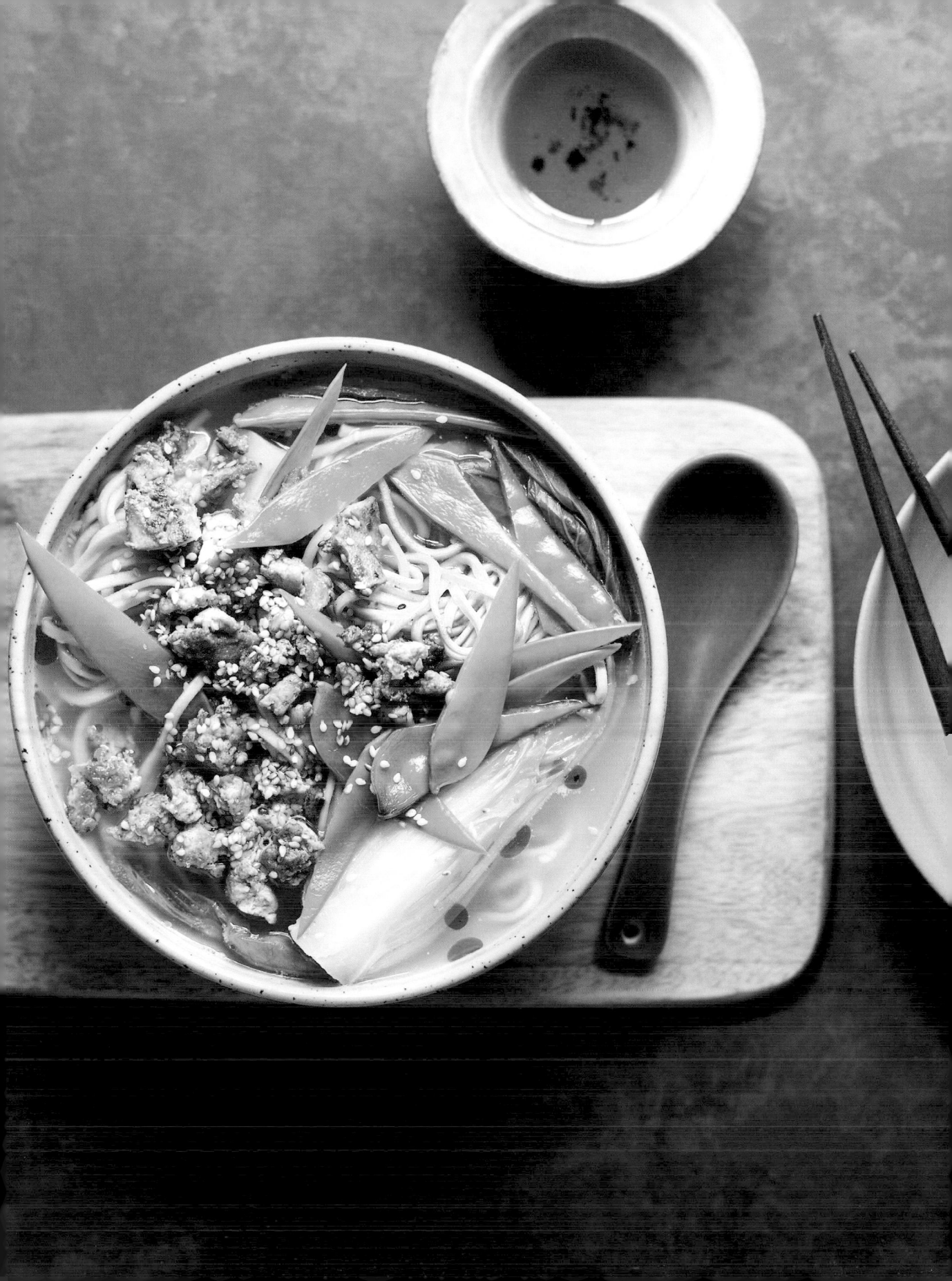

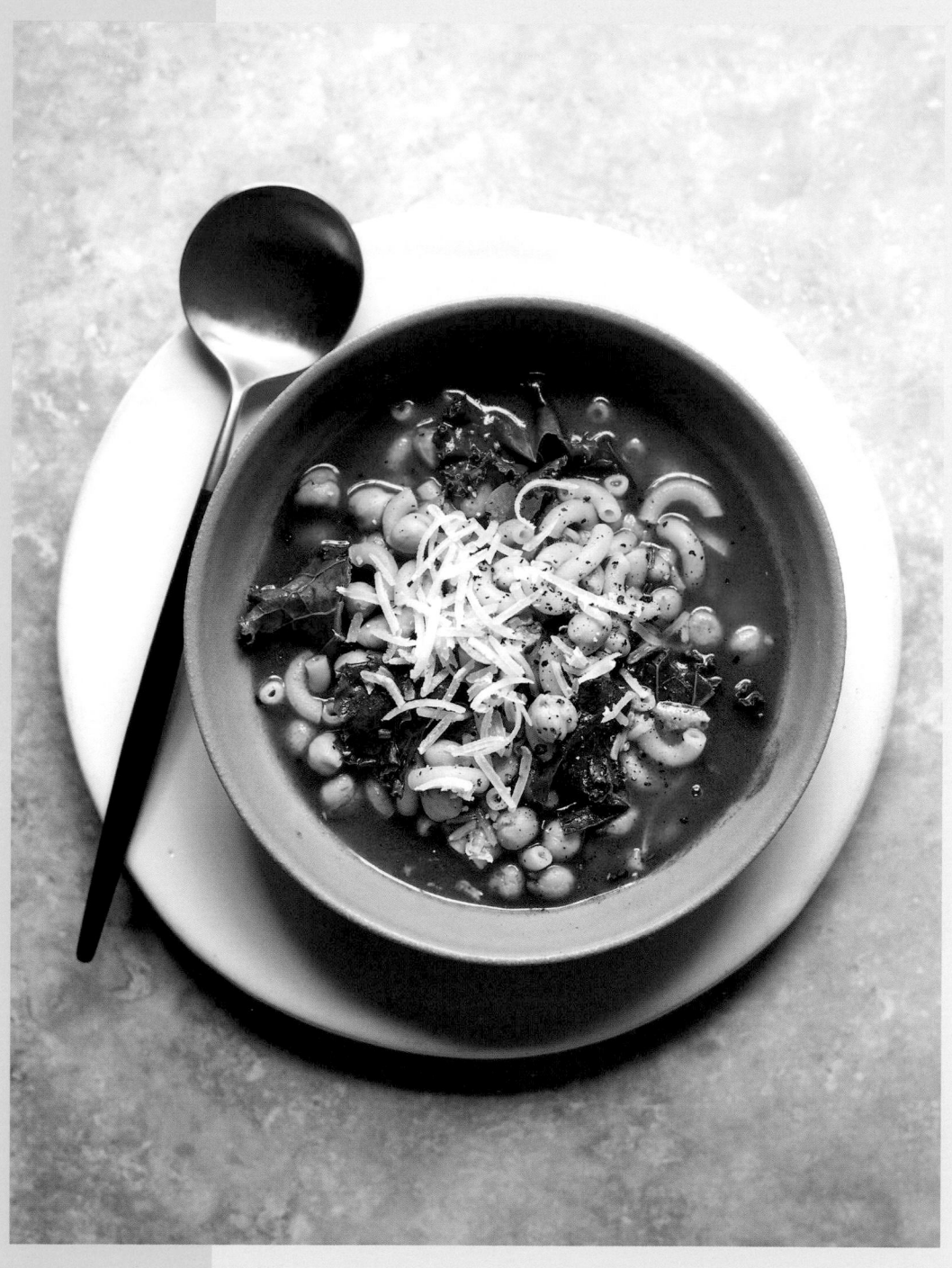

PASTA AND CHICKPEA STEW

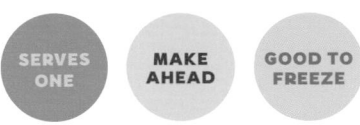

INGREDIENTS

1 large sprig of rosemary
1 fat clove garlic
1 chicken stock cube
½ tbsp olive oil
big pinch of dried chilli flakes
1 tbsp tomato puree
1 x 210g tin of chickpeas, drained
    and rinsed
50g macaroni
salt and pepper
2 handfuls of kale
grated parmesan, to serve

1. Bring a kettle of water to the boil.

2. Meanwhile, strip the leaves from the sprig of rosemary and finely chop along with the garlic clove.

3. Put the chicken stock cube into a jug, measure in 300ml boiling water and whisk with a fork to dissolve.

4. Heat a saucepan over a medium heat. Pour in the olive oil, add the chopped garlic, rosemary and dried chilli flakes. Cook, stirring, for 30 seconds then spoon in the tomato puree and cook for 30 seconds more.

5. Tip in the drained chickpeas and macaroni. Give everything a good mix then pour in the chicken stock. Bring to the boil, season with salt and pepper, place a lid on the pan then leave to bubble away for 8–10 minutes until the macaroni is cooked, stirring halfway to stop the pasta from sticking.

6. When the macaroni is cooked, drop in the kale. Once wilted, spoon the pasta and chickpea broth into a bowl and sprinkle over some grated parmesan to serve.

Veggie Swap

I love the richness of chicken stock in this recipe, but simply swap for a veggie stock cube and use vegetarian hard cheese if you prefer.

INGREDIENTS

knob of butter

4 slices of parma ham

1 tbsp basil pesto (fresh is best)

50g frozen peas

1 egg

1 bagel

salt and pepper

PARMA HAM AND PESTO POACHED EGG BAGEL

SERVES
ONE

1. Bring a kettle of water to the boil. Pour the water into a pan over a medium heat.

2. Meanwhile melt the butter in a frying pan over a medium to high heat. When bubbling, peel the parma ham slices straight out of their packaging into the frying pan. Fry for 1–2 minutes until the ham shrivels and crisps. Turn down the heat to low, spoon in the pesto and chuck in the frozen peas. Give everything a mix, leave for the peas to gently warm through.

3. Come back to the pan of water. Carefully crack your egg into the hot water, reducing the heat until the water is just 'burping'. Cook the egg for about 3 minutes for a runny yolk, then carefully lift it out with a slotted spoon and drain on paper towels.

4. While the egg is poaching, toast your bagel.

5. Spoon the pesto peas and parma ham onto your toasted bagel, place the poached egg on top, sprinkle over some salt and pepper, dive in.

Veggie Swap

Swap the parma ham for 100g asparagus tips, each cut in half lengthways and cooked in the same way as the parma ham.

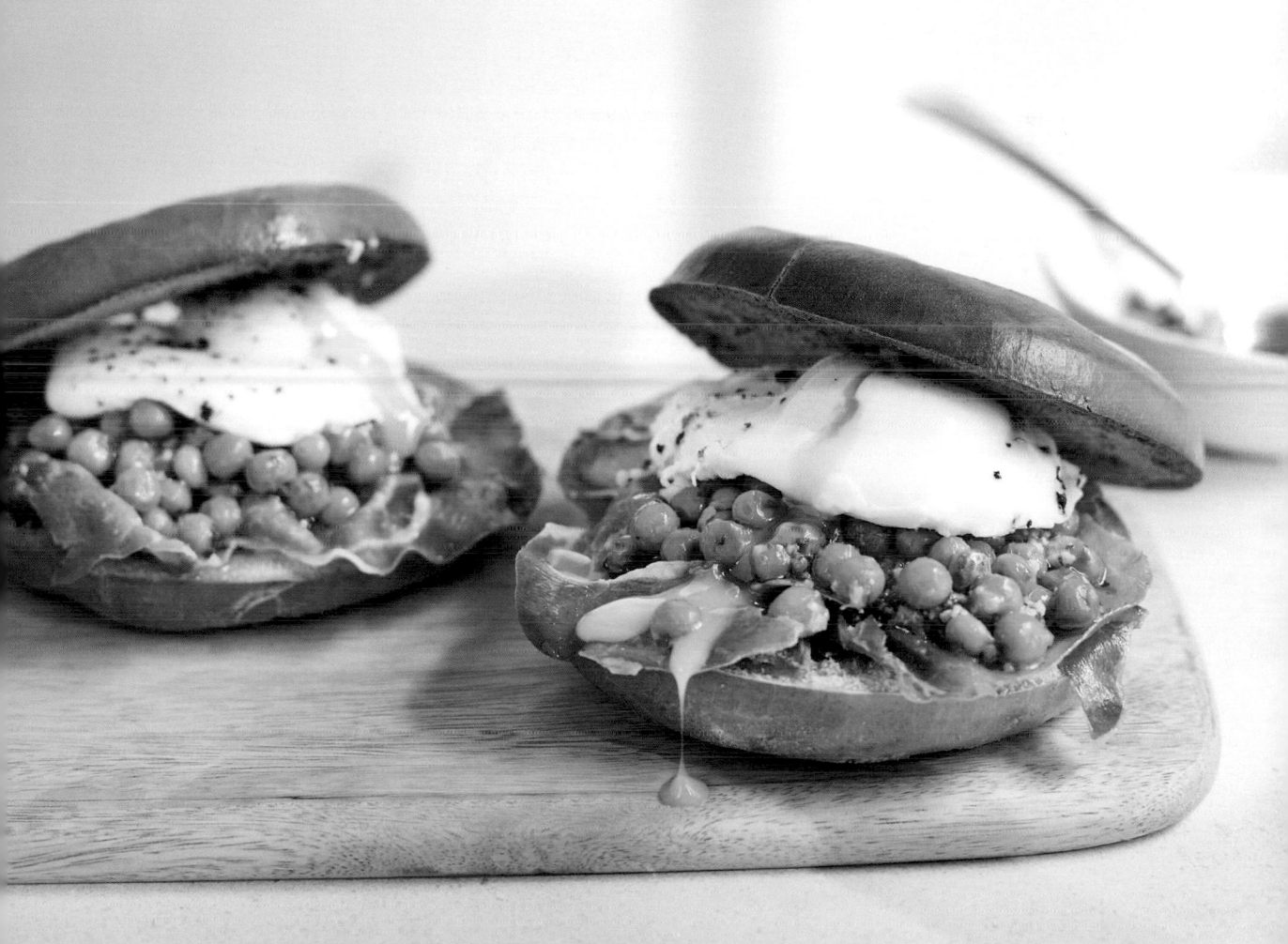

HOISIN TURKEY PANCAKES

INGREDIENTS

1 tbsp coconut oil

200g skinless turkey breast fillets, sliced into 1cm strips

2 spring onions (green and white parts)

½ cucumber

2 tbsp hoisin sauce

1 tsp soy sauce

5–6 Chinese pancakes

SERVES ONE

1. Melt the coconut oil in a wok or large frying pan over a medium to high heat. Chuck in the turkey and fry, stirring occasionally, for around 4 minutes until the turkey is nearly cooked through.

2. Meanwhile cut the spring onions and cucumber into fine matchsticks.

3. Come back to the turkey, pour in the hoisin sauce, soy sauce and 50ml of water. Bring to the boil, bubble away for 1–2 minutes into a sticky sauce. Take the pan off the heat and check to make sure the turkey is cooked through by slicing into one of the larger pieces to make sure the meat is white all the way through, with no raw pink bits left.

4. Once you are happy with the turkey, heat the pancakes in the microwave according to packet instructions.

5. Bring everything to the table for DIY turkey pancakes. Get in.

Veggie Swap

Swap the turkey for 200g sliced mushrooms of your choice, cooked in the same way as the turkey.

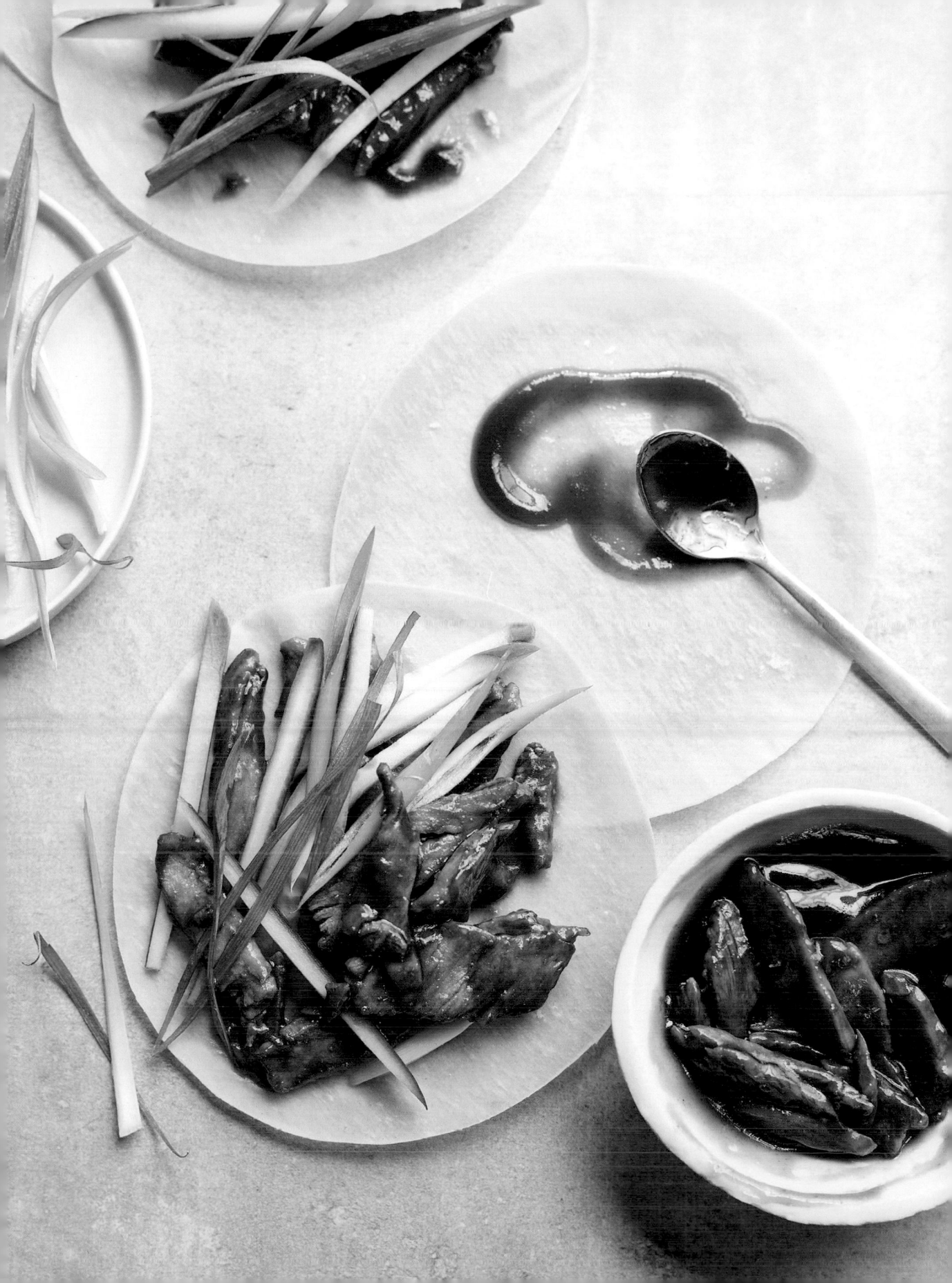

INGREDIENTS

½ chorizo ring (110g)
1 celery stick
½ red onion
½ yellow or orange pepper
½ chicken stock cube
100g orzo
½ tbsp coconut oil
1 tbsp Cajun seasoning
1 x 227g tin of chopped tomatoes
salt and pepper
100g raw king prawns
squeeze of lemon juice
small handful of parsley

PRAWN AND CHORIZO ORZO JAMBALAYA

SERVES ONE

1. Bring a kettle of water to the boil.

2. Meanwhile slice the chorizo, celery, red onion and pepper.

3. Pour the boiling water into a saucepan over a medium heat. Add the chicken stock cube. Drop in the orzo, cook for 3 minutes less than packet instructions.

4. While the pasta is cooking, melt the coconut oil in a large frying pan over a medium to high heat. Chuck in the chorizo, celery, onion and pepper. Fry for 5 minutes until the chorizo is crisp and the veg has softened. Sprinkle in the Cajun seasoning, give everything a good mix and cook for a minute more. Tip in the chopped tomatoes along with some salt and pepper. Bring to the boil, then leave the jambalaya mix to bubble away for a few minutes.

5. Come back to the orzo, drain into a colander, saving half a mugful of pasta water. Tip the orzo into the frying pan along with the sauce, stir well then drop in the prawns. Pour in half of the pasta water and crank up the heat.

6. Cook for 2–3 minutes. The raw grey colour of the prawns will turn pink, which shows you they are cooked. Squeeze over some lemon juice and tear over some parsley leaves. If you like your jambalaya more soupy, stir through the remaining pasta water. I like to eat this one straight from the pan.

Joe's Top Tip

Jambalaya originates from Louisiana, USA, and is traditionally made with sausage, seafood and veg with rice. My take uses tasty orzo instead.

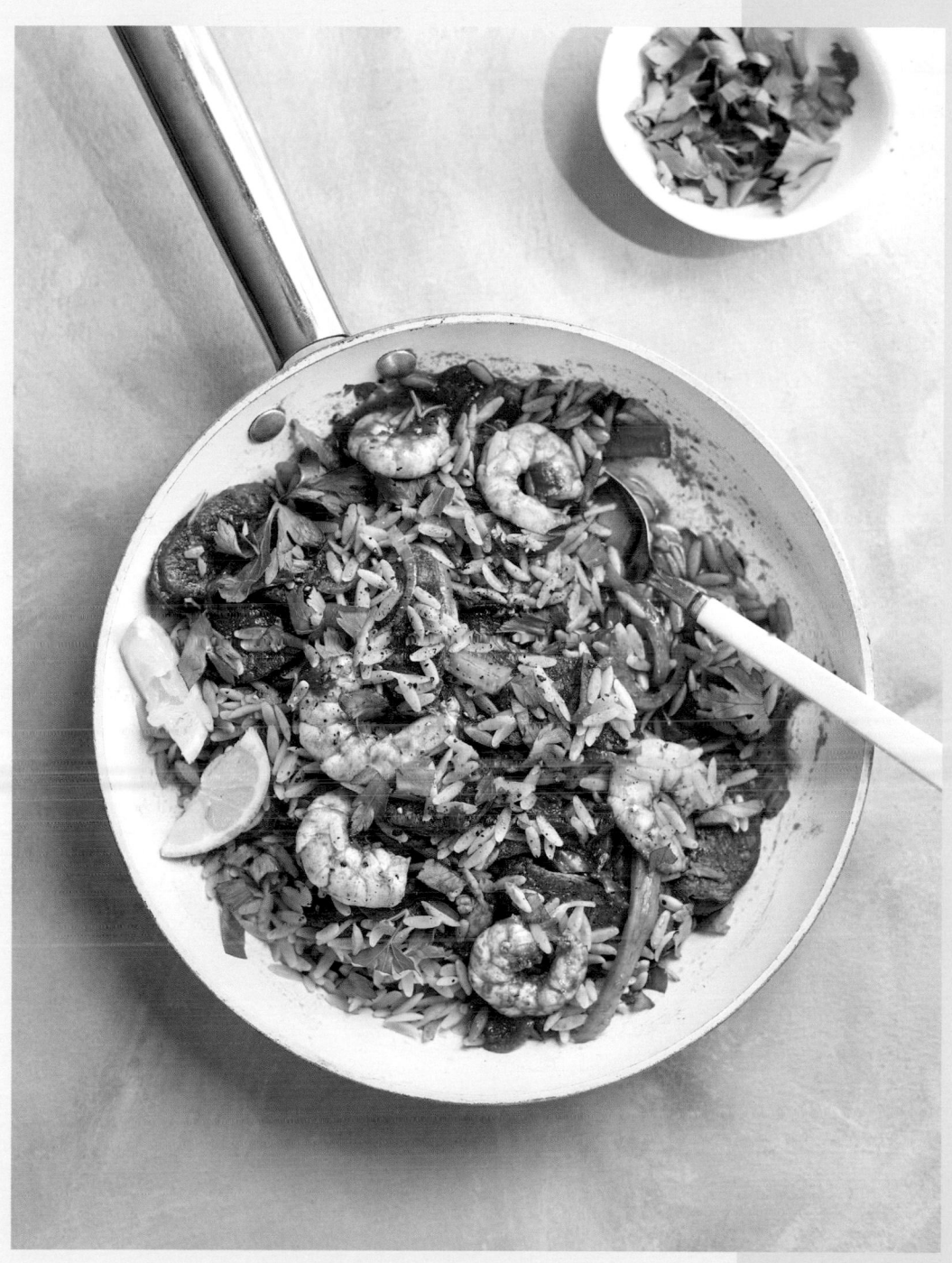

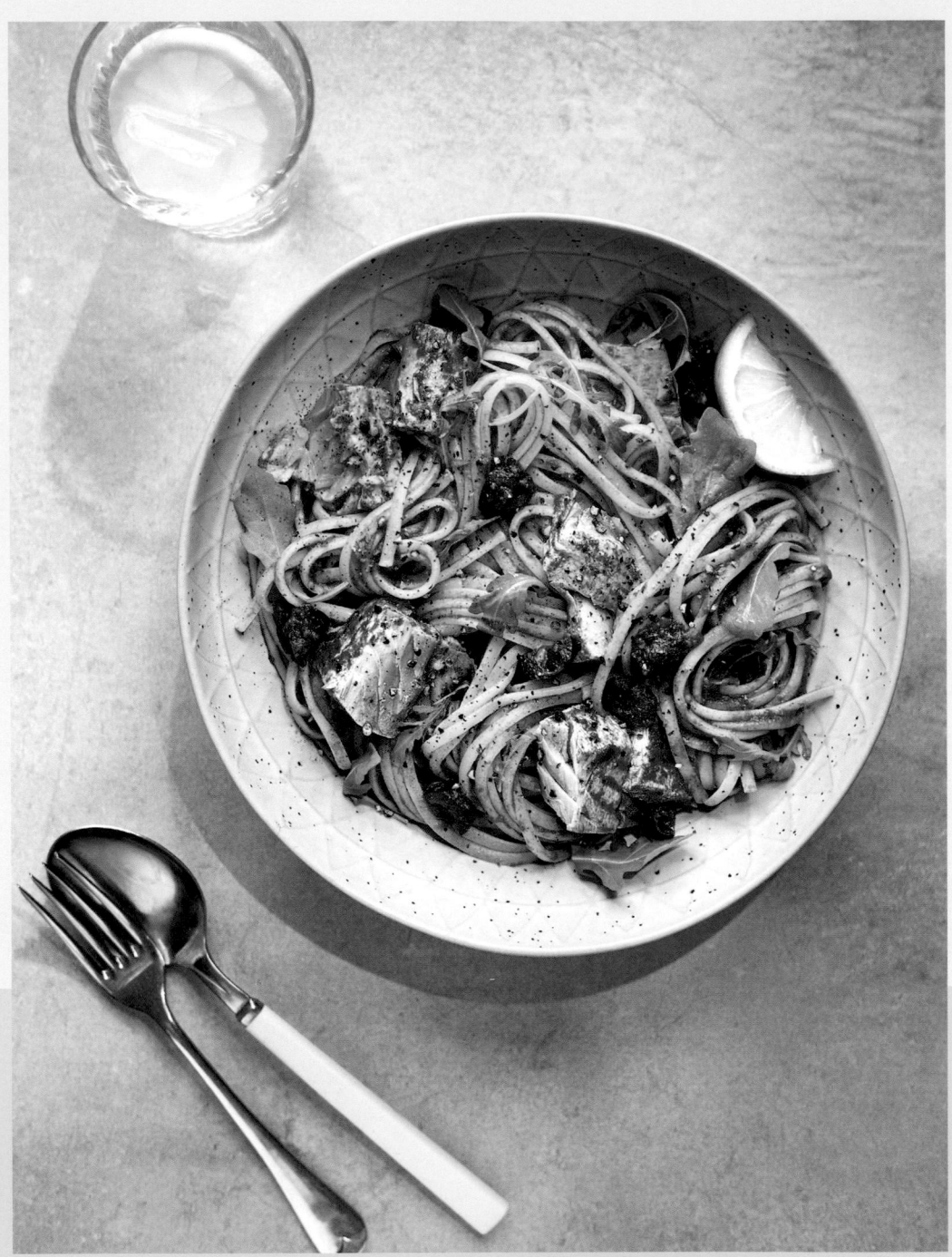

SALMON PUTTANESCA LINGUINE

SERVES ONE

INGREDIENTS

1 tbsp olive oil
1 fat clove garlic
2 anchovies
big pinch of dried chilli flakes
100g passata
salt and pepper
100g linguine
1 x 140g skinless boneless
    salmon fillet
5 pitted black olives
juice of ½ lemon
large handful of rocket

1. Bring a kettle of water to the boil.

2. Meanwhile heat a frying pan over a medium to high heat.
    Pour in the olive oil, crush in the garlic clove, add the
    anchovies and chilli flakes. Cook, stirring, until the anchovies
    have 'melted' into the oil then pour in the passata. Stir, leave
    to bubble away.

3. Pour the boiling water into a saucepan over a medium heat.
    Salt the water, drop in the linguine. Cook for 1 minute less
    than packet instructions.

4. Season the salmon fillet with salt and pepper. Lay the salmon
    into the tomato sauce, place a lid on the pan and cook for
    around 5–6 minutes until the salmon is cooked through,
    flipping halfway. Check by slicing into the thick end of the fillet
    to make sure the flesh has turned matt pink in colour.

5. Meanwhile roughly chop the olives. Once you are happy that
    the salmon is cooked, use a wooden spoon to break up the
    fillet into large pieces. Scrape the olives into the sauce.

6. Drain the linguine into a colander, saving half a mugful
    of pasta water, then tip it into the pan with the salmon
    and sauce. Squeeze in the lemon juice, add a good splash
    of pasta water and dump in the rocket. Toss everything
    together and serve up.

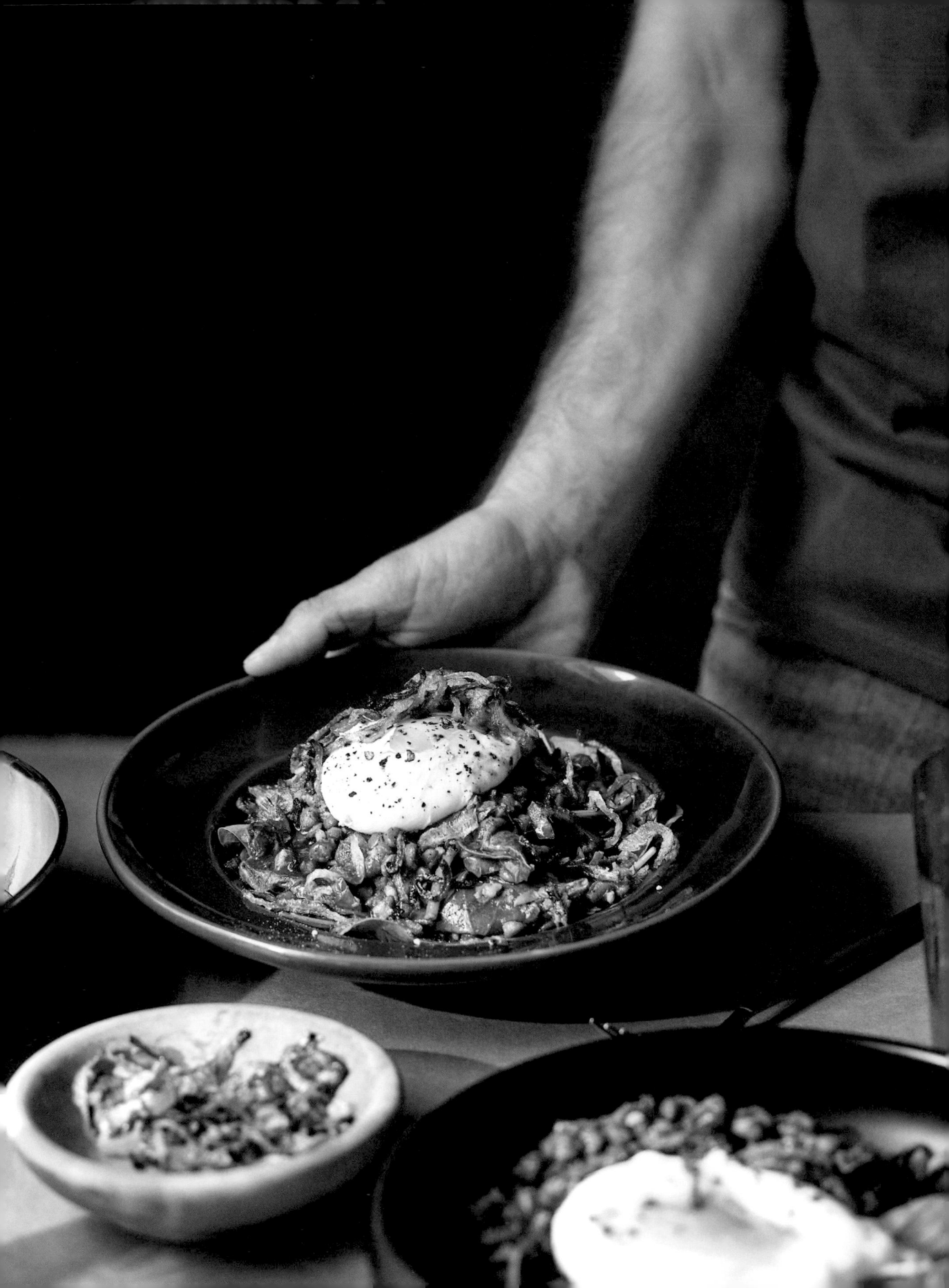

GREEN LENTIL SPINACH DAAL WITH POACHED EGG AND CRISPY ONIONS

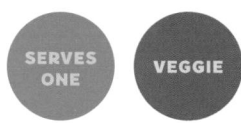

SERVES ONE

VEGGIE

INGREDIENTS

½ tbsp coconut oil

2 tsp garlic-ginger paste

½–1 tbsp medium curry powder, depending on how spicy you like it

1 x 400g tin of green lentils

salt and pepper

1 egg

2 large handfuls of baby spinach leaves

drizzle of hot sauce

2 tbsp crispy onions

1. Bring a kettle of water to the boil.

2. Meanwhile melt the coconut oil in a saucepan over a medium heat. Spoon in the garlic-ginger paste. Cook, stirring for 30 seconds, then sprinkle in the curry powder. Cook for 30 seconds more. Tip in the tin of green lentils, along with its water. Stir, season with a big pinch of salt and pepper, then leave the quick-cook daal to bubble away.

3. Pour the boiling water into a saucepan over a medium heat. Once re-boiled, carefully crack your egg into the hot water, reducing the heat until the water is just 'burping'. Cook the egg for 3 minutes for a runny yolk, then carefully lift it out with a slotted spoon and drain on paper towels.

4. While the egg is poaching, drop the spinach into the daal. Once the spinach is wilted, dish up the daal into a bowl.

5. Place the poached egg on top of the daal, drizzle over some hot sauce and scatter over the crispy onions to serve.

INGREDIENTS

240g basmati rice

1 chicken stock cube

2 onions, sliced

2 tbsp mango chutney, plus
    extra to serve – optional

1 tbsp cumin seeds

3 bay leaves

2 tsp ground turmeric

salt and pepper

6 large bone-in, skin-on chicken
    pieces – I like thighs and
    drumsticks (around 750g)

2 tbsp olive oil

50g pistachios

handful of coriander

dollop of low-fat yoghurt,
    to serve – optional

*** DEFROST THOROUGHLY AND
REHEAT UNTIL PIPING HOT
THROUGHOUT.**

BAKED AROMATIC CHICKEN AND PISTACHIO PILAU

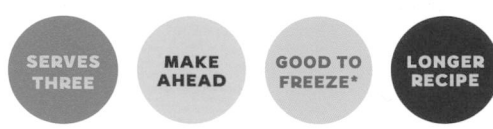

SERVES THREE · MAKE AHEAD · GOOD TO FREEZE* · LONGER RECIPE

1. Preheat the oven to 200°C (fan 180°/gas mark 6).

2. Wash the basmati rice in a bowl of cold water, using your fingers to rub the grains together. Drain off the water, then repeat until the water is no longer cloudy. Tip the drained rice into a large shallow ovenproof dish or casserole pot.

3. Bring a kettle of water to the boil. Put the chicken stock cube into a jug, measure in 600ml of boiling water and whisk with a fork to dissolve.

4. Pour the stock into the rice. Add the sliced onions, mango chutney, cumin seeds, bay leaves and ground turmeric, mix well to combine. Season with a generous pinch of salt and black pepper.

5. Season the chicken pieces all over with salt and pepper then place in a single layer, skin side up, into the rice mixture. Drizzle over the olive oil then cook in the oven, uncovered, for 40–45 minutes until the liquid has been absorbed by the rice and the chicken is cooked through and golden.

6. After 30 minutes, toast the pistachios in a dry frying pan over a medium heat until they smell nutty. Leave to cool then roughly chop, along with the coriander.

7. Scatter the pistachios and coriander over the baked chicken pilau. I like to serve this out of the pan, with some yoghurt and mango chutney, if you like.

Veggie Swap

Swap the chicken pieces for
1 large aubergine, cut into
small chunks and mixed
through the rice with all the
other ingredients before
cooking in the same way.
Serve with 3 boiled eggs,
cooked for 6½ minutes then
peeled and halved on top.

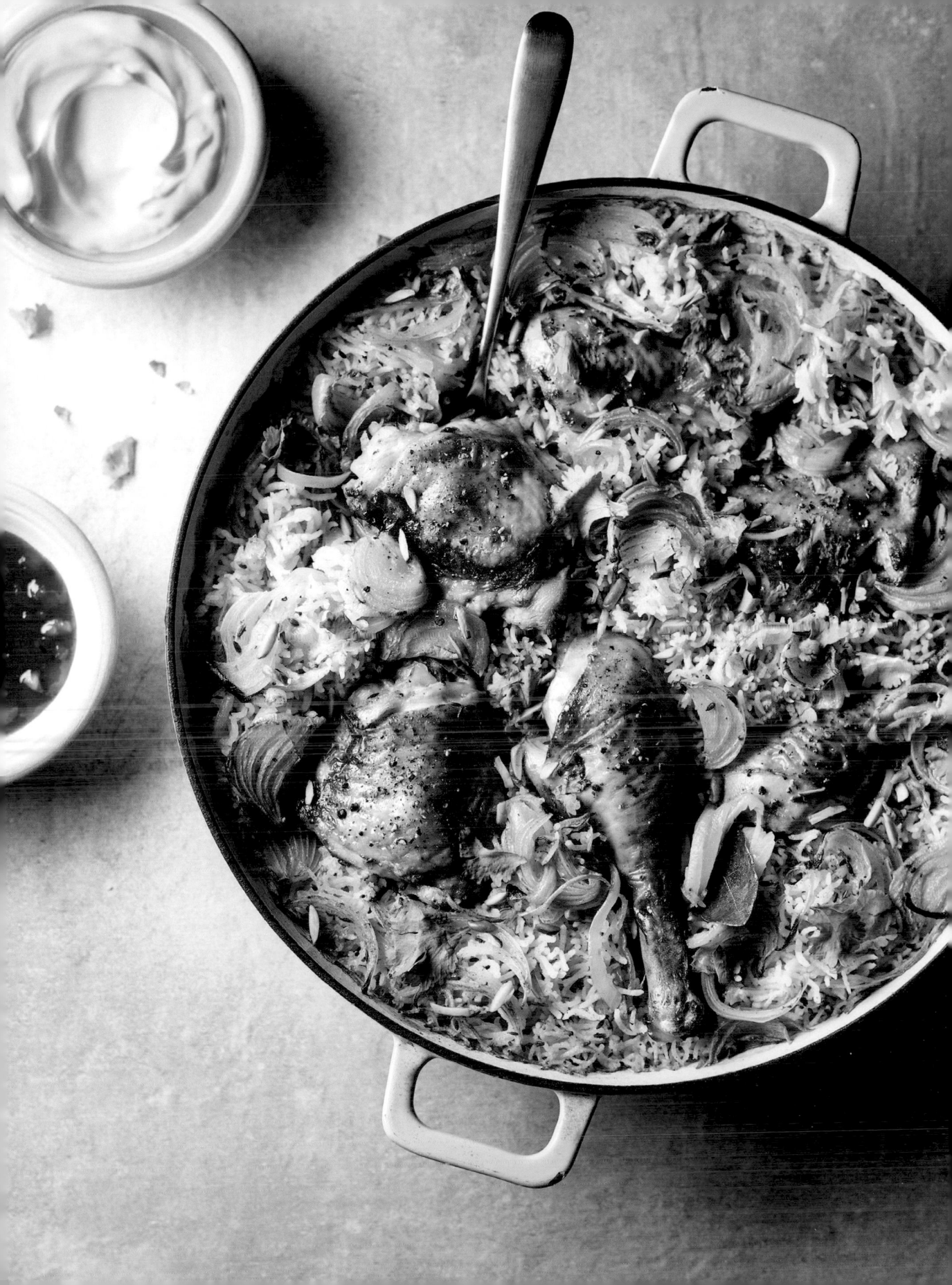

INGREDIENTS

8 pitted mixed olives
1 tsp capers
small handful of parsley
    leaves
1½ tbsp olive oil
zest and juice of ½ lemon
80g couscous
1 fat clove garlic
big pinch of fennel seeds
10 cherry tomatoes
1 x 200g skinless boneless
    cod fillet
salt and pepper

* TAPENADE ONLY.

COD WITH OLIVE TAPENADE, TOMATOES AND COUSCOUS

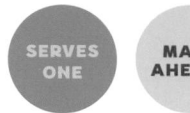

SERVES ONE   MAKE AHEAD*

1. Bring a kettle of water to the boil.

2. Meanwhile make the tapenade. Put the mixed olives, capers, most of the parsley, 1 tablespoon olive oil and a squeeze of lemon juice into a small food processor, blitz to a chunky paste. Don't worry that it is a little salty: with the couscous and cod it will be balanced out and taste mega.

3. Put the couscous into a serving bowl. Measure 100ml boiling water into a jug and pour over the couscous. Cover with a plate or cling film and leave to steam for 10 minutes.

4. While the couscous is steaming, heat a non-stick frying pan over a medium heat. Pour in the remaining oil, crush in the garlic and sprinkle in the fennel seeds. Cook, stirring for 30 seconds then chuck in the cherry tomatoes and zest.

5. Season the cod with salt and pepper then place into the hot pan with the tomatoes. Cook for about 4 minutes on each side, carefully flipping halfway until it is cooked through. Check by cutting into the thickest part to make sure it has turned from raw, pale flesh to cooked bright white.

6. Fluff up the couscous with a fork and squeeze on the remaining lemon juice. Place the cod on top and spoon over the garlicky tomatoes. Dollop in the tapenade and scatter over the remaining parsley leaves.

Veggie Swap

Swap the cod for 1 medium courgette cut into diagonal slices and 30g roughly chopped almonds, fried with the cherry tomatoes for 5 minutes over a high heat.

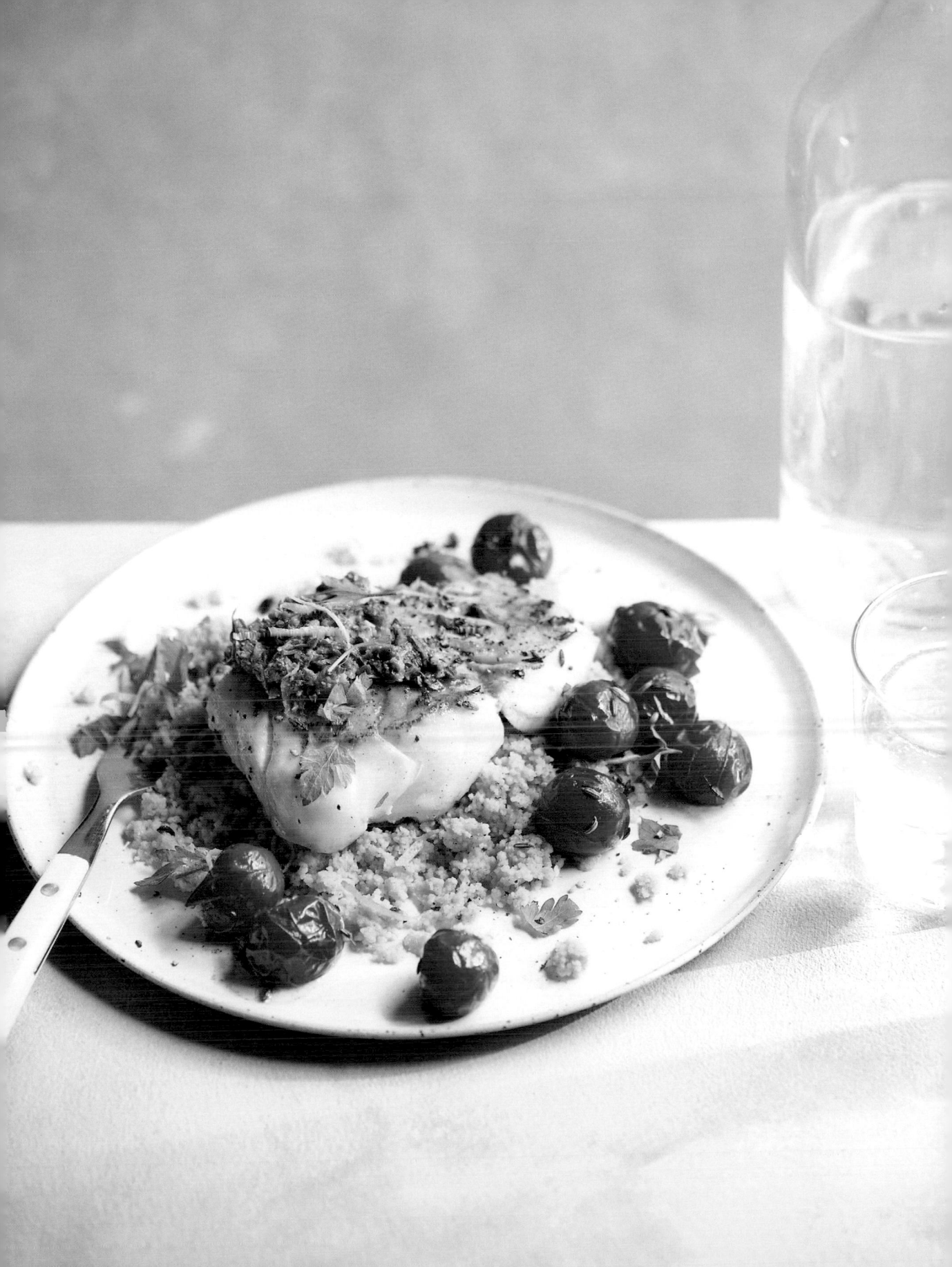

INGREDIENTS

1 tbsp coconut oil
½ head of broccoli
salt and pepper
2 tbsp peanut butter
juice of ½ lime
1 tsp sweet chilli sauce
2 tsp soy sauce
knob of fresh ginger
2 spring onions
1 tsp ground turmeric
1 egg
250g pre-cooked rice

* REHEAT UNTIL PIPING HOT.

SATAY BROCCOLI AND EGG FRIED RICE

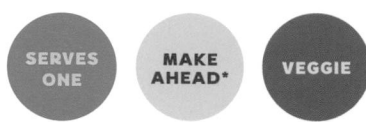

SERVES ONE   MAKE AHEAD*   VEGGIE

1. Preheat the oven to 220°C (fan 200°/gas mark 7). Dollop half the coconut oil onto a roasting tray, then place in the oven to melt.

2. Meanwhile cut the ½ head of broccoli into four wedges. Put in a microwaveable bowl with 1 tablespoon of water, cover and zap on high for 2 minutes.

3. Carefully bring the hot roasting tray out of the oven. Tip in the broccoli wedges and sprinkle over some salt and pepper. Coat the broccoli in the oil using a pair of tongs. Roast in the oven for 12 minutes.

4. While the broccoli is roasting, mix together the peanut butter, lime juice, sweet chilli, 1 teaspoon of soy and 2 tablespoons of water to make your satay sauce.

5. Finely slice the ginger and spring onions (green and white parts). Melt the remaining coconut oil in a wok or large frying pan. Chuck in the ginger and most of the spring onions, cook for 30 seconds then sprinkle in the ground turmeric, stir, then move the veg to one side of the pan and crack in the egg. Fry, stirring for 1 minute to lightly scramble.

6. Add the rice, crumbling it between your fingers as you drop it in, then stir-fry for about 2 minutes, breaking up any clumps with a wooden spoon. Season the egg fried rice with the remaining soy.

7. Dish up the egg fried rice into a bowl. Place the roasted broccoli on top, drizzle over the satay sauce and scatter over the remaining spring onions.

SINGAPORE PRAWN NOODLES

SERVES ONE

knob of fresh ginger
2 spring onions (green and
    white parts)
1 medium carrot
1 egg
1 tbsp sesame oil
150g raw king prawns
1 tbsp medium curry powder
150g 'straight to wok' rice
    noodles
1 tbsp soy sauce
large handful of beansprouts

1. Finely slice the ginger, spring onions and carrot. Crack the egg into a jug and whisk well with a fork until the white and yolk combine.

2. Heat a wok or large frying pan over a high heat. Pour in the sesame oil, scrape in the ginger, carrot and half the spring onion. Stir-fry for 3 minutes, then tip in the prawns. Cook for 2–3 minutes. The raw grey colour of the prawns will turn pink, which shows you they are cooked.

3. Sprinkle in the curry powder and pour in 50ml water. Give everything a good mix then move to one side of the pan. Pour in the beaten egg. Fry, stirring for 1 minute, to lightly scramble then stir the egg into the prawn mixture.

4. Add the noodles, breaking up the clumps with your fingers as you drop them in. Pour in the soy sauce and chuck in the beansprouts. Toss to mix the noodles with the other ingredients, then stir-fry for a minute until the noodles are warmed through and soft.

5. Pile the noodles into a bowl, scatter over the remaining spring onion to serve.

Veggie Swap

Swap the prawns for ½ small head of broccoli, cut into smallish florets, and 2 tbsp cashews, both chucked into the pan at the same time as the carrot.

POST WORKOUT

INGREDIENTS

1 tbsp coconut oil
200g turkey mince
salt and pepper
2 tbsp tomato puree
2 tsp chipotle paste
⅛ small red cabbage
juice of 1 lime
½ avocado, de-stoned
3 small corn tortillas
small handful of coriander

CHIPOTLE TURKEY TACOS

SERVES
ONE

1. Melt the coconut oil in a frying pan over a medium to high heat. Tip the turkey mince into the pan. Use the back of a wooden spoon to break the mince into small pieces. Season with salt and pepper and fry for 3 minutes.

2. Meanwhile, stir together the tomato puree, chipotle paste and 50ml water in a small bowl. Pour into the pan with the turkey, mix well then leave the turkey to bubble away in its sauce for 5 minutes.

3. While the turkey is cooking, finely slice the red cabbage, chuck into a bowl, squeeze over half the lime juice and season with salt and pepper. Mix together.

4. Scoop the avocado into another bowl, squeeze in the remaining lime juice, season, then use your fork to roughly mash. Heat the tortillas.

5. Come back to the turkey, check it is cooked by making sure the meat is white all the way through, with no raw pink bits left.

6. Once you're happy with the meat, assemble your tacos. Spoon the turkey mince between each tortilla along with the avocado and red cabbage. Tear over the coriander leaves, gobble down.

Veggie Swap

Swap the turkey mince for ½ small head of cauliflower, cut into smallish florets and cooked in the same way.

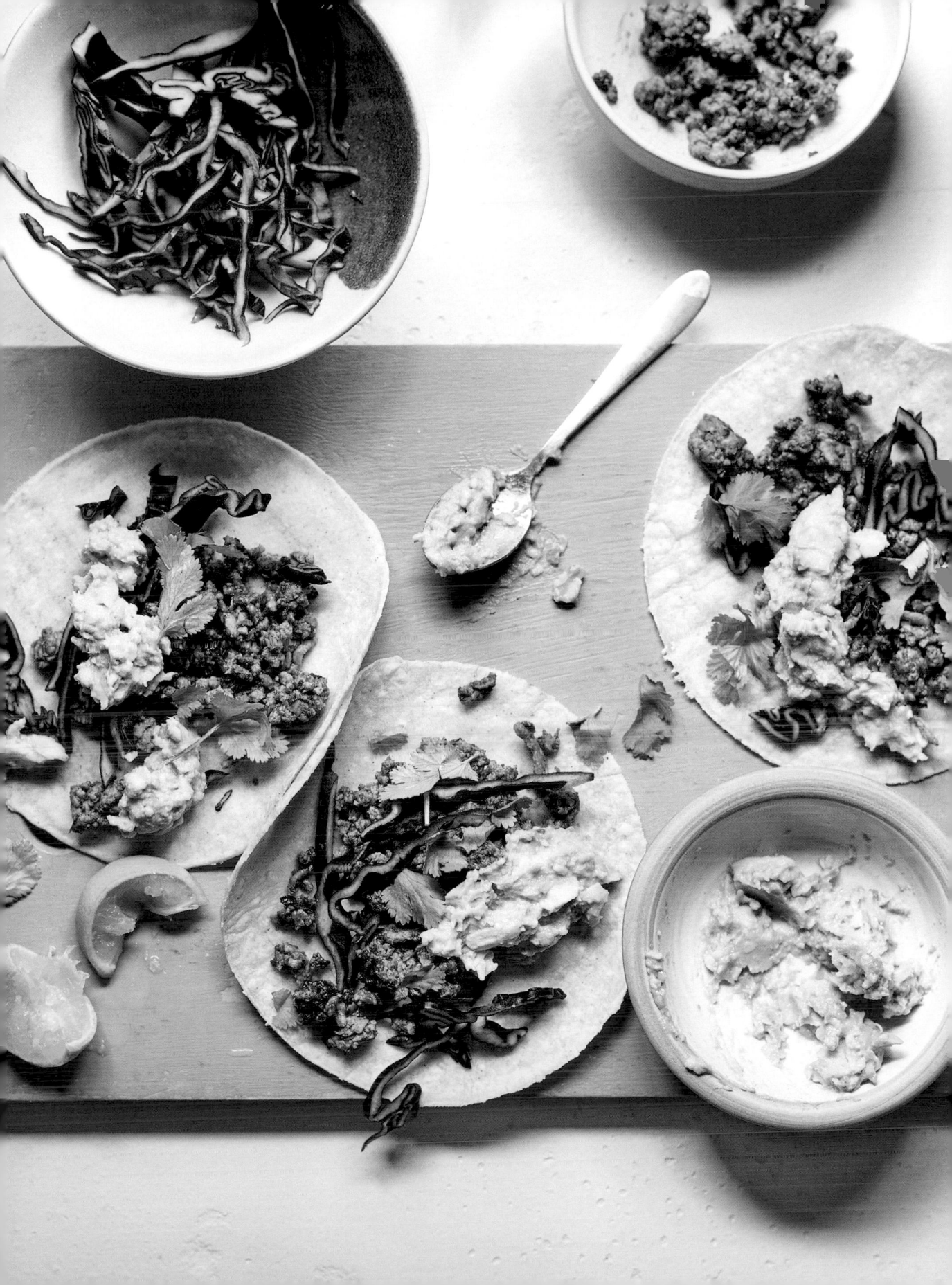

INGREDIENTS

150g trimmed Brussels sprouts,
    cut in half
½ red onion, sliced
drizzle of oil
6–7 pork chipolatas (200g)
knob of butter
salt and pepper
200g pre-cooked puy lentils
1 fat clove garlic
a few sprigs of thyme
1–2 tsp wholegrain mustard
2 tbsp balsamic vinegar

CHIPOLATAS WITH BALSAMIC LENTILS

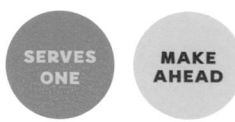

SERVES ONE · MAKE AHEAD

1. Put the Brussels sprouts and red onion into a microwaveable bowl with 1 tablespoon of water. Cover and zap on high for 3 minutes.

2. Meanwhile heat a frying pan over a medium to high heat. Drizzle in a little olive oil, add the chipolatas. Cook for about 7 minutes, turning regularly with tongs. Once cooked, turn down the heat to low and keep warm.

3. Melt most of the butter in a second non-stick frying pan over a medium to high heat. When bubbling, carefully uncover the microwaved sprouts and onion and tip into the pan. Season with a little salt and pepper, fry for 5 minutes until all the water has evaporated and the sprouts are starting to crisp.

4. Dump the lentils into the sprout pan. Crush in the garlic clove, strip the leaves off the thyme sprig. Add the final bit of butter and crank up the heat. Mix everything together, cook for 1–2 minutes until the lentils are warmed through, then stir in the mustard and balsamic vinegar.

5. Once the balsamic has bubbled off, season the lentils to taste then spoon into a bowl and pile the cooked chipolatas on top.

Veggie Swap

Swap the chipolatas for 3 ready-cooked beetroot, cut into wedges and fried in a little olive oil for 2–3 minutes until warmed through.

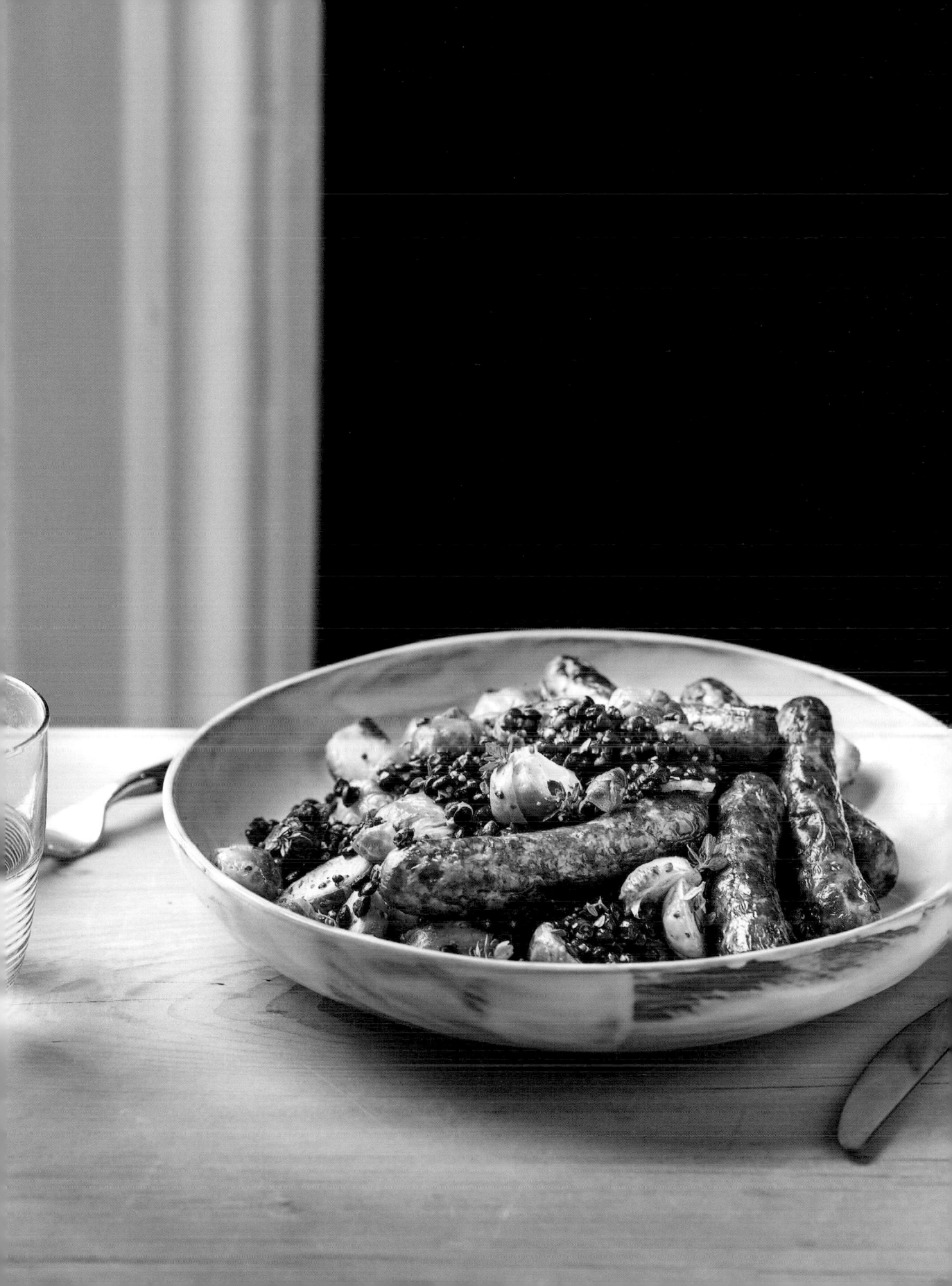

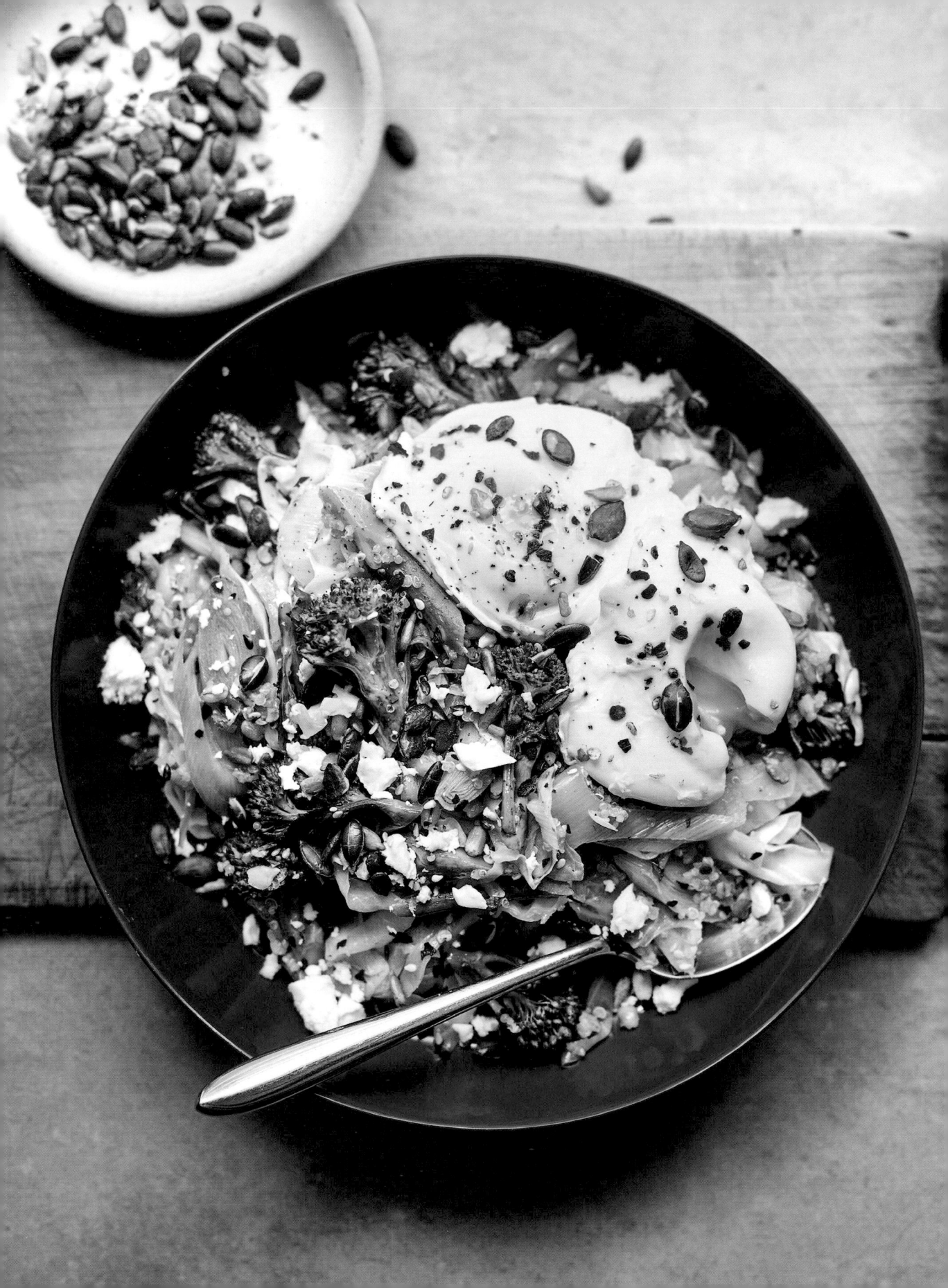

GARLICKY GREENS AND POACHED EGG GRAIN BOWL WITH TOASTED SEEDS

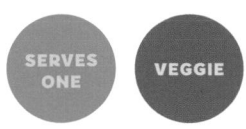

SERVES ONE

VEGGIE

1. Bring a kettle of water to the boil.

2. Meanwhile toast the seeds in a dry frying pan over a medium to high heat until they begin to pop. Tip the seeds into a bowl and put the pan back onto the heat.

3. Pour the water into a saucepan over a medium heat.

4. Melt the coconut oil in the frying pan, dump in the sliced leek. Cook, stirring occasionally, for 2 minutes until it begins to collapse and soften. Add the garlic and chilli flakes to the pan, cook for 30 seconds more then chuck in the cabbage and little trees along with 50ml of water. Leave to bubble away.

5. Come back to the pan of water. Carefully crack your eggs into the hot water, reducing the heat until the water is just 'burping'. Cook the eggs for 3 minutes for a runny yolk, then carefully lift them out with a slotted spoon and drain on paper towels.

6. While the eggs are poaching, ping the grains in the microwave according to packet instructions. Crank up the heat on the greens and fry until tender and bright green, around 2–3 minutes. Sprinkle over some salt and pepper and squeeze over the lemon juice.

7. Mix the greens with the heated grains in a serving bowl. Place the poached eggs on top and sprinkle over the mixed seeds, a few more chilli flakes and the feta if you like, then get stuck in.

INGREDIENTS

1 tbsp mixed seeds
1 tbsp coconut oil
½ medium leek, finely sliced
2 cloves garlic, sliced
½ tsp dried chilli flakes, plus extra to serve – optional
¼ spring or sweetheart cabbage, sliced
100g little trees (tenderstem broccoli), each cut into three pieces, any bigger stalks sliced in half lengthways
2 eggs
200g pre-cooked grains
salt and pepper
juice of ½ lemon
30g feta, crumbled – optional

INGREDIENTS

drizzle of olive oil

½ onion, finely sliced

salt and pepper

knob of butter

1 fat clove garlic, finely chopped

1 heaped tsp smoked paprika

200g pork loin steaks, sliced into 1cm strips

1 x 400g tin of chopped tomatoes

splash of red wine vinegar

2 jarred roasted red peppers, drained and finely sliced

250g pre-cooked wholegrain rice

dollop of reduced-fat sour cream, to serve – optional

* PORK STEW ONLY.

PORK WITH ROASTED RED PEPPER AND RICE

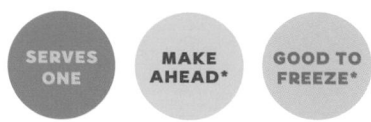

1. Heat a non-stick frying pan over a medium to high heat. Drizzle in the olive oil, chuck in the onion along with a pinch of salt. Fry, stirring almost constantly, for 4–5 minutes until the onion is collapsed and starting to brown.

2. Melt the butter into the pan. When bubbling, add the garlic and smoked paprika. Cook for 30 seconds then chuck the pork loin slices into the pan. Sprinkle everything with some salt and pepper. Fry, stirring for 1 minute to coat the pork in the spices, then tip in the chopped tomatoes.

3. Crank up the heat. Splash in some red wine vinegar and tip in the sliced red peppers. Cook for 4 minutes until the pork is cooked through. Check by slicing into one of the larger pieces to make sure the meat is white all the way through, with no raw pink bits left. Take the pan off the heat.

4. Ping the rice in the microwave according to packet instructions. Season the stew to taste. Tip the rice into a serving bowl and spoon over the stew. Swirl through the sour cream, if you like.

Veggie Swap

Swap the pork for 150g mushrooms of your choice, added into the pan at the same time as the onion.

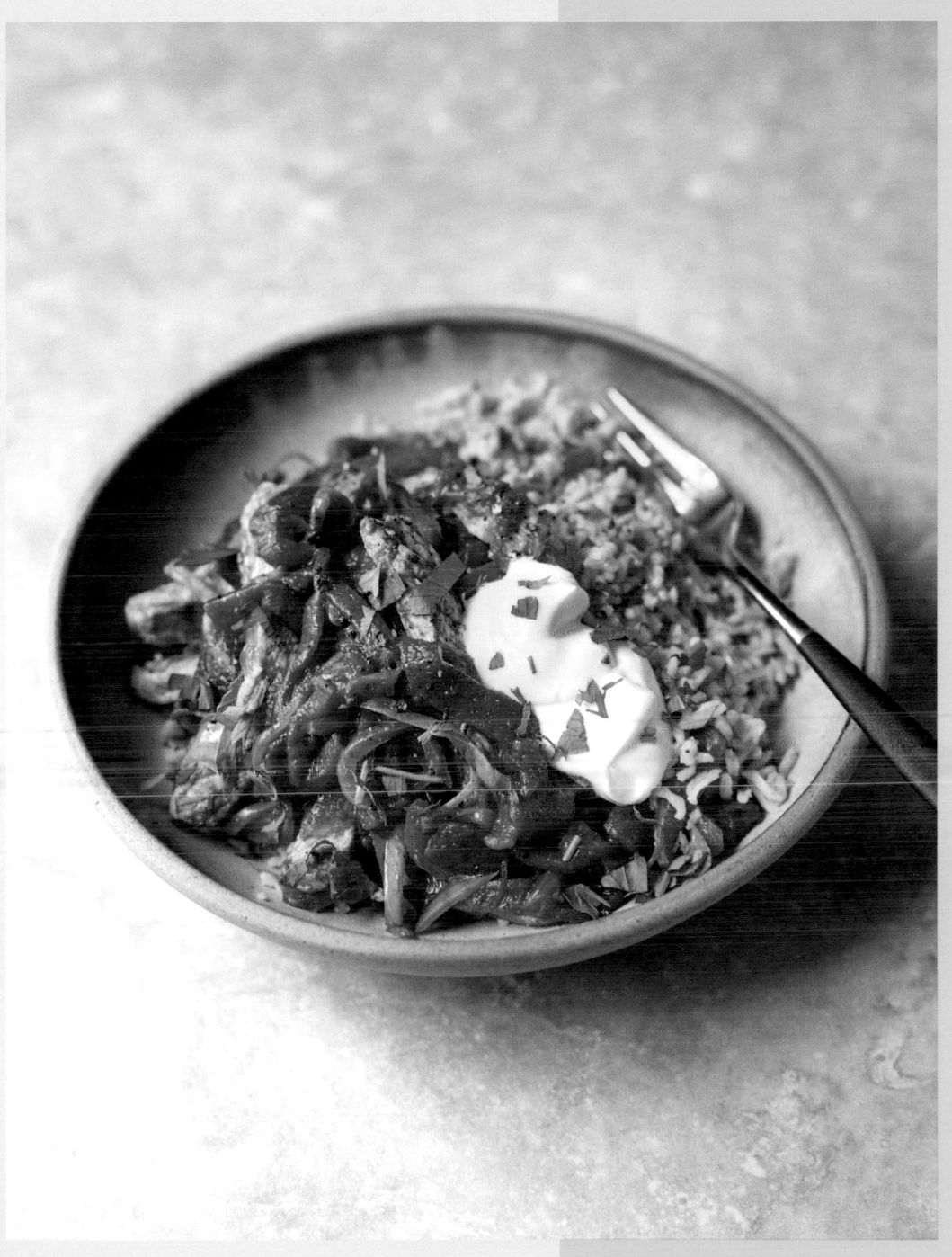

INGREDIENTS

1 x 200g skinless chicken
    breast fillet
drizzle of olive oil
2 tsp ras el hanout
salt and pepper
2 tbsp tahini
juice of ½ lemon
¼ cucumber
8 radishes
½ yellow pepper
small handful of mint leaves
handful of parsley
200g pre-cooked mixed grains

CHICKEN SHAWARMA AND MIXED GRAIN TABBOULEH

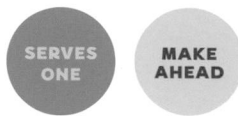

1. Place the chicken between two pieces of cling film or baking parchment on a chopping board. Using a rolling pin, meat mallet or any other blunt instrument, bash the chicken until it is about 1cm thick all over. Drizzle the chicken breast with a little olive oil, sprinkle over the ras el hanout and a good pinch of salt and pepper, then rub the spices into the flesh.

2. Heat a griddle pan over the highest heat. Once searingly hot, carefully lay the chicken in the pan. Cook for about 4 minutes on each side.

3. Meanwhile mix together the tahini, lemon juice and 2 tablespoons of water in a small bowl to a creamy dressing. Season with salt and pepper to taste. Roughly chop the cucumber, radishes, pepper, mint and parsley. Scrape all the vegetables and most of the herbs into a serving bowl.

4. Ping the grains in the microwave according to packet instructions. Once warmed, tip into your serving bowl. Pour in the tahini dressing, give everything a good mix.

5. Come back to your chicken, which should now be cooked. Check by slicing into a thicker part to make sure the meat is white all the way through with no raw pink bits left. Slice the grilled chicken on a diagonal, place on top of the tabbouleh and scatter over the remaining herbs.

Veggie Swap

Swap the chicken for
4 slices of halloumi, coated
in ras el hanout and olive
oil, then fried in a non-stick
frying pan for 1–2 minutes on
each side until crisp.

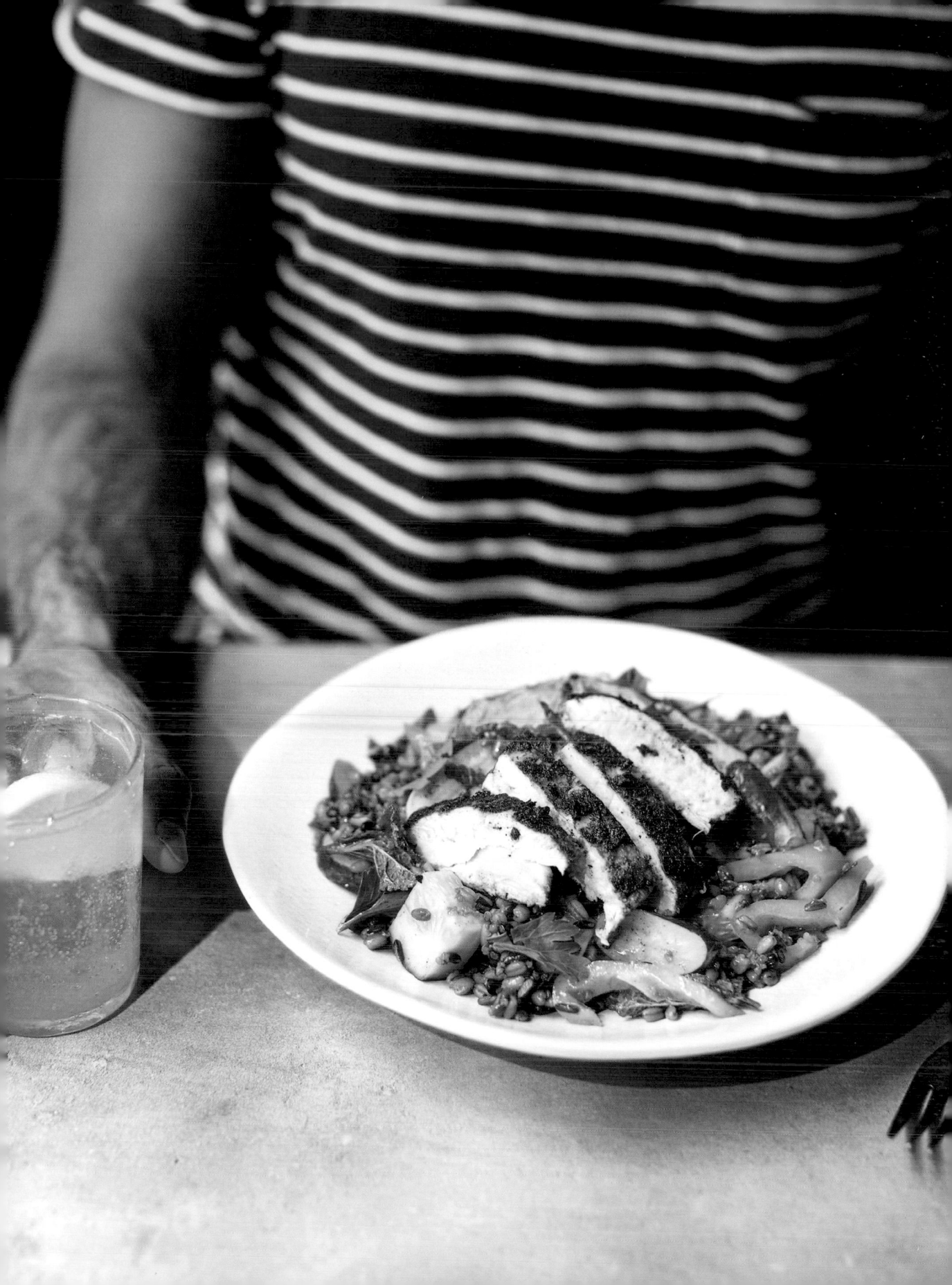

INGREDIENTS

6–8 new potatoes (200g)
1 x 200g skinless boneless
  salmon fillet
drizzle of olive oil
salt and pepper
2 spring onions
¼ small savoy or sweetheart
  cabbage
30g butter
juice of ½ lemon
2 tsp wholegrain mustard

SALMON AND NEW POTATO COLCANNON

SERVES ONE

1. Preheat the grill to maximum.

2. Halve the new potatoes, leaving the skin on. Put in a large microwaveable bowl with 1 tablespoon of water, cover and zap on high for 10 minutes until completely soft.

3. Place the salmon fillet on a baking tray, drizzle with a little oil and season with salt and pepper. Slide under the grill for 5 minutes.

4. While the salmon is grilling, finely slice the spring onions (green and white parts) and the cabbage. Melt the butter in a frying pan over a medium heat. When bubbling, chuck in the spring onions and cabbage. Cook, stirring regularly, for 3–4 minutes until the veg has collapsed and softened. Take the pan off the heat.

5. Come back to your salmon. Mix half the lemon juice with the mustard in a small bowl. Spoon the mustardy mixture over the top of the salmon and slide back under the grill for 3 minutes, until cooked through. Check by slicing into the thick end of the fillet to make sure the flesh has turned matt pink in colour, then turn off the grill and leave the salmon to keep warm until you're ready to eat.

6. Carefully uncover the potatoes, pour in the buttery juices from the cabbage mixture, roughly mash then tip in the greens, mix together and season with salt, pepper and a squeeze of lemon juice to taste.

7. Spoon the colcannon mash onto a plate and lay the mustardy salmon fillet alongside to serve.

Veggie Swap

**Swap the salmon for
2 poached eggs. See p. 190
for my way of poaching.**

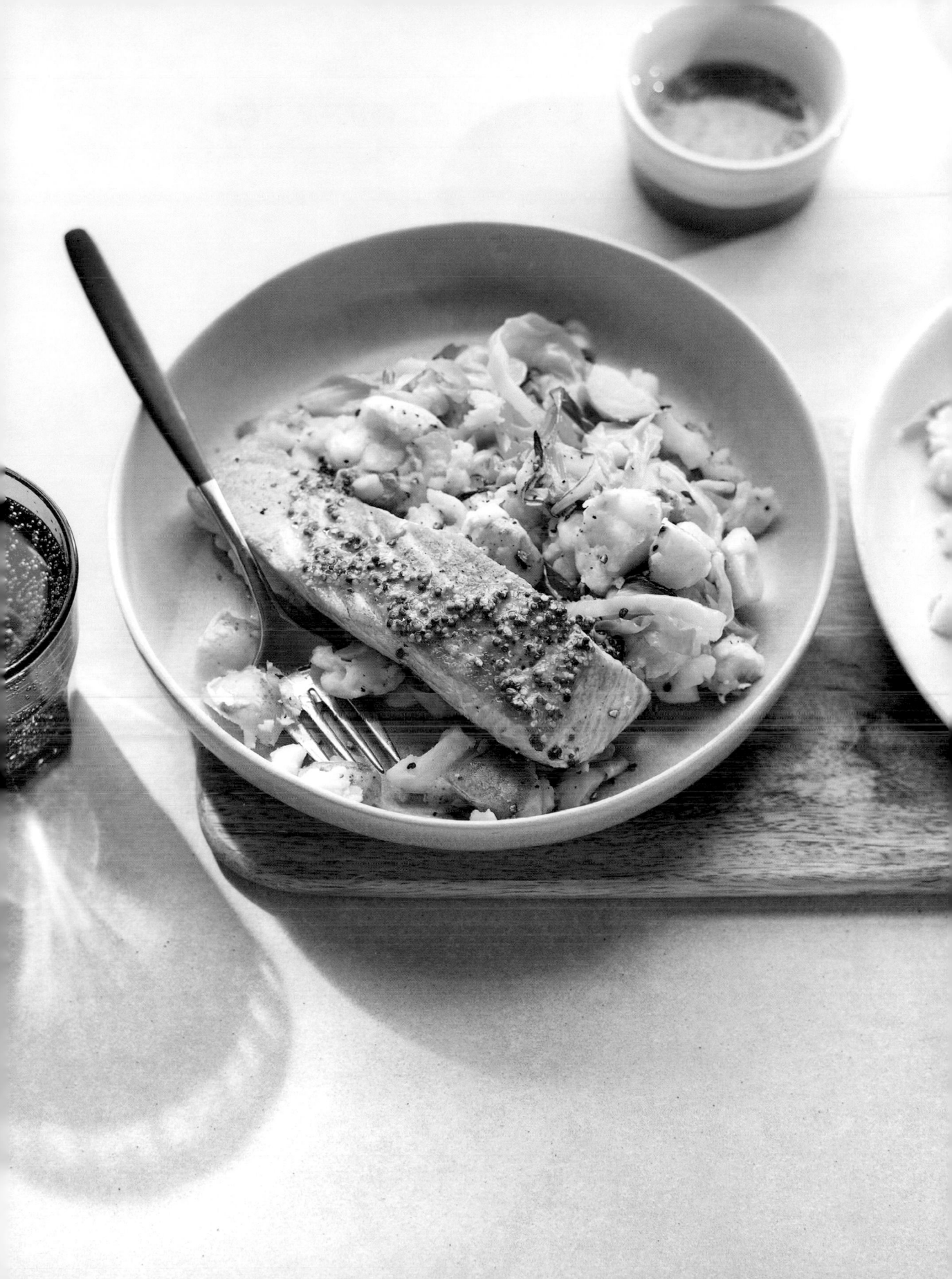

INGREDIENTS

½ red onion
1 small carrot
½ medium courgette
1 tbsp coconut oil
salt and pepper
1 fat clove garlic
1 tsp chilli powder
1 tsp ground cumin
1 x 400g tin of green lentils,
    drained and rinsed
200g passata
1 square of dark chocolate
2 wholegrain burger buns

* LENTILS ONLY.

LENTIL SLOPPY JOE

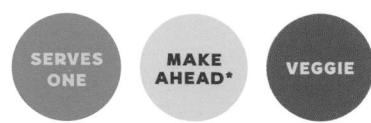

SERVES ONE · **MAKE AHEAD*** · **VEGGIE**

1. Grate the red onion, carrot and courgette.

2. Melt the coconut oil in a frying pan over a medium heat. Scrape in the grated vegetables along with a pinch of salt. Cook, stirring, for 2–3 minutes until softened then crush in the garlic clove. Sprinkle in the chilli powder and ground cumin. Cook for 30 seconds more.

3. Tip in the green lentils, passata and 50ml water. Crank up the heat. Mix everything together and drop in the dark chocolate. Leave to bubble away for 5 or so minutes until you have a nice thick lentil-style chilli. Season to taste.

4. Cut the buns in half, pile in your lentil chilli and tuck in!

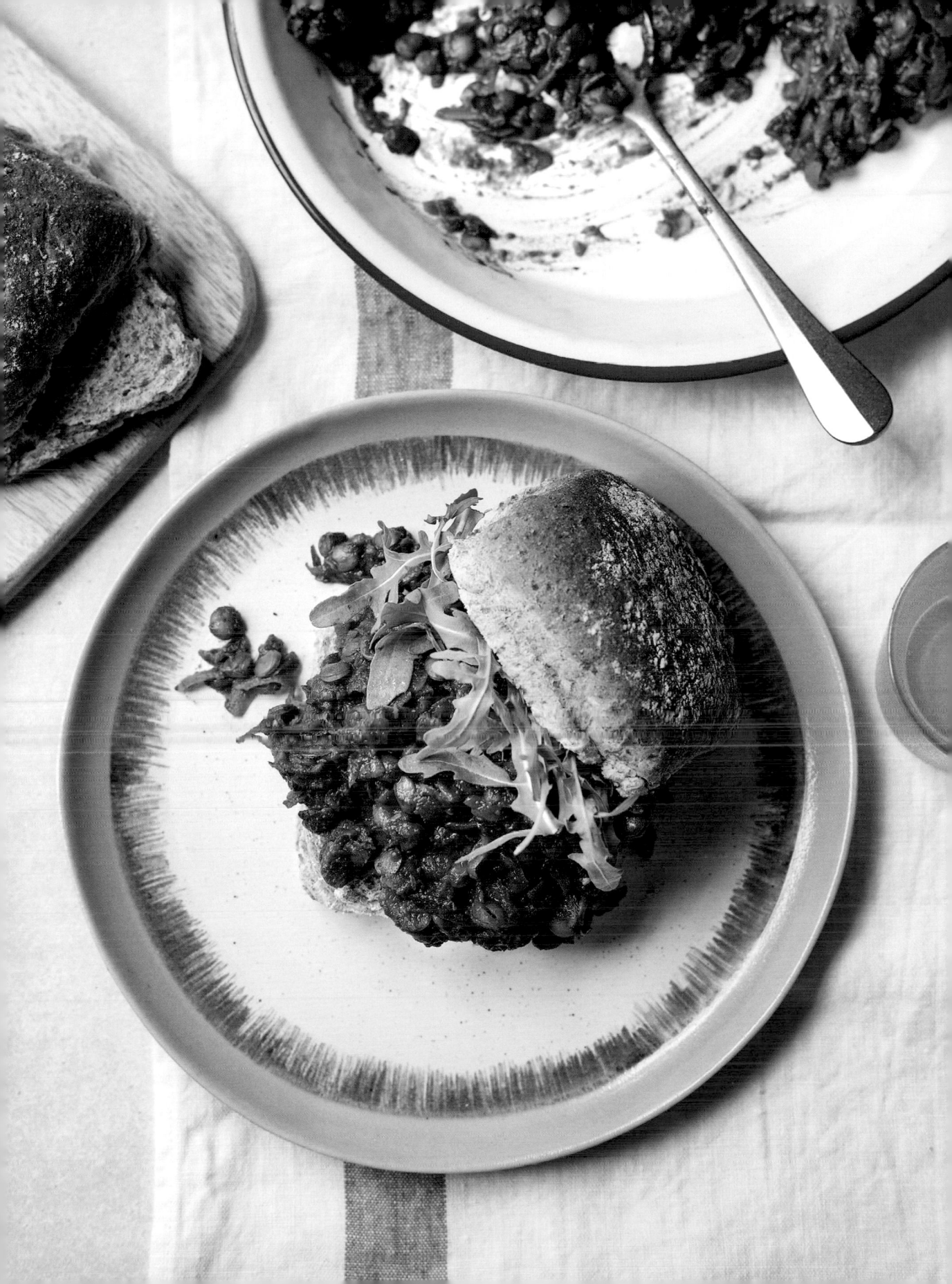

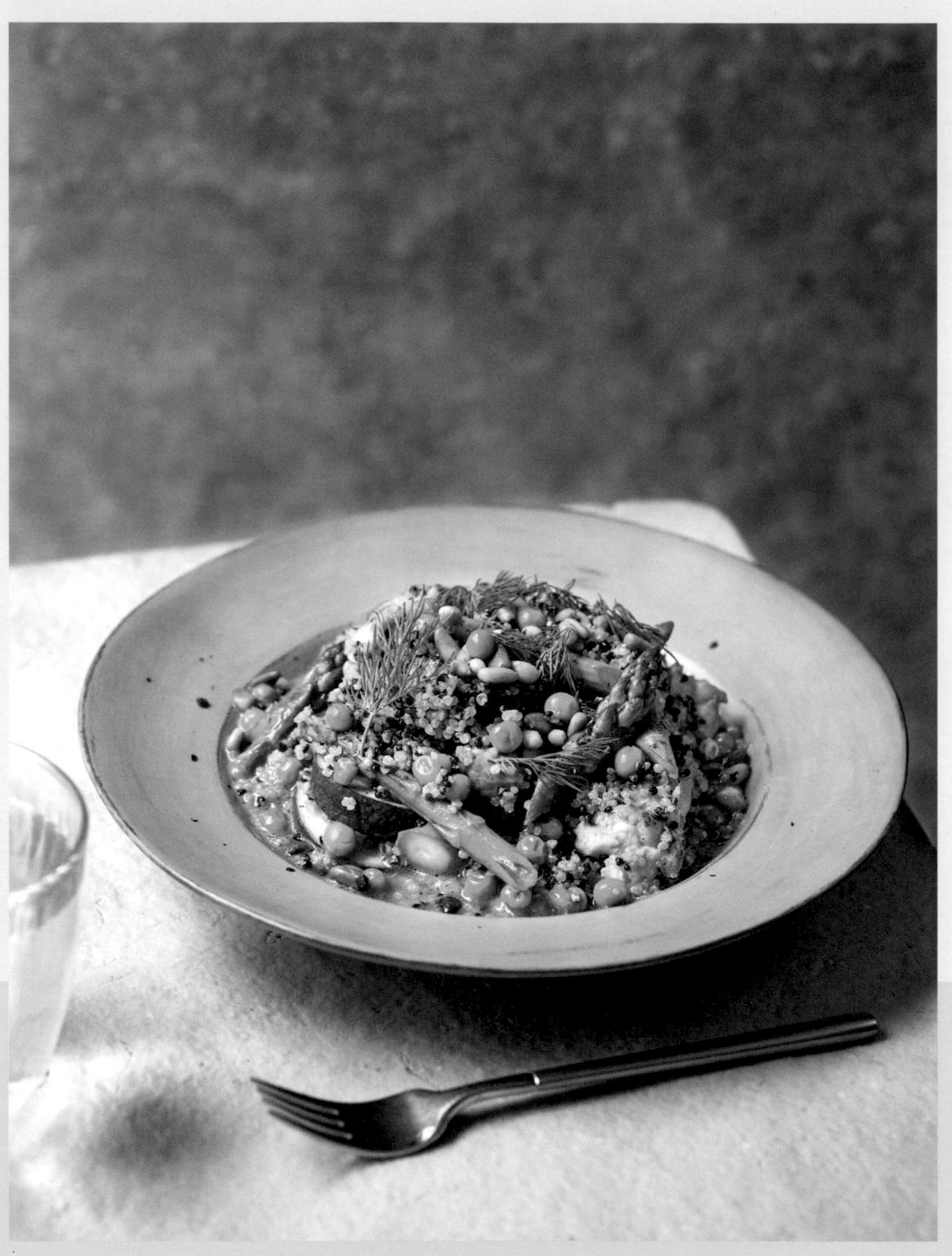

CHICKEN QUINOA PRIMAVERA

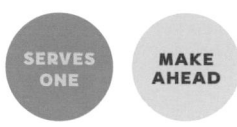

SERVES ONE   MAKE AHEAD

knob of butter
200g skinless, boneless chicken thighs, cut into large, bite-sized pieces
1 medium courgette, sliced
salt and pepper
½ chicken stock cube
200g pre-cooked quinoa
100g asparagus tips, cut into three
50g frozen peas
juice of ½ lemon
1 tbsp toasted pine nuts
small handful of dill or mint, roughly chopped

1. Melt the butter in a frying pan over a medium to high heat. When bubbling, chuck in the chicken and sliced courgette, sprinkle over some salt and pepper. Fry, stirring regularly, for around 5 minutes until the chicken has started to brown.

2. Meanwhile bring a kettle of water to the boil. Put the chicken stock cube into a jug, measure in 150ml boiling water and whisk with a fork to dissolve.

3. Come back to the chicken and courgette, add the quinoa, asparagus and frozen peas to the pan. Pour in the chicken stock, give everything a good stir and place a lid on the pan. Cook for a further 3–4 minutes, until the asparagus is tender and the chicken is cooked through. Check by slicing into one of the larger pieces – the knife should cut through easily and the meat will have turned from pink to a whitish brown.

4. Squeeze in the lemon juice and season the quinoa primavera to taste – it should be a nice soupy risotto consistency. Spoon into a bowl, finish with a scattering of toasted pine nuts, a good crack of black pepper and some roughly chopped dill or mint sprinkled over the top.

Veggie Swap

Omit the chicken and stir 30g crumbled feta mixed into 2 tbsp low-fat Greek yoghurt. Dollop on top of the primavera before eating.

THE
TRAINING
PLAN

THE TRAINING PLAN

I have included 6 home workouts in this plan to choose from:

2 X BEGINNERS HIIT

2 X INTERMEDIATE

2 X ADVANCED WORKOUTS

Of the two for each fitness level one of them is a body weight HIIT session using no equipment and the other is a strength-based resistance workout using dumbbells. This means the workouts are accessible to everyone and you can choose the type of workout you like depending on your fitness levels and preferences.

**LISS CARDIO OPTIONS
(LOW-INTENSITY STEADY STATE)**

If you don't fancy the HIIT workouts, feel free to select any of the following exercises for a less intense workout at your own pace. Aim to do one or a combination of exercises for around 30–60+ minutes at a moderate intensity. Choose either a HIIT, weight session or LIIS session in a day. One workout per day is enough.

- **Walking**
- **Jogging**
- **Stairclimber**
- **Cycling**
- **Rowing**
- **Cross trainer**
- **SkiErg**
- **Swimming**

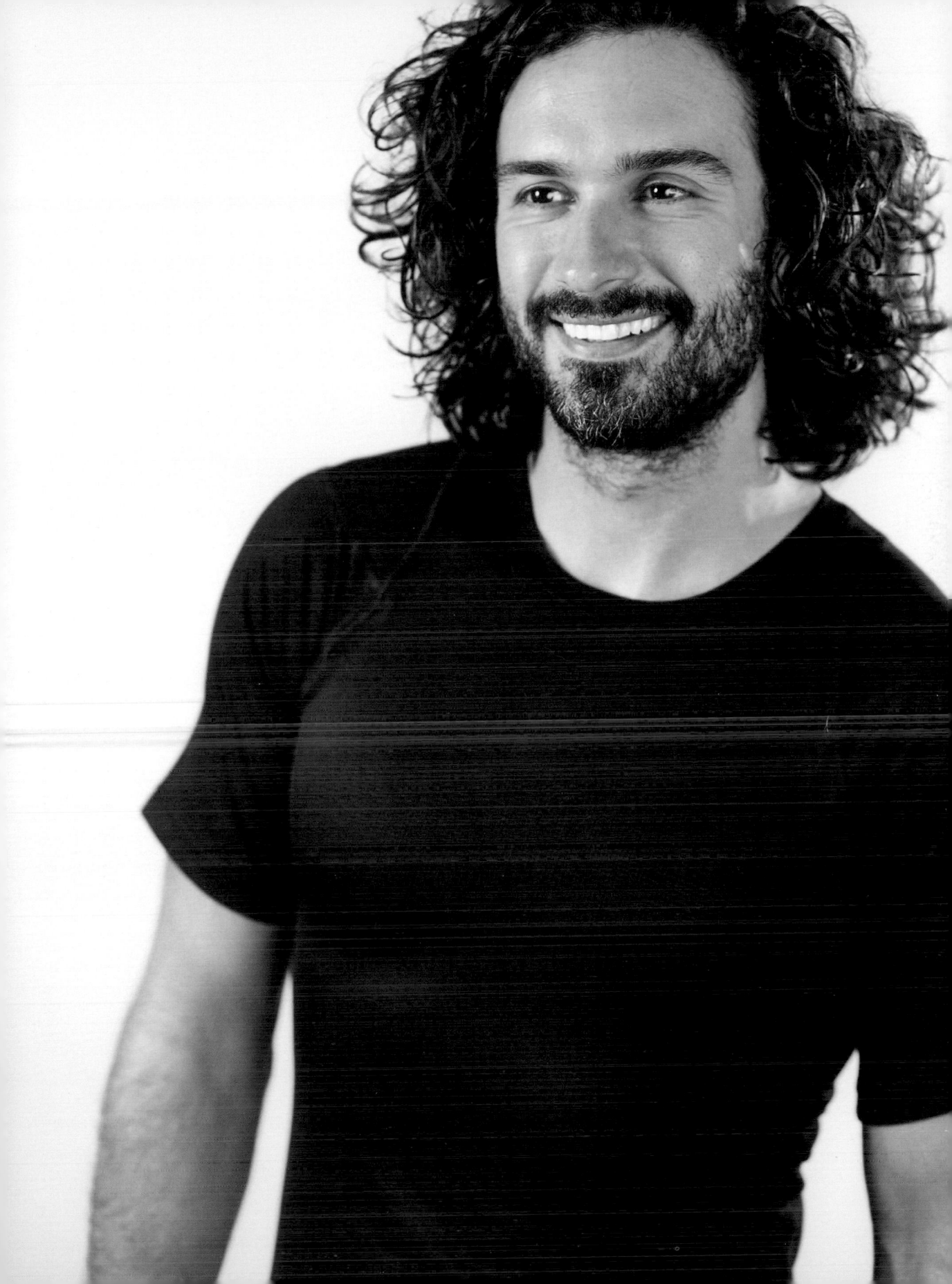

"

Working out every morning with Joe kick started a fitness regime that continues to benefit our whole family. We've used it to structure our daily routine.

Fitness is a priority for us now and that's extended into nutrition too. Those 20-minute workouts have completely changed us for the better and we are so grateful.

"

FLO, 42

> "
>
> **Following your HIIT sessions and dining on some of your delicious recipes helped me get through some big transitions in my life.**
>
> **Now I have a crazy happy year ahead as I become a dad. I have the energy and mental wellbeing due to the positivity you spread.**
>
> "

LEVI, 28

BEGINNER HIIT 1: BODYWEIGHT

(24 MINUTES)

30 SECONDS WORK / 30 SECONDS REST

X 3 ROUNDS IN TOTAL

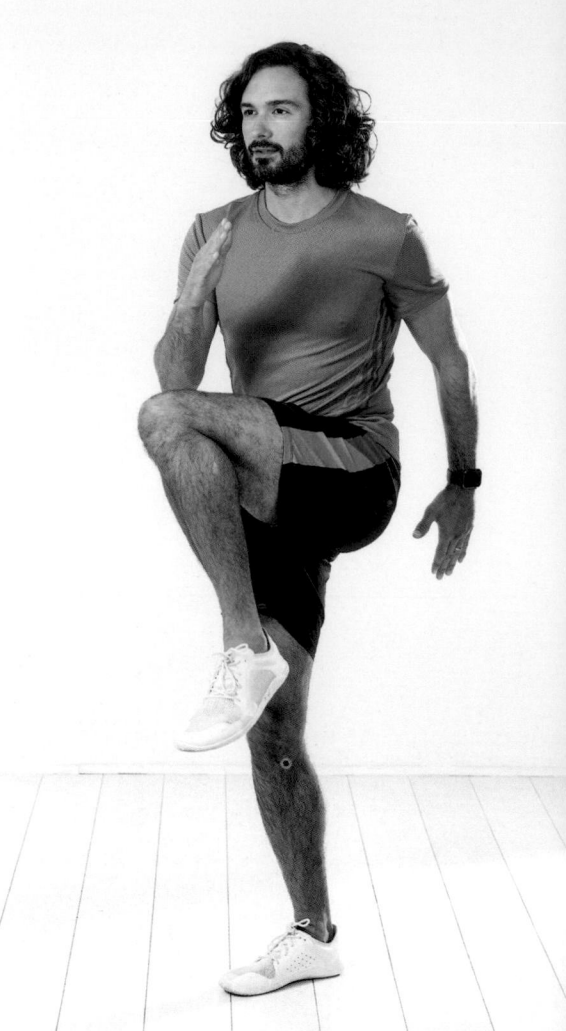

1. MARCH ON SPOT / JOG

Jog or march up and down on the spot. Lift knees high, keep your back straight and pump your arms to accelerate.

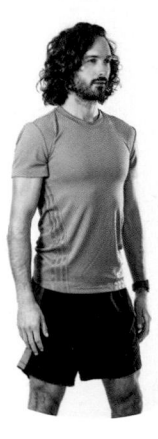

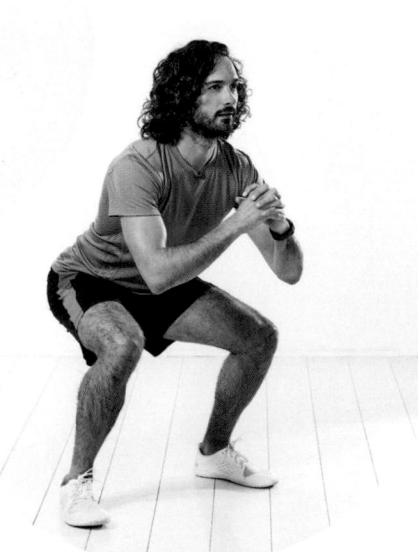

2. SQUATS

Place your feet in a comfortable position that will allow you to squat down while keeping them firmly flat on the ground. Sit low and drive through the heels to stand up. Repeat fast.

3. STAR JUMPS

A PE with Joe favourite! Stand tall with your arms by your side. Jump up, extending your arms and legs out into a star shape in the air. Land with your knees together and hands by your side.

ENGAGE YOUR CORE AND KEEP YOUR BACK STRAIGHT.

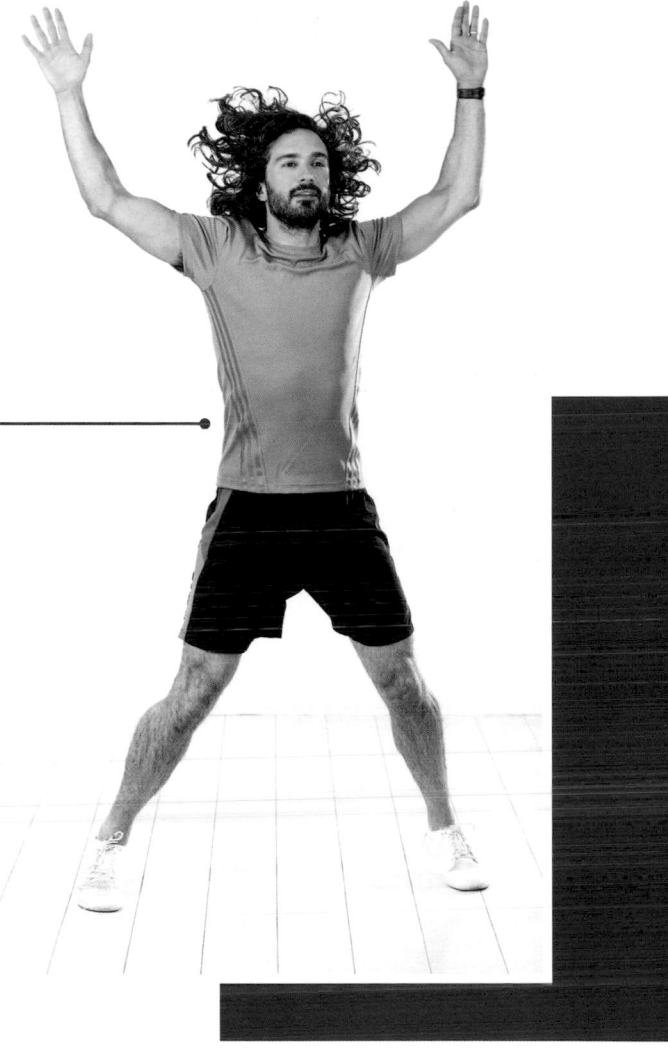

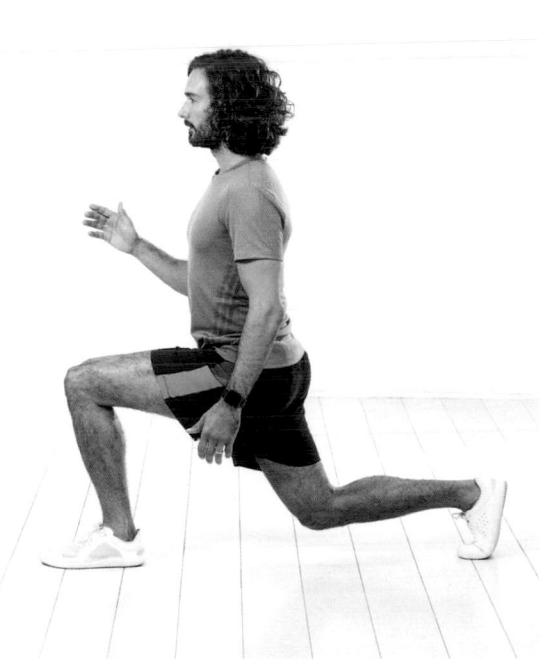

4. REVERSE LUNGES

Start with both feet together, then step backwards with one foot and bend both knees into a reverse lunge. Aim to keep your back straight. Alternate each leg.

THE TRAINING PLAN

5. CLIMB THE LADDER

Start by running on the spot. Imagine you are reaching up above your head to pull yourself up a ladder. Do this as fast as possible.

LIFT UP YOUR KNEES AS HIGH AS YOU CAN.

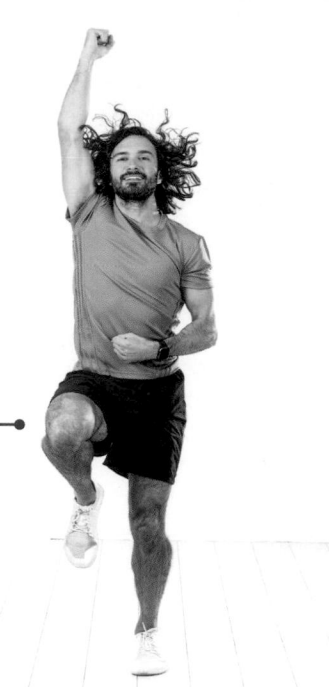

6. WALK OUTS

Stand with your feet hip-width apart. Bend your knees and place your palms on the floor in front of your feet. Shift your weight onto your hands and walk them forward until your body is in a straight line from your head to your heels. Walk back and repeat.

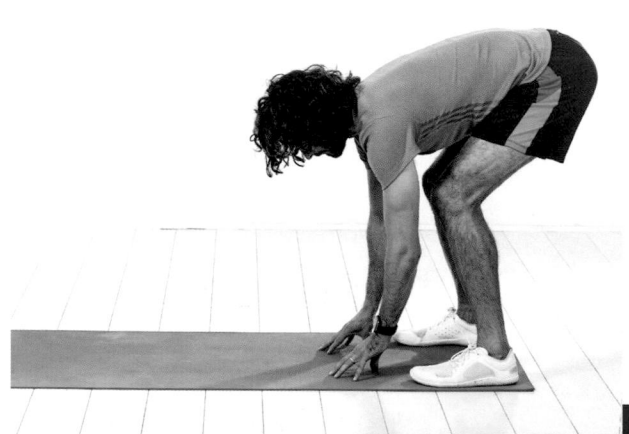

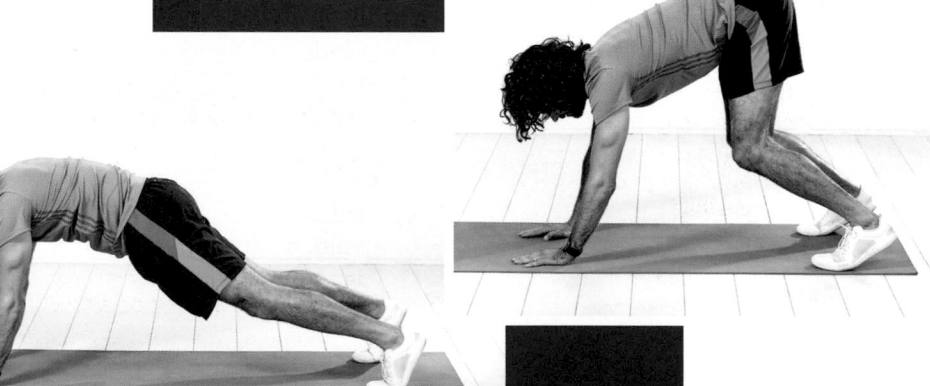

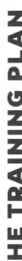

7. MOUNTAIN CLIMBERS

Start in a high plank position. Look down towards your hands and keep your back flat. Then drive your knees towards your chest as fast as possible one at a time.

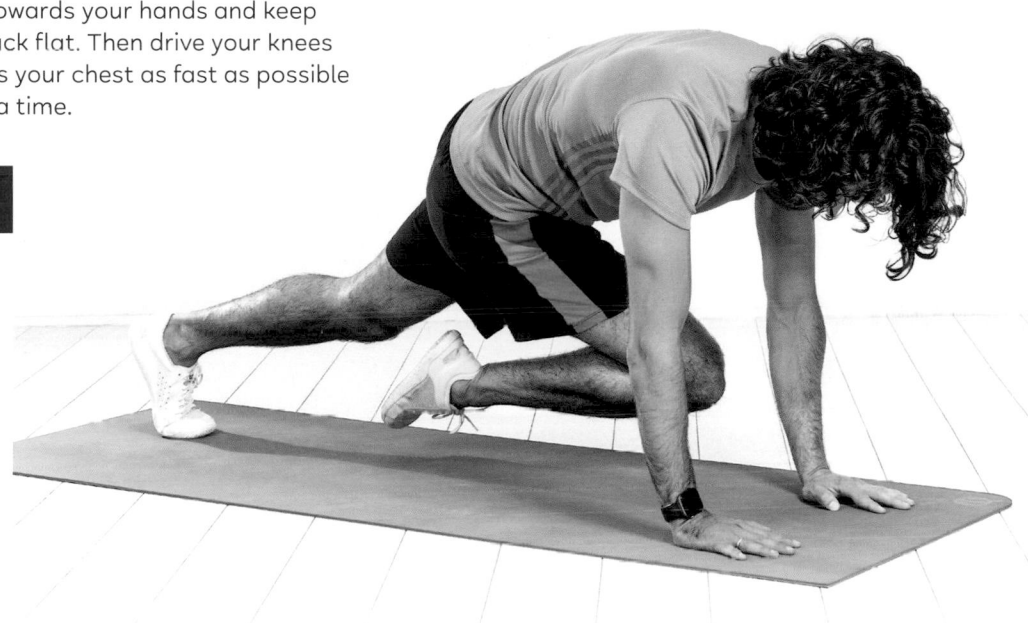

8. ELBOW PLANK

Lift and hold your torso and legs off the ground with your elbows on the floor directly under your shoulders. Aim to keep a flat back and active abs and glutes.

MAKE SURE YOUR ELBOWS ARE DIRECTLY BELOW YOUR SHOULDERS.

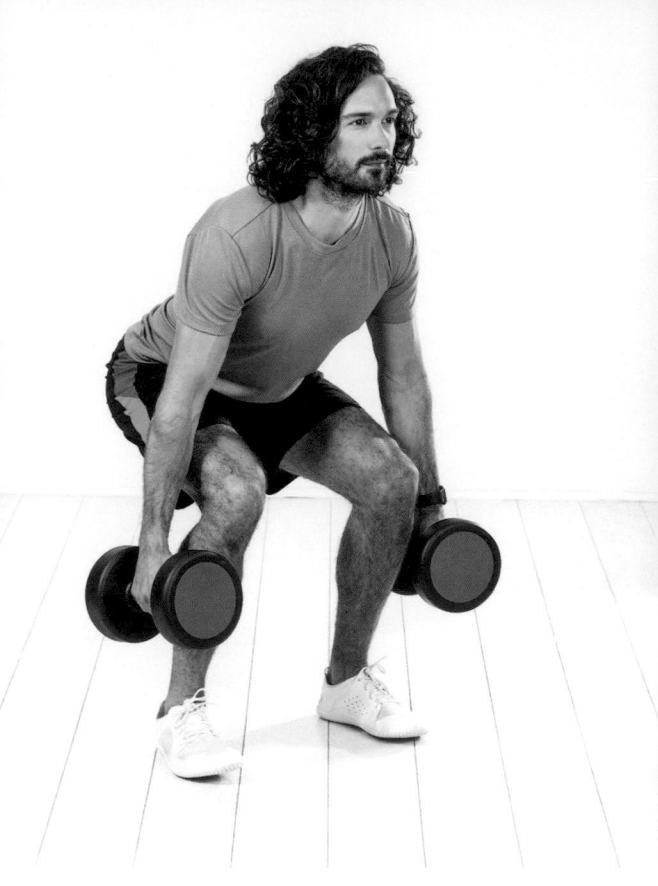

1. SQUATS WITH DUMBBELLS

Hold the the dumbells at your sides. Keep your core engaged as you lower down into a squat. Drive through the heels back up into a standing position and repeat.

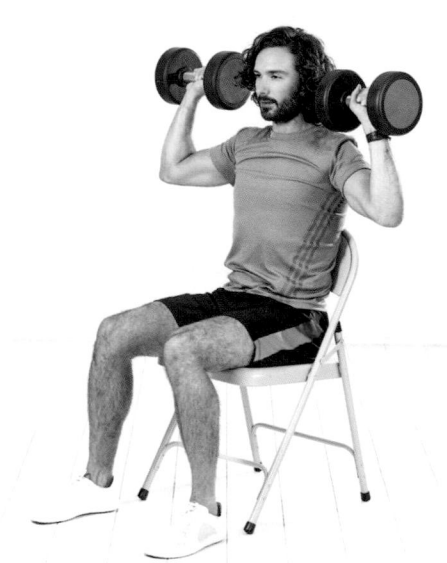

2. SHOULDER PRESS

Hold one dumbbell in each hand at your shoulders with elbows pointing out. Then drive the hands up until the dumbbells meet. Slowly lower and repeat in a controlled way.

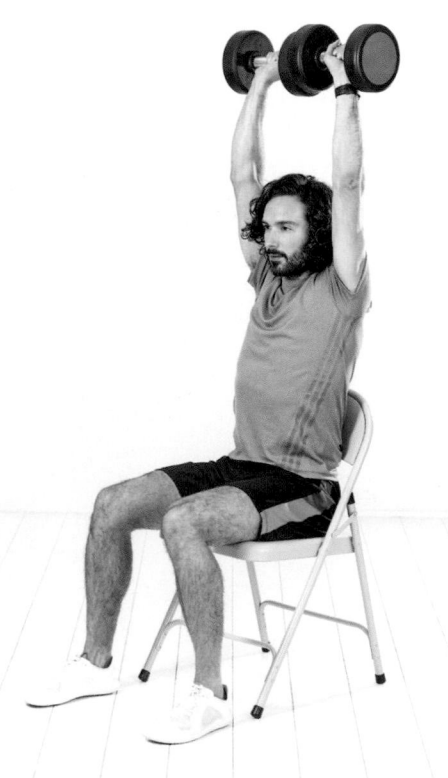

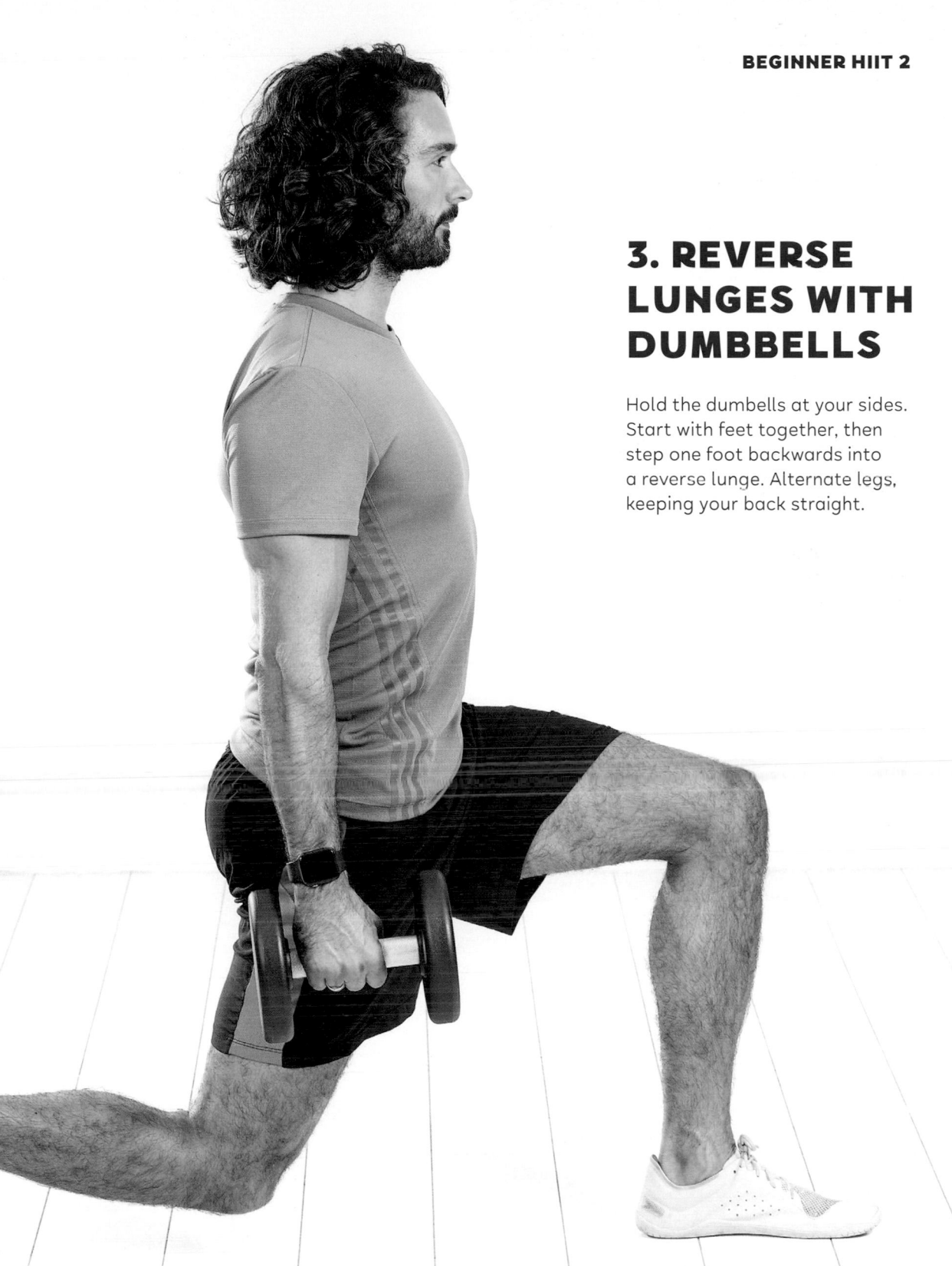

3. REVERSE LUNGES WITH DUMBBELLS

Hold the dumbells at your sides. Start with feet together, then step one foot backwards into a reverse lunge. Alternate legs, keeping your back straight.

THE TRAINING PLAN

4. BOX PUSH UPS

Start in a high plank position. Lower your knees. Keep hands narrow and elbows close to the body. Lower yourself down towards the ground and push back up.

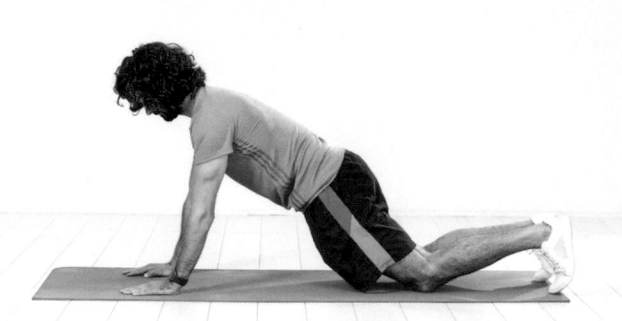

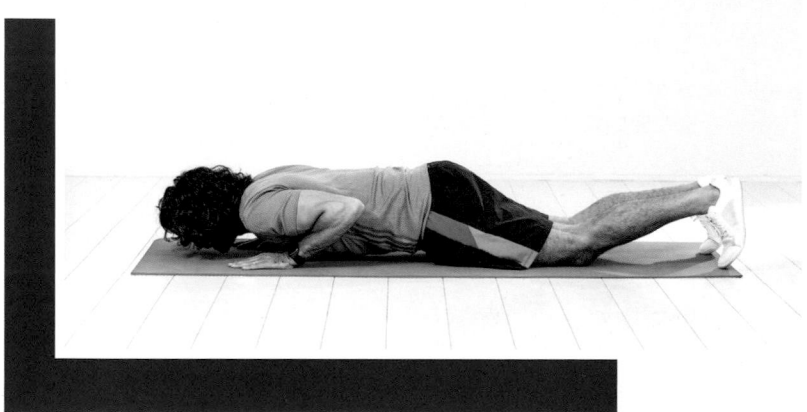

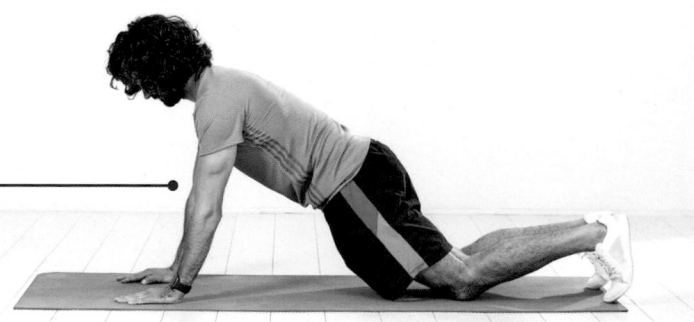

FULLY EXTEND YOUR ARMS WHEN YOU PUSH BACK UP.

5. BICEP CURLS

Standing up straight with one dumbbell in each hand, one at a time slowly curl up each dumbbell towards your shoulder.

ROTATE YOUR HANDS TOWARDS YOU AS YOU CURL EACH DUMBBELL.

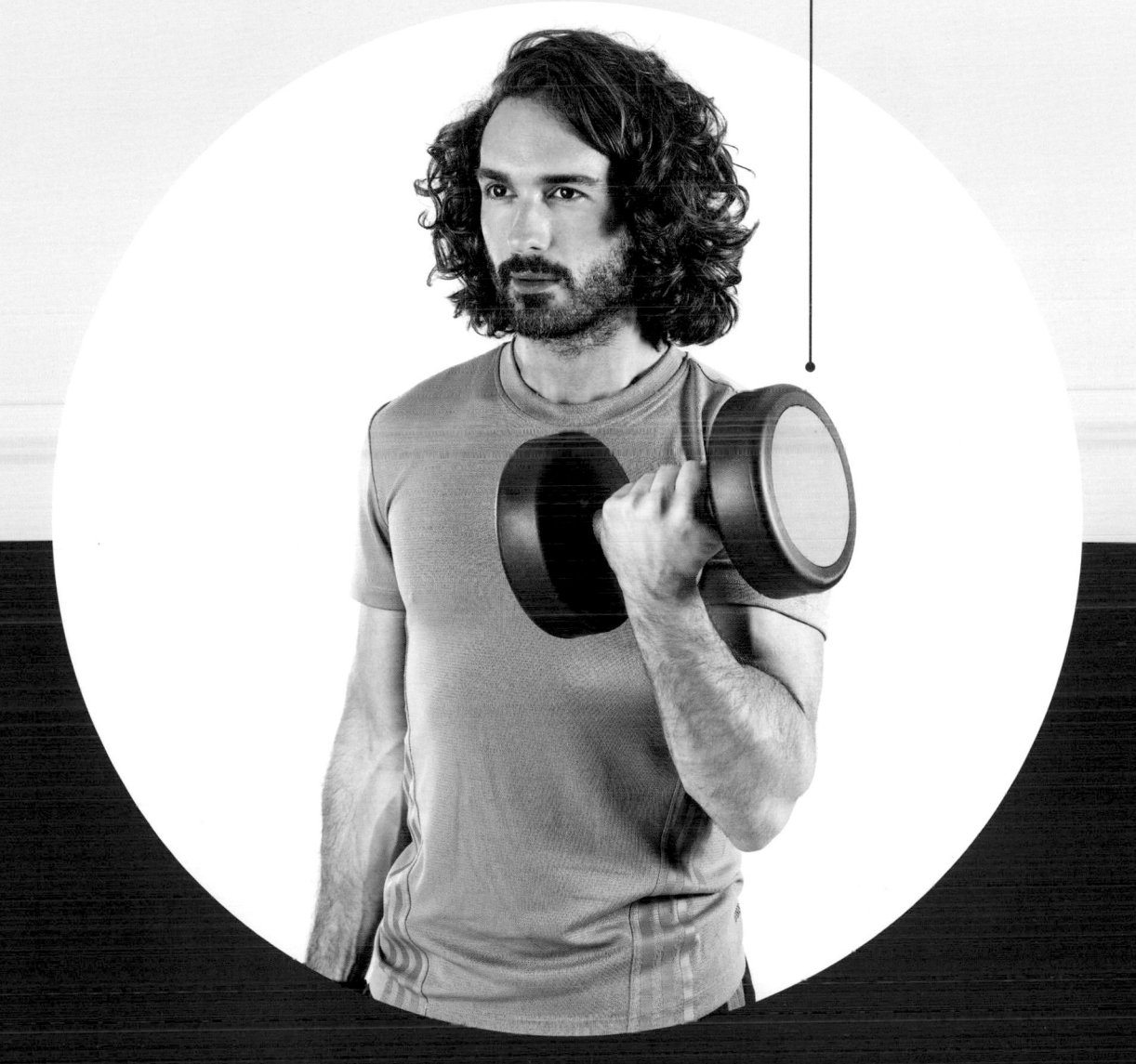

6. TRICEP DIPS ON CHAIR

Lean against a chair with your legs in front of you. Keeping elbows tucked in, lower yourself towards the ground, then push back up to fully extend your arms.

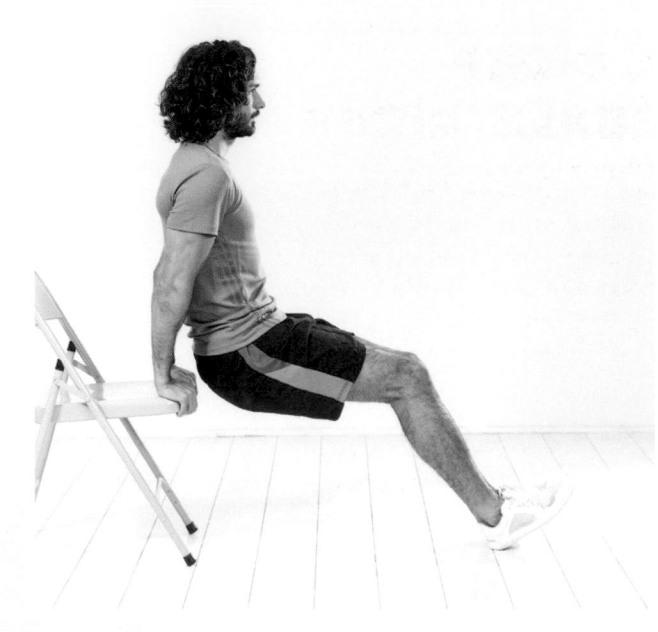

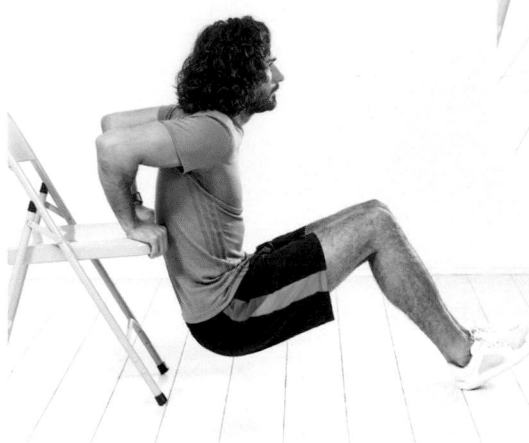

STAY LOW TO KEEP THE TENSION ON YOUR QUADS.

7. SUMO SQUAT PULSES

Hold one dumbbell in front of you as pictured. Place your feet a comfortable distance apart and lower yourself as if you're about to sit into a chair. Rather than standing up fully, just pulse up and down.

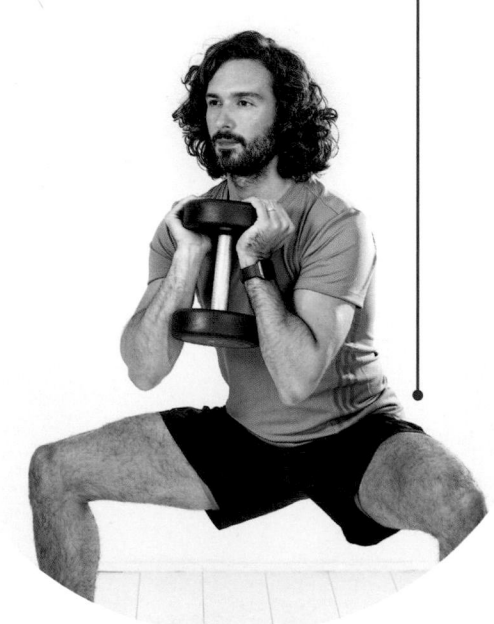

8. OVER HEAD TRICEP EXTENSION

Stand up straight with one dumbbell in both hands. Slowly lower it behind you. Drive the dumbbell back up by extending your triceps.

KEEP YOUR ELBOWS CLOSE TO YOUR EARS.

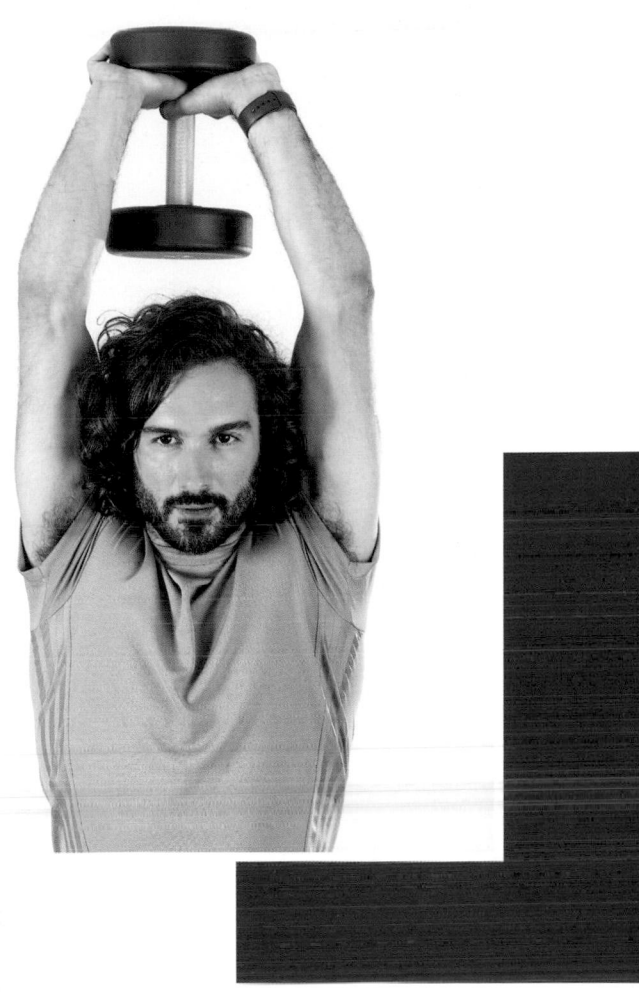

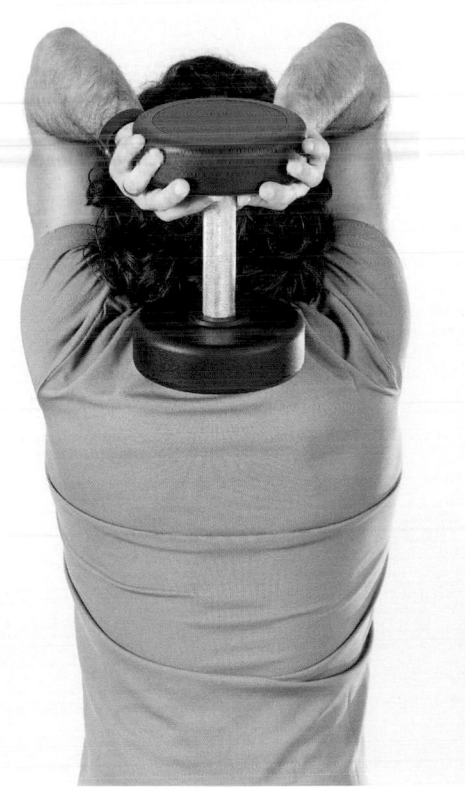

INTERMEDIATE HIIT 1: BODYWEIGHT

(28 MINUTES)

35 SECONDS WORK / 25 SECONDS REST

X 4 ROUNDS IN TOTAL

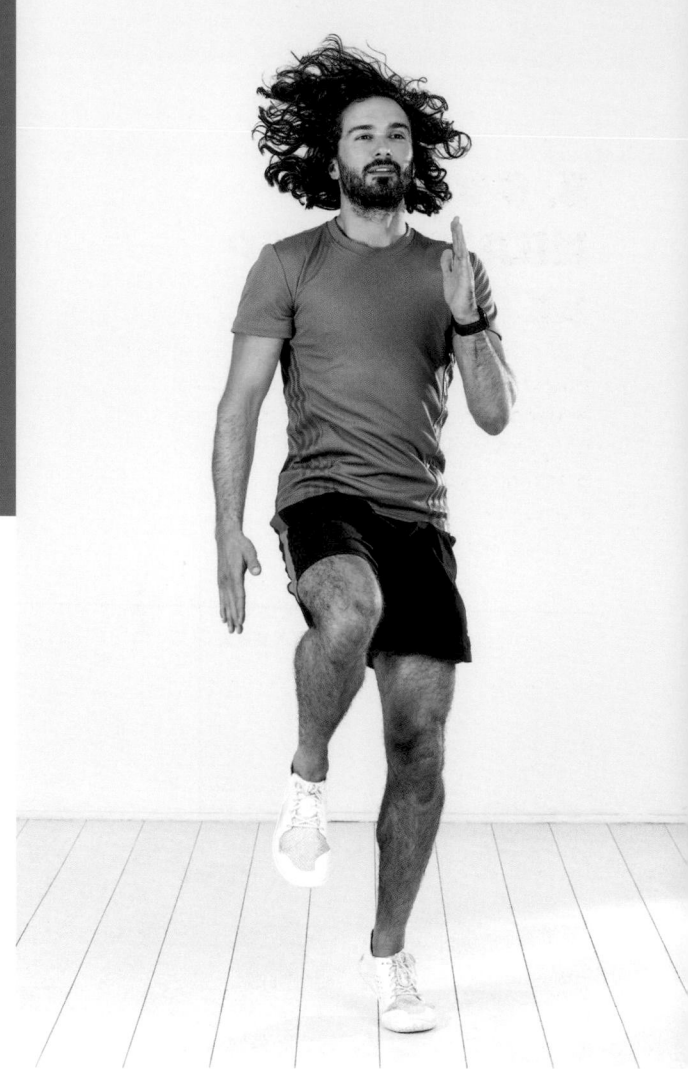

1. SPRINT

Run up and down on the spot as fast as you can. Lift knees high, keep your back straight and pump your arms to accelerate.

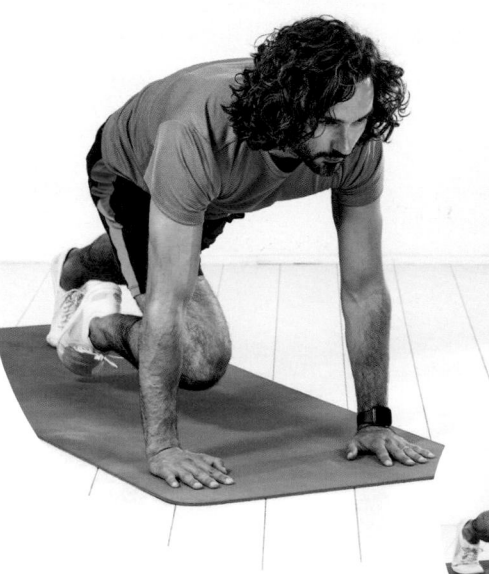

2. MOUNTAIN CLIMBERS

Start in a high plank position. Look down towards your hands and keep your back flat. Then drive your knees towards your chest as fast as possible one at a time.

3. SQUAT KICKS

Keep your core engaged as you lower down into a squat. As you push up to stand with one leg, bring your other knee up and kick your foot out in front of you. Place your feet back on the ground and repeat with the opposite legs.

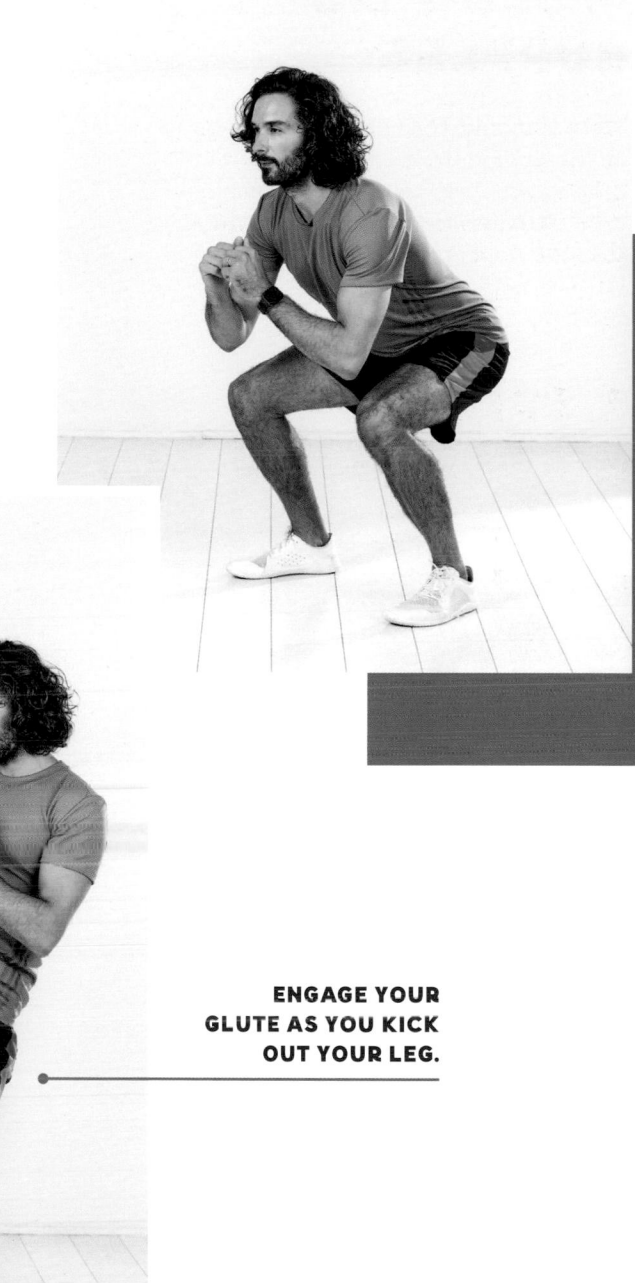

ENGAGE YOUR GLUTE AS YOU KICK OUT YOUR LEG.

4. SLOW MO BURPEES

Start standing, then place your hands on the floor in front of you. Slowly walk both of your feet back into a high plank. Walk both feet forward and then stand up straight. Repeat as fast as you can.

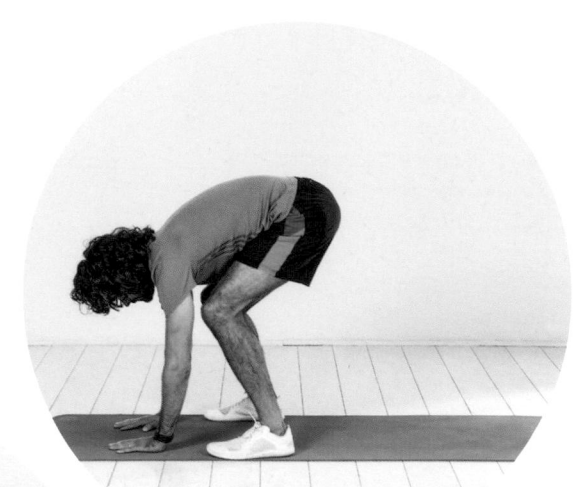

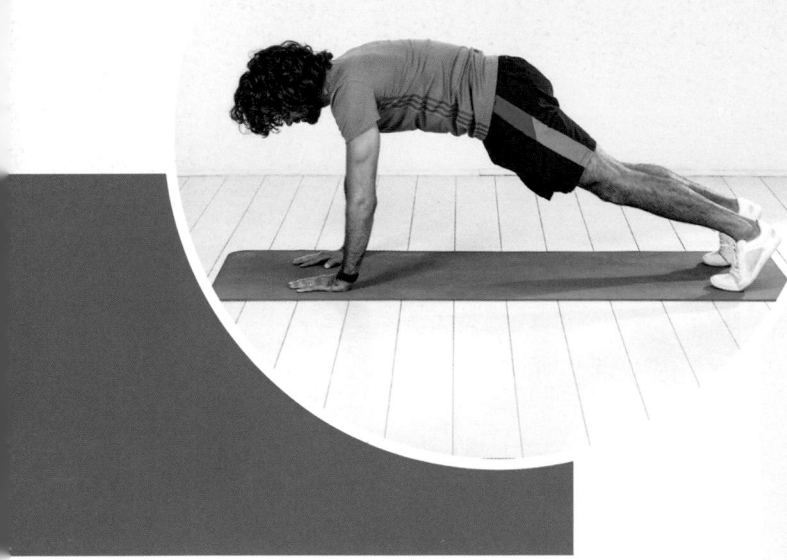

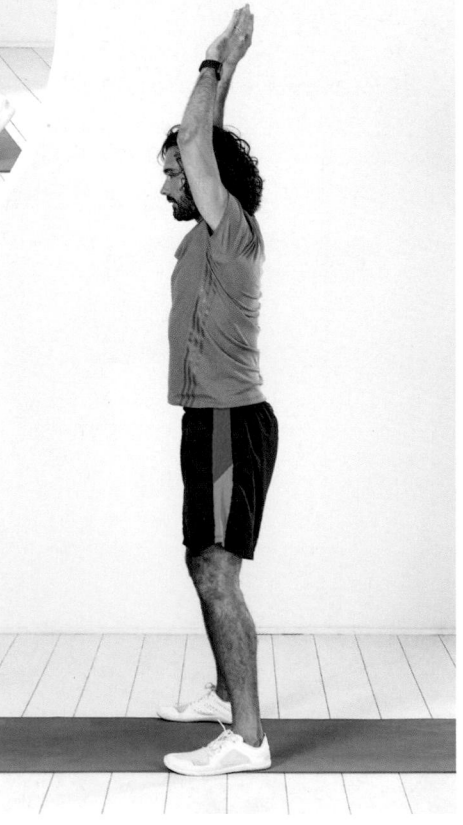

5. LATERAL LUNGES

Start with your legs shoulder-width apart. Take a big step to the side, keeping your back straight, and lower your standing leg. Push back up to starting position and repeat on the other side.

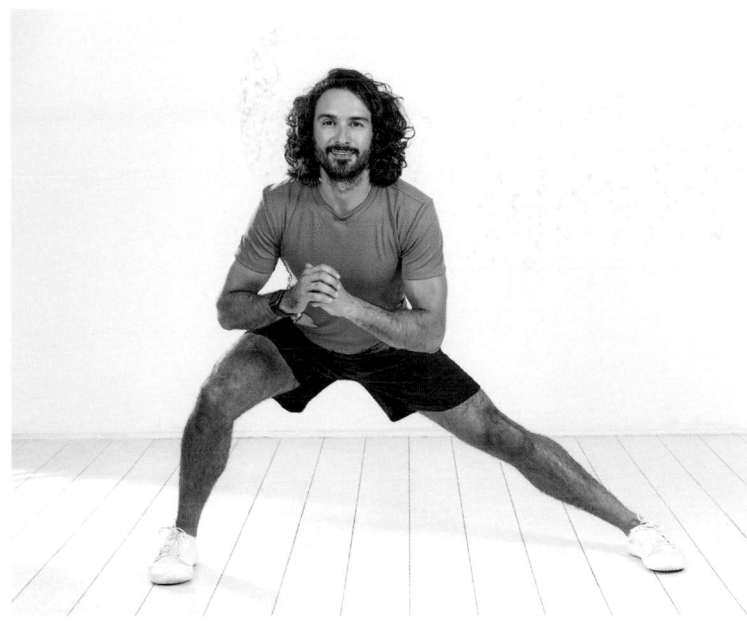

6. SQUAT LUNGE LUNGE

Start with your legs shoulder-width apart. Complete one slow and controlled squat then go straight into two reverse lunges. Repeat this sequence of one squat and two lunges.

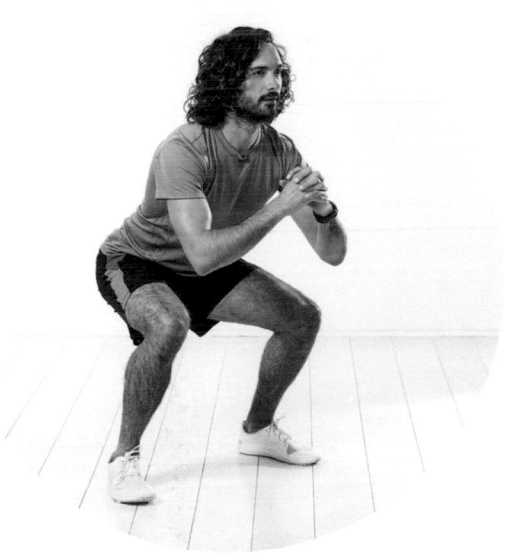

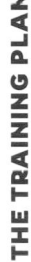

SINK DOWN LOW AS YOU KEEP YOUR BACK STRAIGHT.

THE TRAINING PLAN

7. JAB CROSS HOOK UPPERCUT KICKS

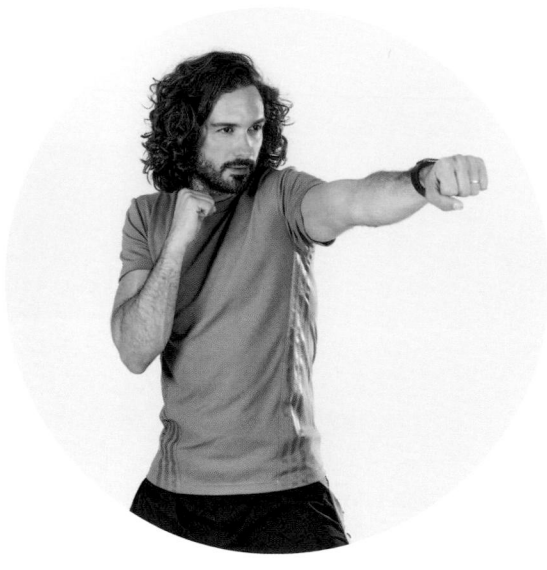

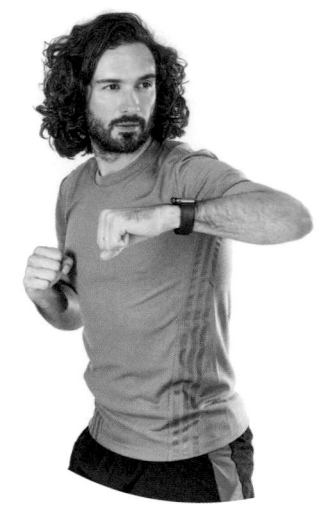

Stand with feet slightly wider than shoulder-width apart with one foot in front of the other. Keeping the hands up by the chin throw two straight punches. One left and one right directly in front of you.

Rotate the hips and bring the elbow up as you throw one hook punch to the chin.

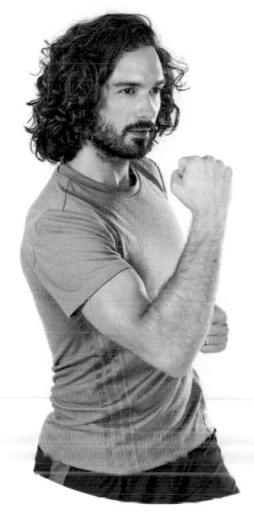

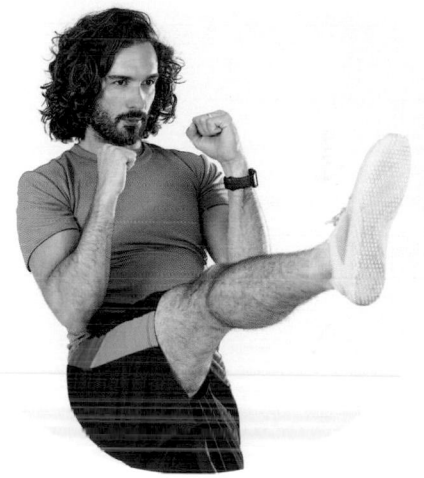

Follow up with an uppercut: come from low down and up to aim for the chin.

Finally kick your back standing leg forward once. Keep repeating this jab, cross, hook, uppercut and kick combo as fast as you can.

INTERMEDIATE
HIIT 2: RESISTANCE

(28 MINUTES)

**35 SECONDS WORK
/ 25 SECONDS REST**

X 4 ROUNDS IN TOTAL

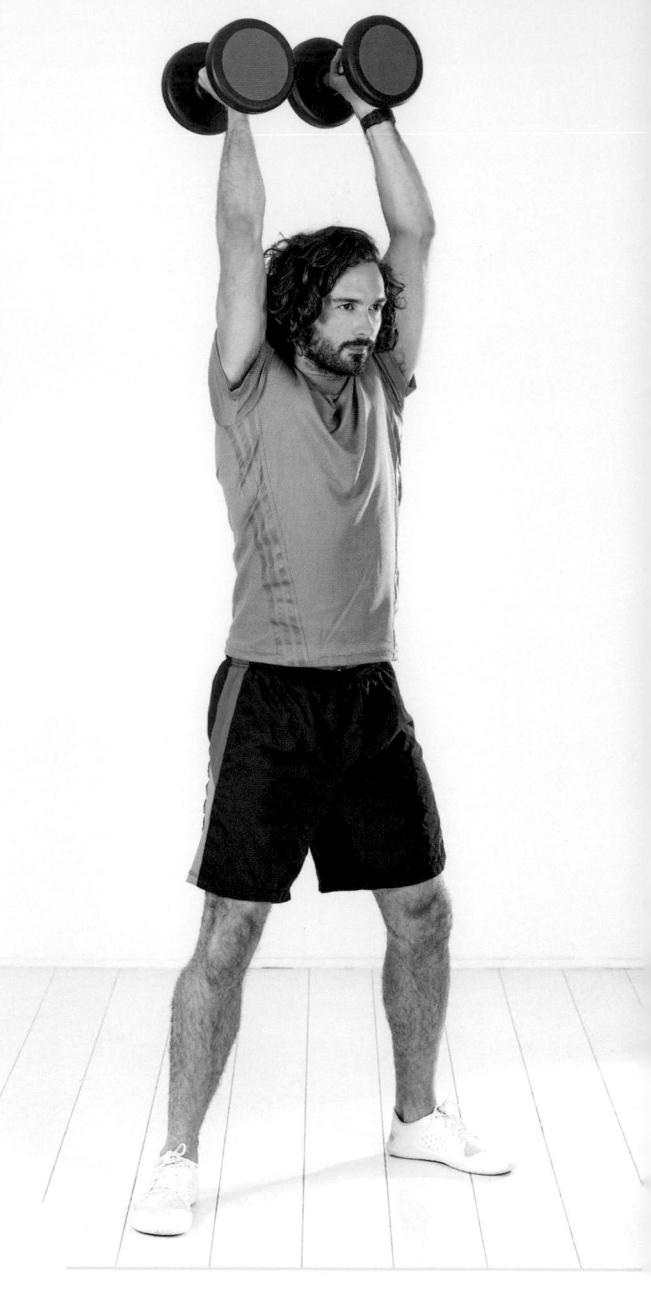

1. THRUSTERS

Hold your dumbbells at shoulder height. Squat down, keeping back straight, and thrust up to standing with your arms extended over your head. Lower the dumbbells to your shoulders and repeat.

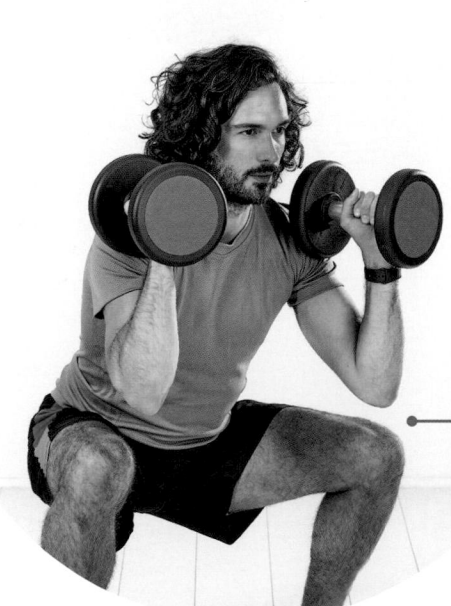

**AIM FOR YOUR THIGHS
TO BE PARALLEL
TO THE FLOOR.**

2. BICEP CURLS TO SHOULDER PRESS

This exercise combines two moves that target the biceps and your shoulders. First hammer curl the dumbbells and push straight up above the head.

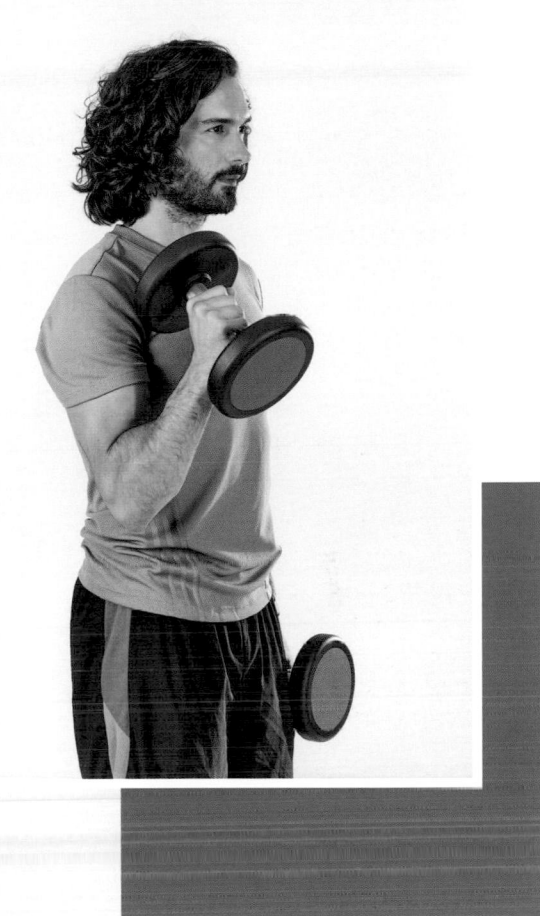

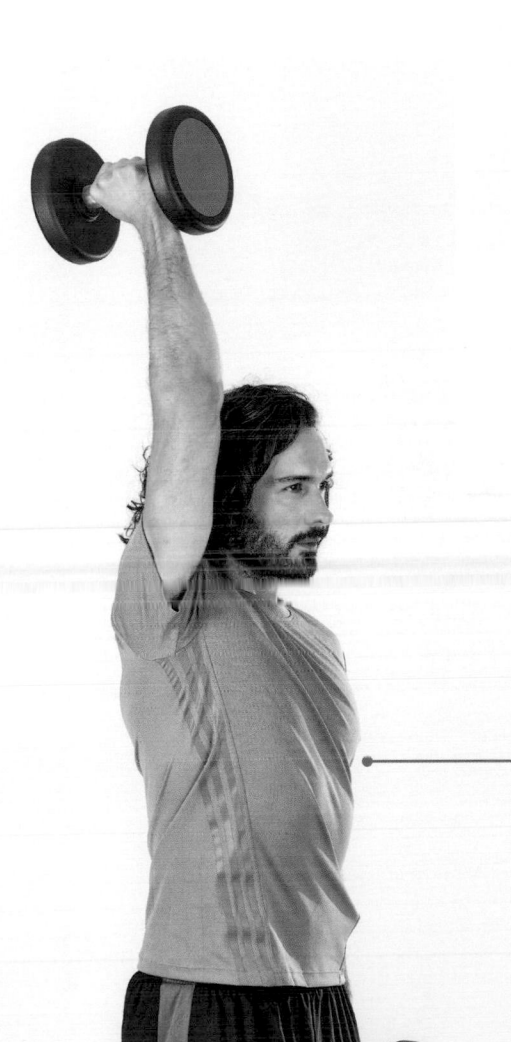

FULLY STRAIGHTEN YOUR ARMS AS YOU PUSH UP.

3. PRESS UPS

Start in a high plank position. Keep hands narrow and elbows close to the body. Lower yourself down towards the ground and push back up, fully extending your arms.

KEEP YOUR BACK STRAIGHT AS YOU GO DOWN.

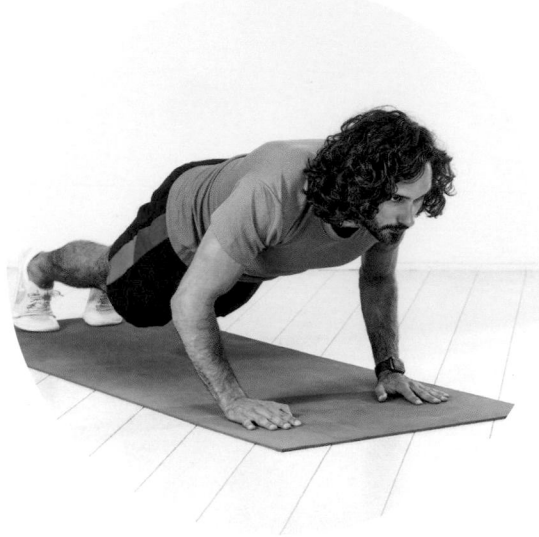

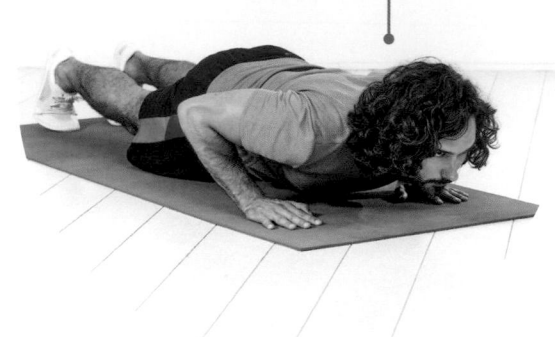

4. GOBLET SQUATS

Hold the kettlebell in both hands close to the chest as you lower down into a squat. Aim to keep your core engaged and back straight.

5. SINGLE ARM CLEAN AND PRESS

Standing with your legs shoulder-width apart, lift a dumbbell above your head, then bring it down to shoulder level before bending your knees and bringing it down to the floor in front of you. Bring it back up to shoulder height, then lift above your head. Repeat the whole sequence, swapping arms for the next round.

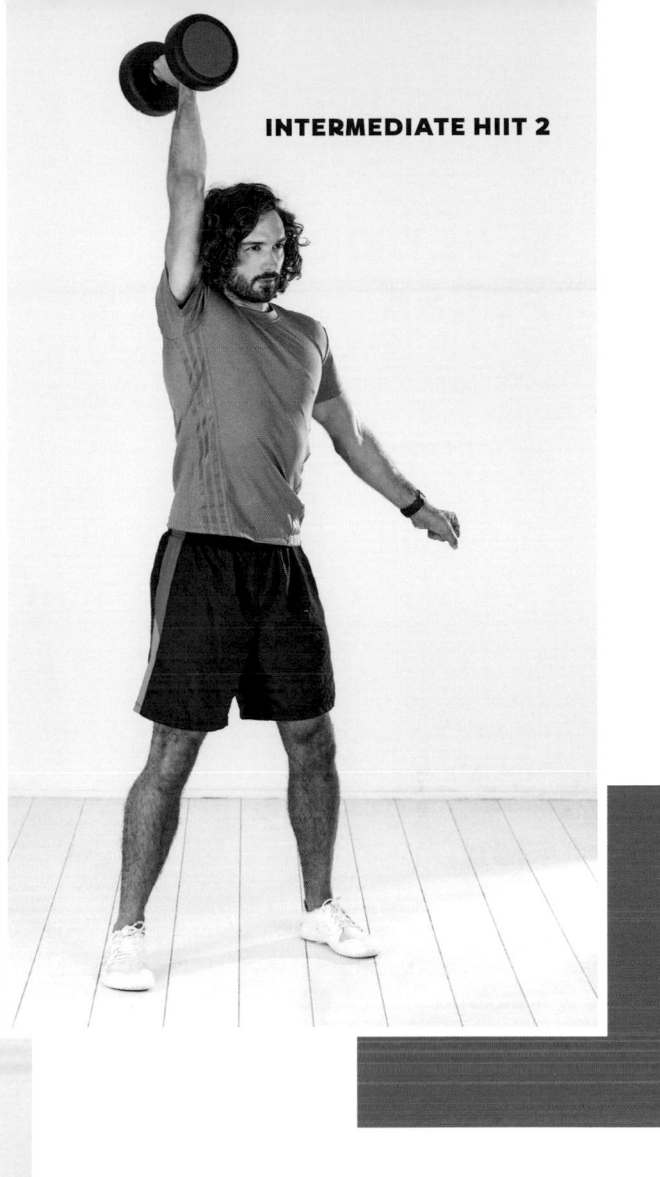

INTERMEDIATE HIIT 2

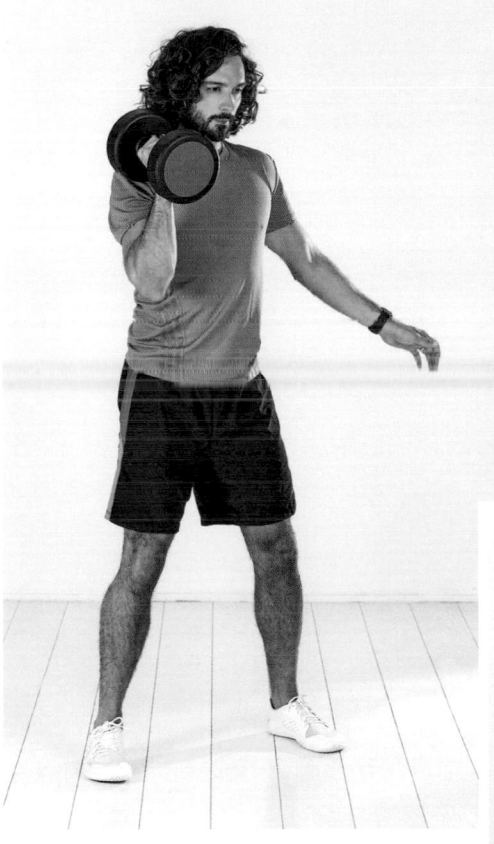

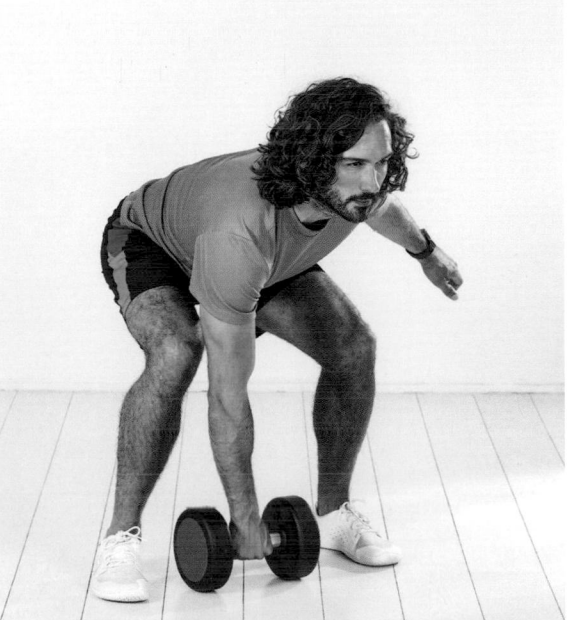

6. FLOOR PRESS

Lower the dumbbells slowly towards your chest and press upwards bringing the weights together.

KEEP YOUR LEGS BENT FOR EXTRA SUPPORT.

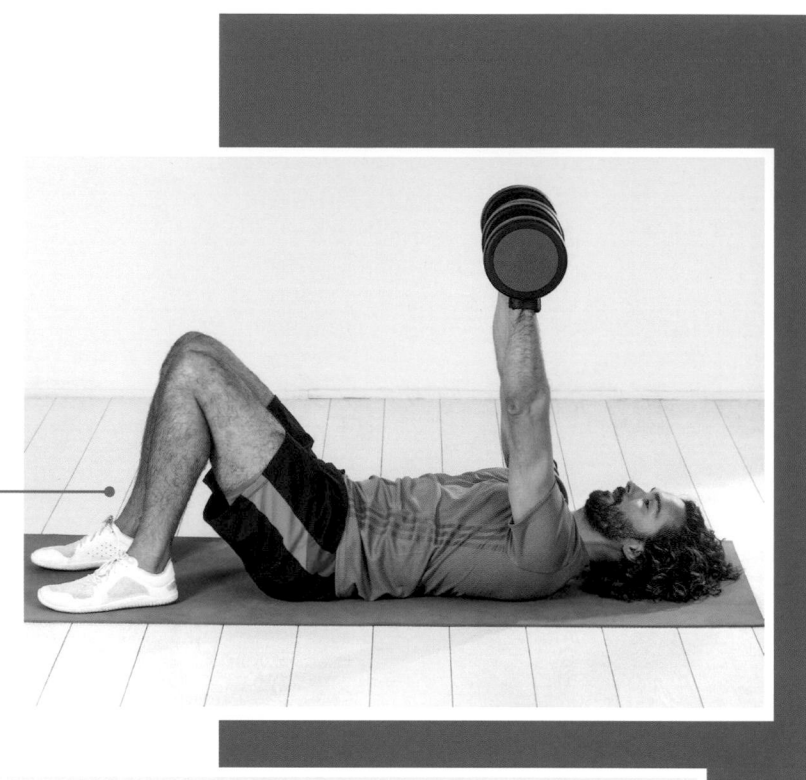

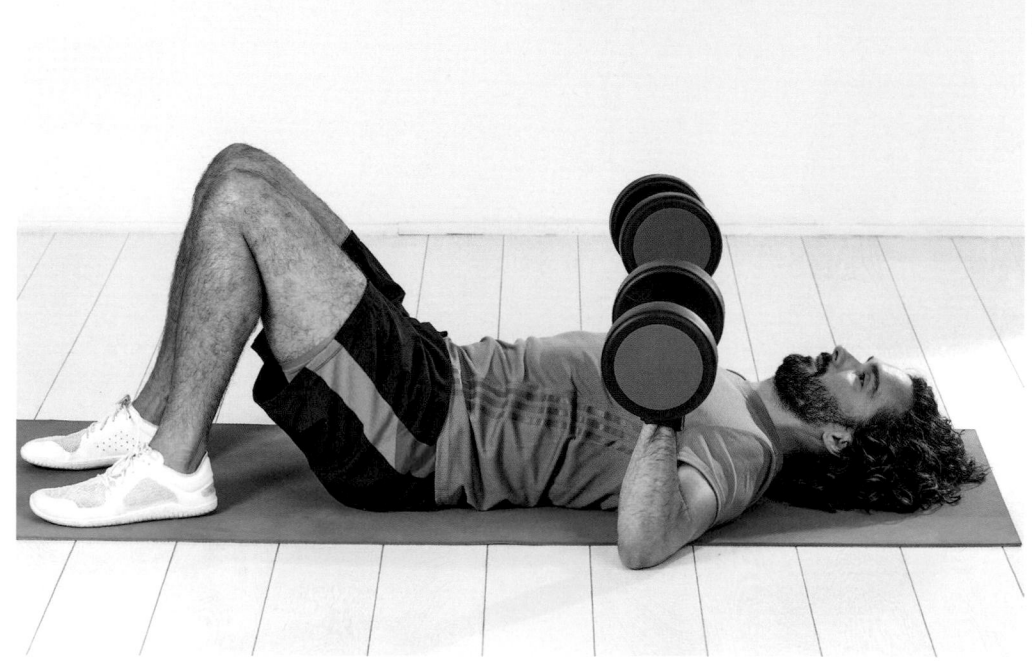

7. CURTSEY LUNGE

Stand up straight holding the dumbbells in each hand. Draw a semicircle with one foot, moving it clockwise until it crosses behind your other foot. Lunge, then slowly return to standing. Repeat on the other side.

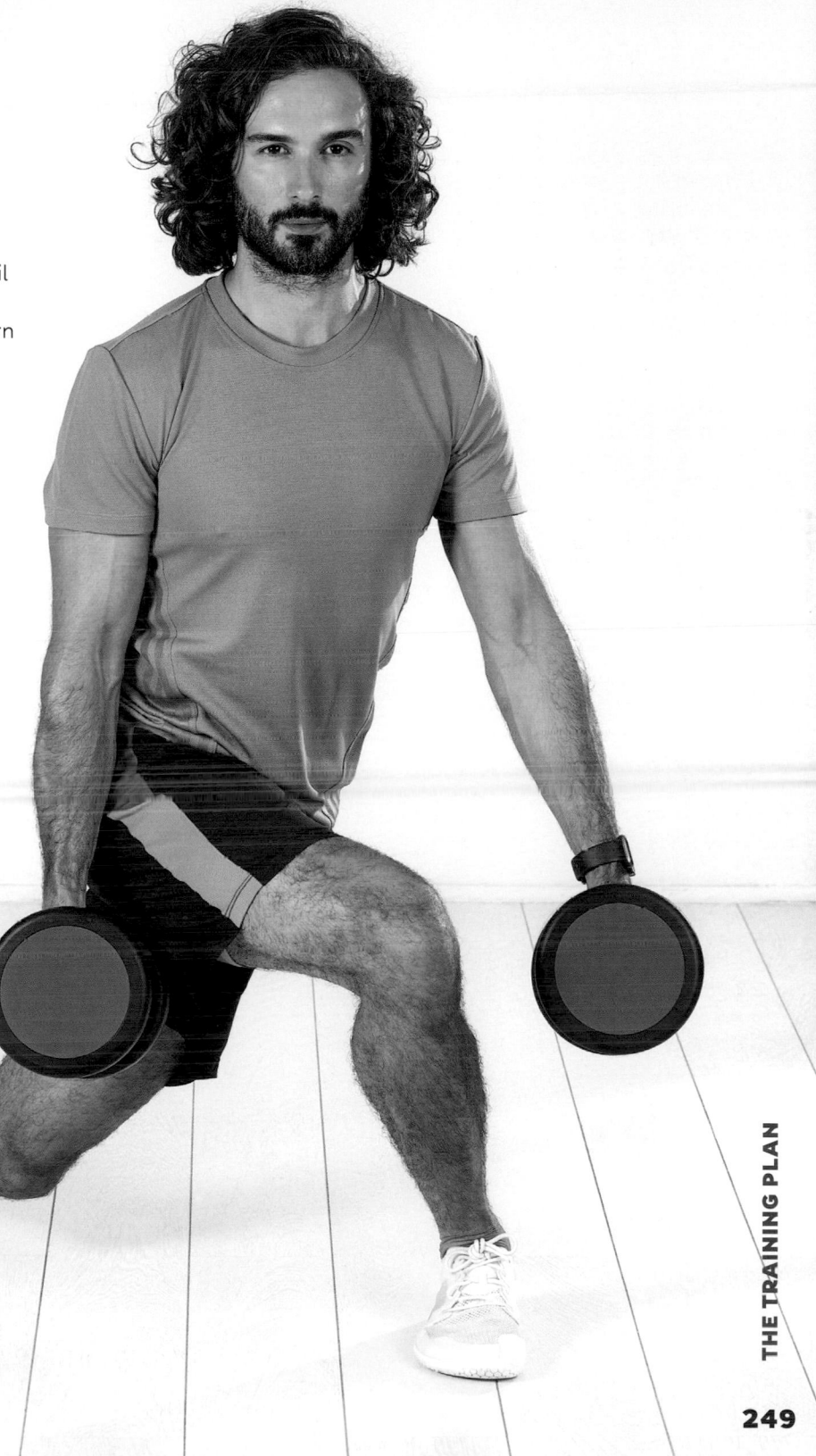

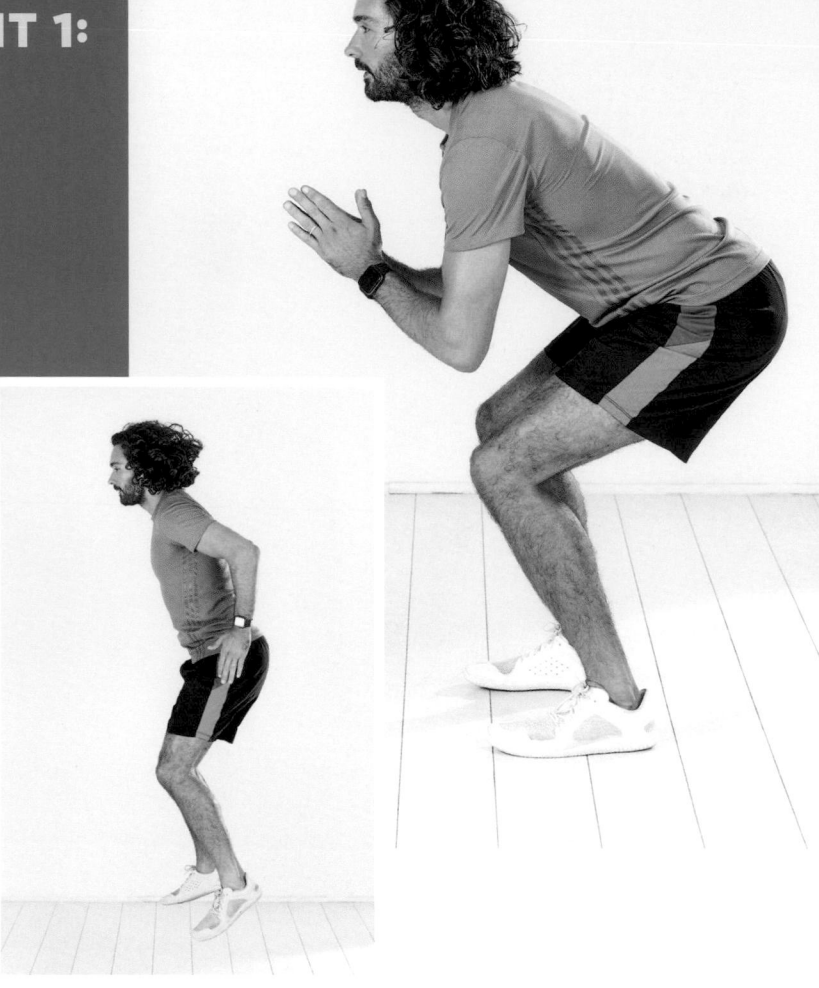

ADVANCED HIIT 1: BODYWEIGHT

(30 MINUTES)

40 SECONDS WORK / 20 SECONDS REST

X 3 ROUNDS IN TOTAL

1. SQUAT JUMPS

Place your feet in a comfortable position that will allow you to squat down while keeping them firmly flat on the ground. Sit low and drive through the heels to jump up. Repeat.

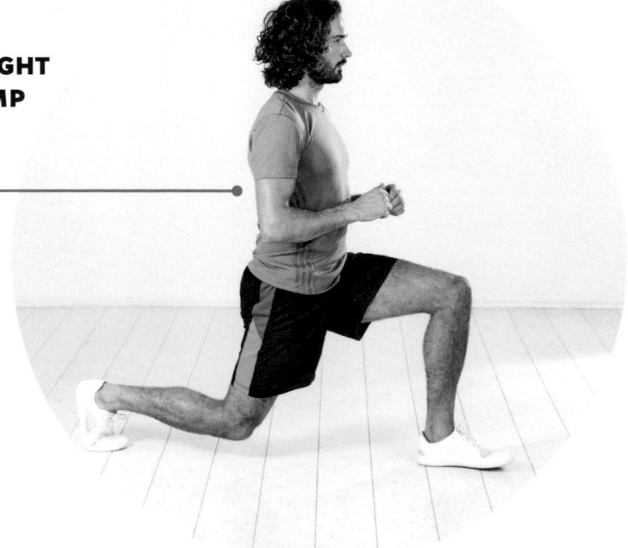

KEEP YOUR BACK STRAIGHT AS YOU JUMP INTO EACH LUNGE.

2. LUNGE JUMPS

Start with both feet together, then step forward with one foot and bend both knees into a lunge. Drive through your feet to jump straight into a lunge on the other side. Alternate each leg.

3. BURPEES

Start standing, then place your hands on the floor in front of you. Quickly kick back your legs into a high plank, then lower your chest to the ground. Push up, jump feet forward and jump up into a standing position. Repeat as fast as you can.

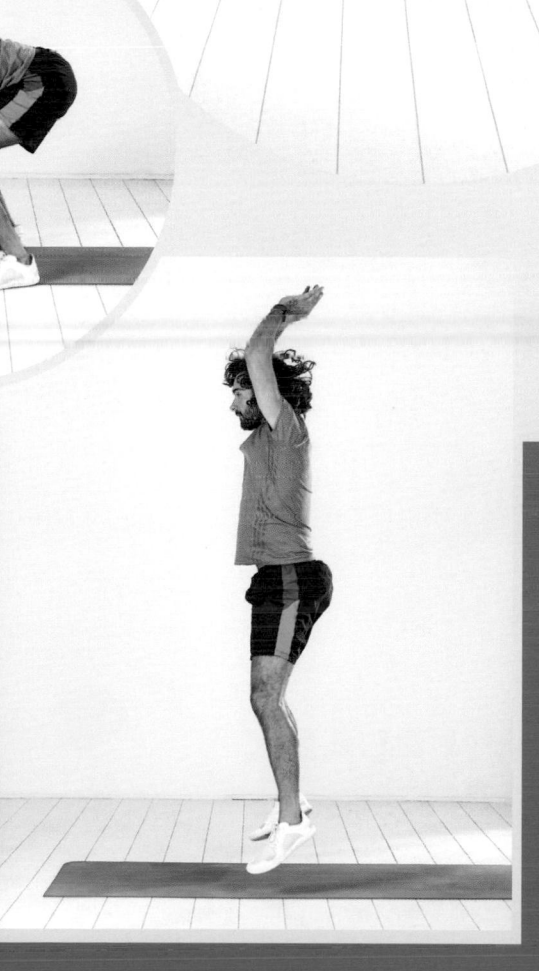

4. MOUNTAIN CLIMBERS

Start in a high plank position. Look down towards your hands and keep your back flat. Then drive your knees towards your chest as fast as possible one at a time.

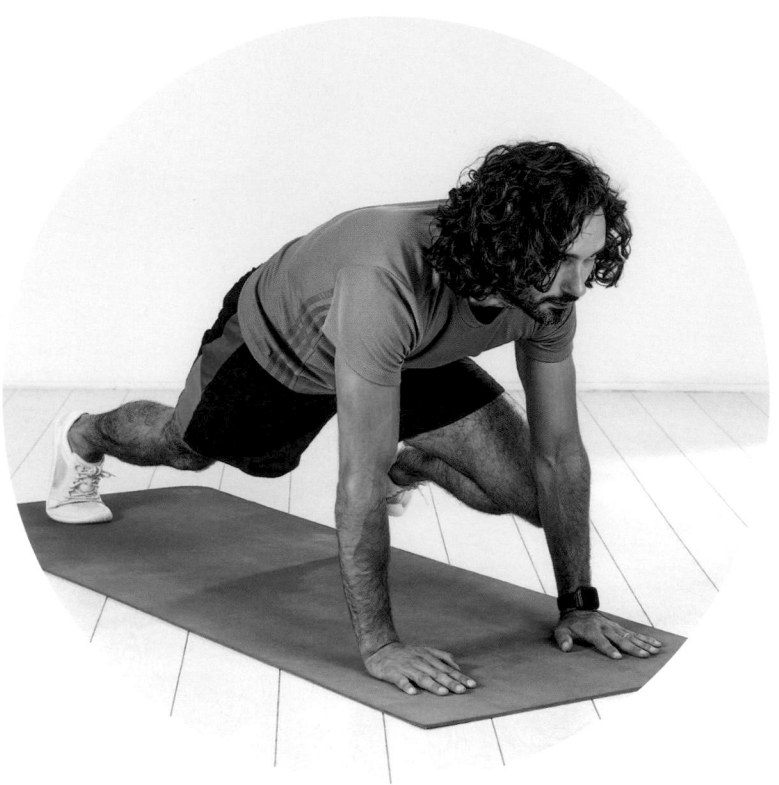

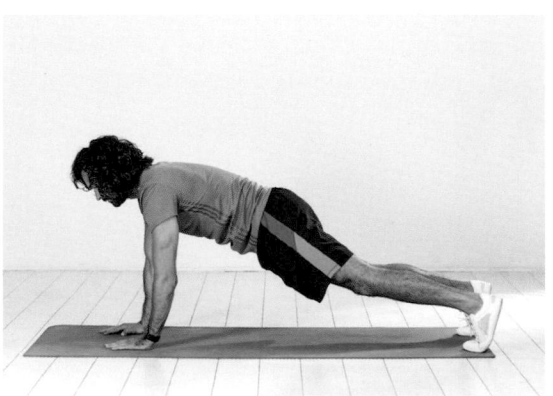

5. UP DOWN PLANK

Start by holding yourself up in the push-up position and lower your body down one elbow at a time. Then push yourself up to the start position with one hand at a time. Repeat as many times as you can.

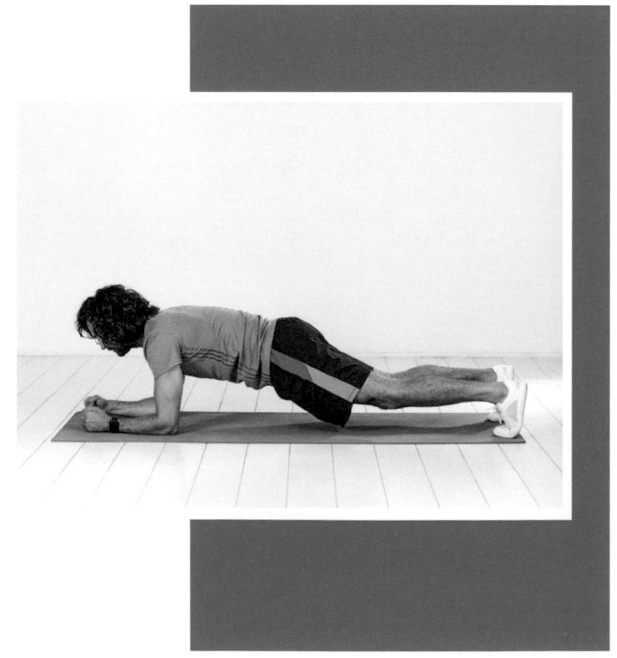

6. SPRINTS

Run up and down on the spot as fast as you can. Lift knees high, keep your back straight and pump your arms to accelerate.

7. BICYCLE CRUNCHES

Place your hands on your temples. As you crunch, try to twist so your opposite elbow touches your opposite knee.

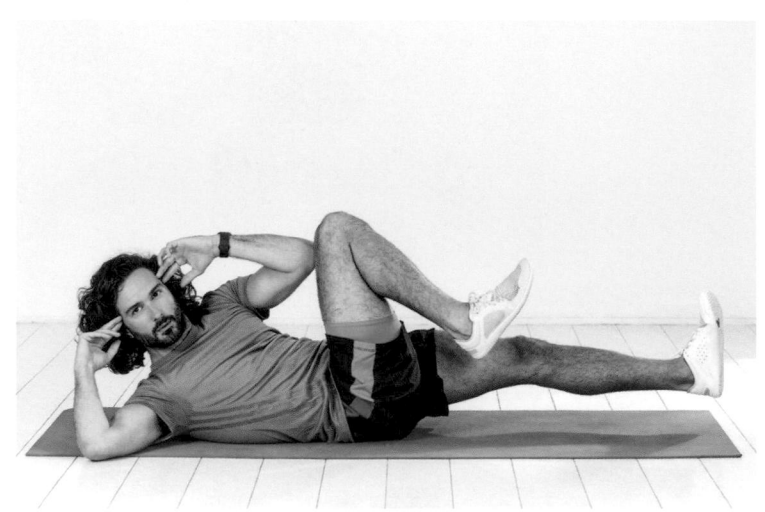

8. SPIDER CLIMBERS

Get down to plank position. Lift your left leg up and move it to the outside of your left foot. Move it back to plank and move your right leg to the outside of your right leg. Repeat.

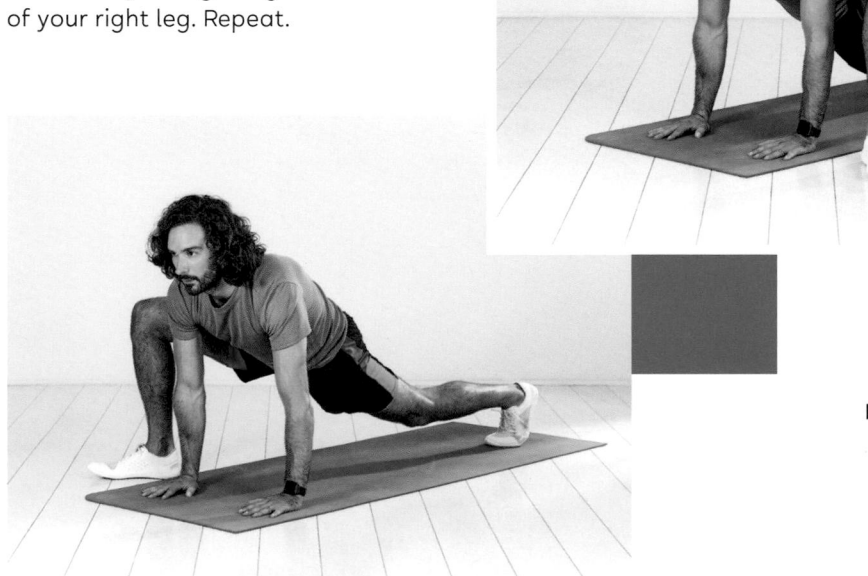

KEEP YOUR BACK LEG ENGAGED.

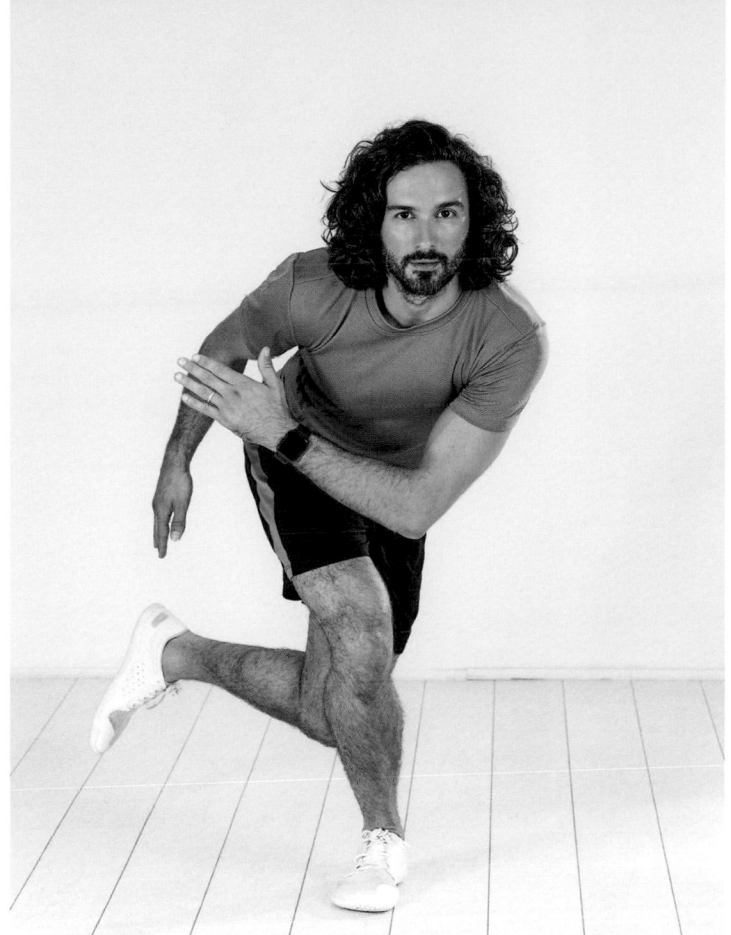

9. ICE SKATERS

Stand straight. Bring one leg behind the other and stretch out your leg diagonally behind you. Swing your arms as if you are ice-skating. Tap your toe, then jump to swap legs and move your arms in the opposite direction. Repeat.

10. CRAB TOE TOUCHES

Aim to lift your body off the ground and alternate between kicking your foot up to touch your toes. Left hand meets right foot and vice versa.

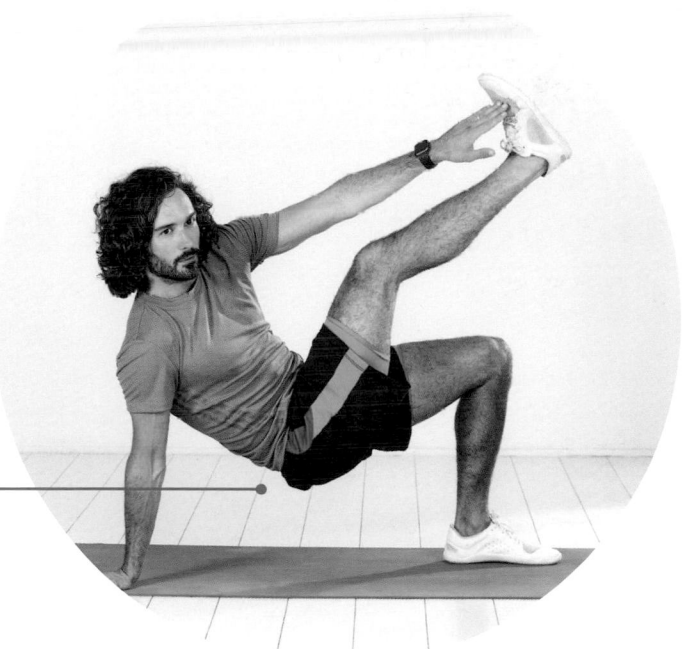

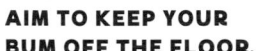

AIM TO KEEP YOUR BUM OFF THE FLOOR.

THE TRAINING PLAN

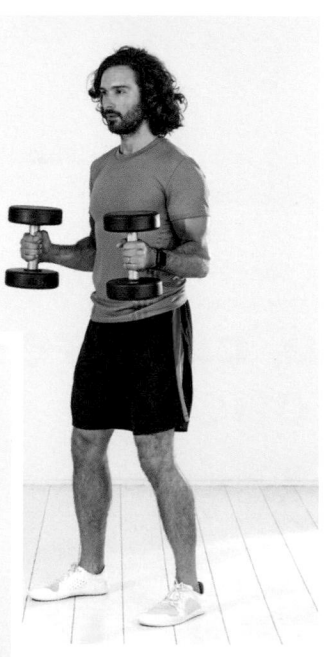

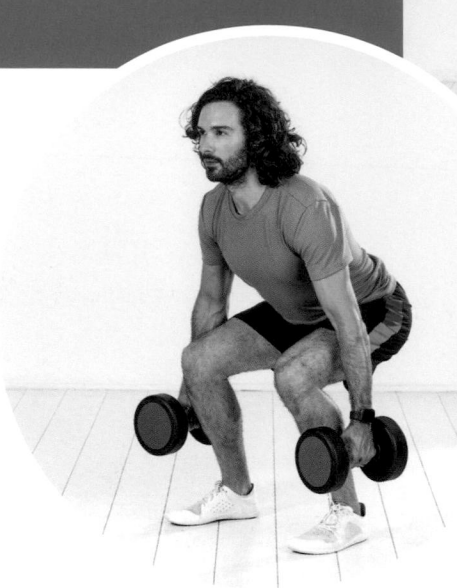

1. SQUAT, CURL, SHOULDER PRESS

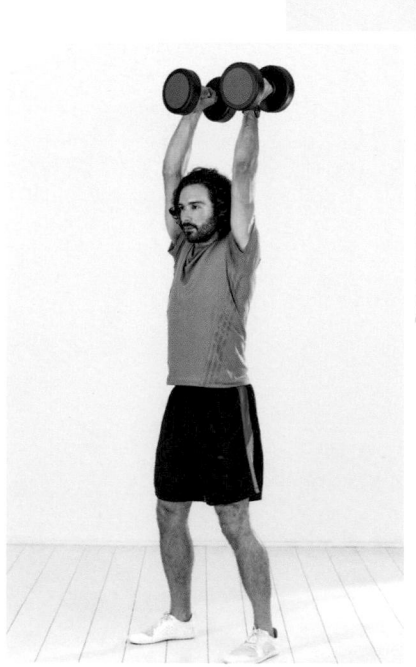

This move brings together three separate exercises in one. Begin by squatting down holding the dumbbells at your side. Push up and curl the dumbbells in front before lifting them above your head. Bring the dumbbells down and repeat.

2. LATERAL SHOULDER RAISE

Hold one dumbbell in each hand and, using your shoulders, raise them up each side until they are parallel with the ground. Repeat.

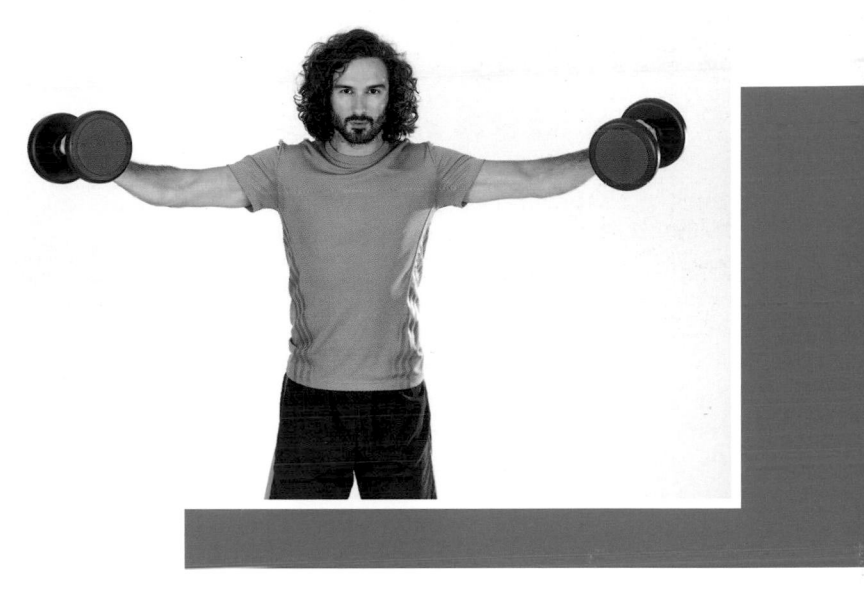

3. FRONT DUMBBELL SQUATS

Hold one dumbbell in each hand and lift to your shoulders. Bend your knees to lower yourself into a squat position. Keep your back straight and chest up, then stand. Repeat.

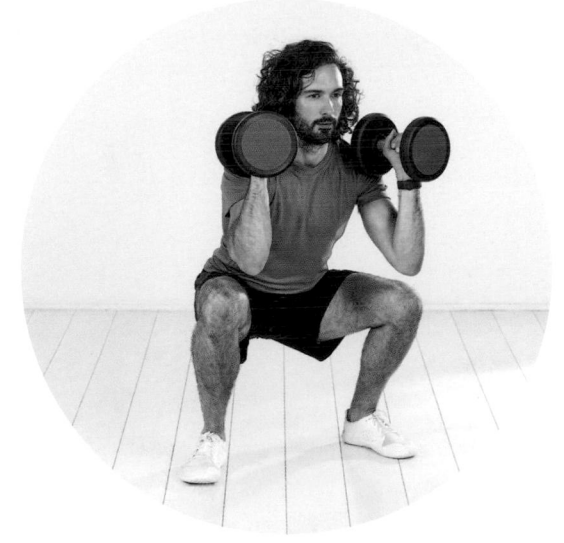

DRIVE THROUGH THE HEELS OF YOUR FEET TO STAND.

4. FLOOR PRESS X 10 INTO 10 PUSH UPS

Start on your back. Lower the dumbbells slowly towards your chest and press upwards bringing the weights together. Repeat 10 times. Turn over into a plank position. Start in a high plank position. Keep hands narrow and elbows close to the body. Lower yourself down towards the ground and push back up, fully extending your arms. Repeat 10 times.

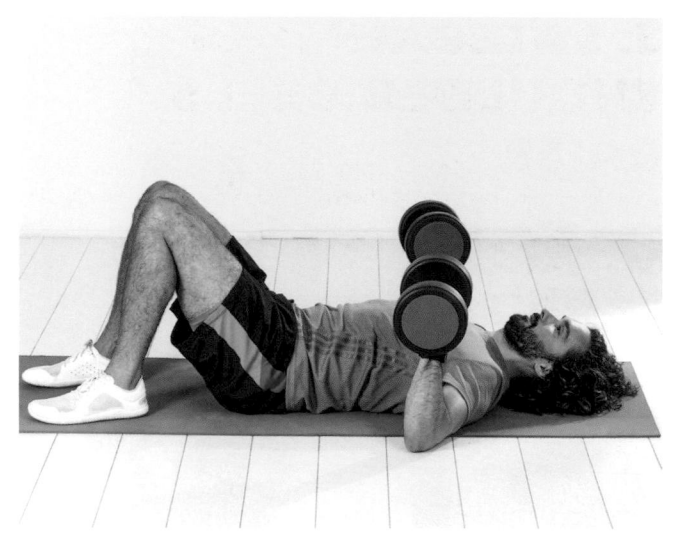

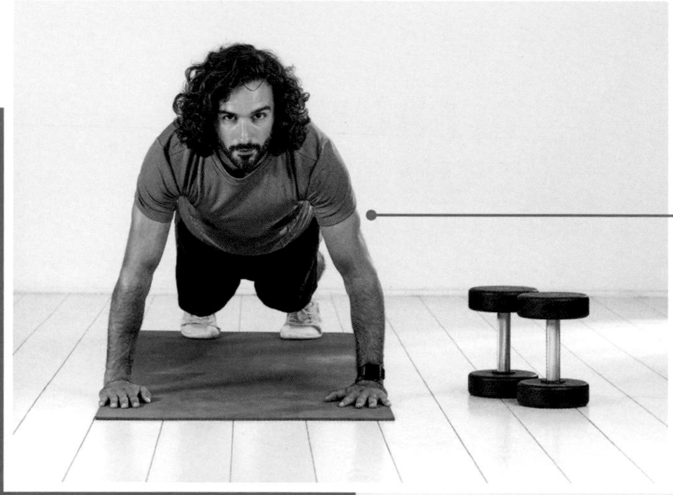

KEEP YOUR GLUTES AND ABS ENGAGED IN HIGH PLANK.

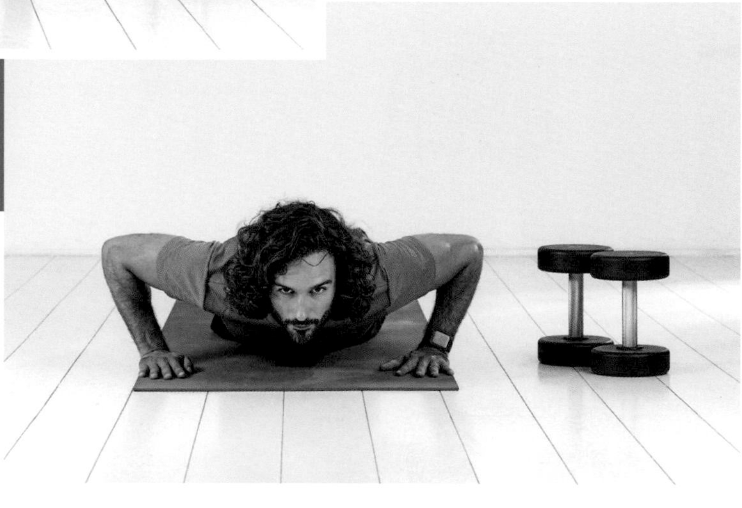

5. SQUAT PULSES WITH DUMBBELLS

Hold the dumbbells at your sides. Place your feet a comfortable distance apart and lower yourself as if you're about to sit into a chair. Rather than standing up fully, just pulse up and down.

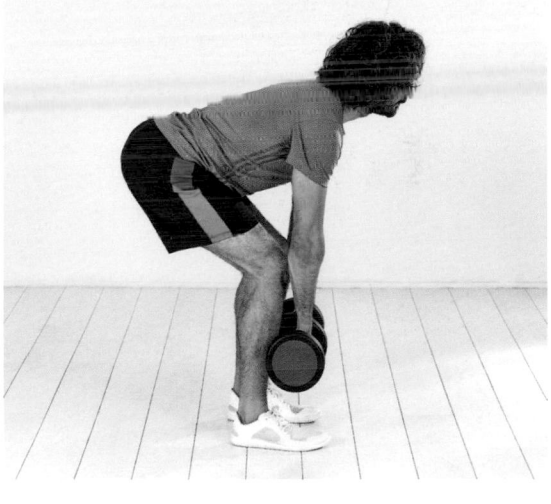

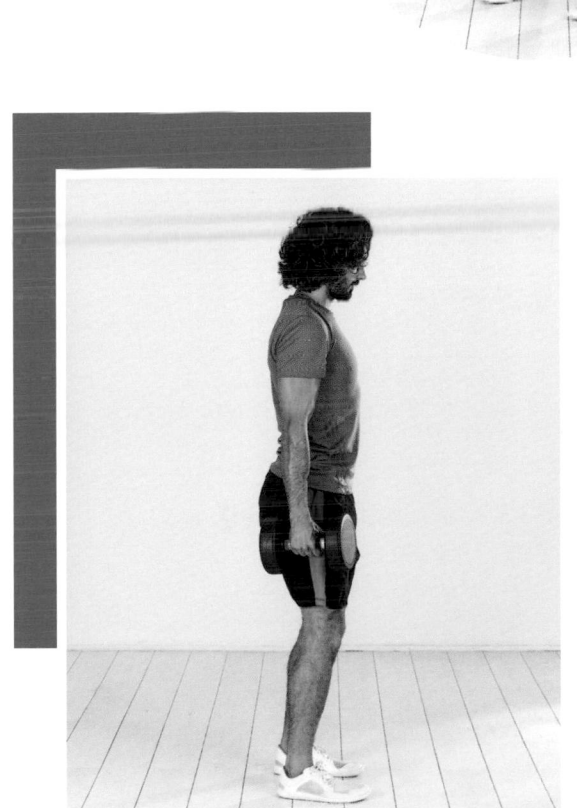

6. ROMANIAN LIFTS

Keep your back straight, bend at the hips and lower the dumbbells towards the ground, keeping tension on the hamstrings. Stand up straight and repeat.

THE TRAINING PLAN

THE 30 DAY PLAN

1 On an exercise day you should aim to eat two reduced-carb meals (RC), one post-workout meal (PW) and two snacks. On a rest day you could aim to eat three reduced-carb meals and two snacks.

2 This is a 30 day sample plan split into weeks to show you how your routine may look if you decided to exercise for 5 days and rest for 2 days. Adjust to whatever works for you: you may find it easier with your lifestyle routine to exercise 4 days a week. If you do this, think about your food choices carefully on that extra rest day.

3 On an exercise day, aim to have your carb refuel meal after you workout, as this helps refuel and replenish your muscles. For instance, if you exercise in the morning, for best results have a carb-loaded breakfast. If you train in the evening then save your carb refuel meal for dinner. In the plan I have varied things a bit in case you exercise in the evening, so mix things up and make it work for you. This is a guideline too and doesn't have to be strictly followed each day.

4 Pick and choose your exercise plan according to your level of experience using The Training Plan on pages 222–59. Don't forget you could choose low-intensity steady state (LISS) workouts instead of HIIT. To see results you might want to increase the intensity of these activities so you're doing them every day, but find what works for you. The key is consistently turning up and introducing activity into your routine.

5 For the purposes of this plan and to showcase the tasty food in this book, I've varied meals and mixed things up through the weeks, but feel free to repeat meals you love and don't feel at all limited to this plan. It might be easier for you to repeat lunches through the week or enjoy them on rotation. Some of the recipes in the book serve 2 or 4 so I have made suggestions for eating leftovers the next day: a great way to save time and effort.

6 My portions are generous, so don't forget to adjust them according to your appetite and how active you have been that week. All the more leftovers!

7 Week 2 is a flexible veggie plan. You could choose to have a completely veggie week by following the veggie swaps as detailed in my recipes. If you like a more varied diet, you can mix this up and pick and choose your options.

THE 30 DAY PLAN

WEEK 1	DAY 1	DAY 2	DAY 3	DAY 4	DAY 5	DAY 6	DAY 7
EXERCISE	**MORNING WORKOUT**	**LUNCHTIME WORKOUT**	**MORNING WORKOUT**	**REST**	**MORNING WORKOUT**	**EVENING WORKOUT**	**REST**
BREAKFAST	**PW** Overnight oats/porridge	**RC** Carrot, orange and ginger smoothie (*page 35*)	**PW** Overnight oats/porridge	**RC** PBJ smoothie (*page 32*)	**PW** Overnight oats/porridge	**RC** Elvis pancakes (*page 36*)	**RC** Manchego, chilli jam and olive frittata (*page 38*)
SNACK 1	75g blueberries	Boiled egg protein pot with spinach and tahini (*page 134*)	30g nuts and seeds	An apple	Boiled egg protein pot with spinach and tahini (*page 134*)	30g nuts and seeds	75g blueberries
LUNCH	**RC** Cayenne pollock with minted pea yoghurt sauce and baby gem (*page 64*)	**PW** Chicken pho (*page 146*)	**RC** Seeded chicken schnitzel salad (*page 103*)	**RC** Tuna, white bean, marinated feta and salsa verde (*page 52*)	**RC** Leftover curried cottage pie (*page 82*)	**RC** Chorizo niçoise salad (*page 71*)	**RC** Thai green pork lettuce cups (*page 90*)
SNACK 2	30g nuts and seeds	An apple	Walnut and roasted red pepper dip with crudités (*page 140*)	30g nuts and seeds	A handful of olives	75g blueberries	30g nuts and seeds
DINNER	**RC** Chicken souvlaki with tzatziki, sliced tomato and olives (*page 117*)	**RC** Peanut butter, mushroom, spinach and tomato stew (*page 130*)	**RC** Tikka masala, halloumi and chickpea kachumba (*page 129*)	**RC** Curried cottage pie (*page 82*)	**RC** Soy, five spice and orange chicken with little trees (*page 74*)	**PW** Tandoori chicken burger with cucumber raita (*page 174*)	**RC** Mediterranean halloumi traybake (*page 110*)

WEEK 2	DAY 8	DAY 9	DAY 10	DAY 11	DAY 12	DAY 13	DAY 14
EXERCISE	MORNING WORKOUT	EVENING WORKOUT	REST	MORNING WORKOUT	LUNCHTIME WORKOUT	EVENING WORKOUT	REST
BREAKFAST	PW Overnight oats/porridge	RC Sweetcorn fritters with chorizo, mango and avocado salsa (or to be veggie swap chorizo for feta; page 106)	RC Chai spiced banana smoothie (page 32)	PW Overnight oats/porridge	RC PBJ smoothie (page 32)	RC Elvis pancakes (page 36)	RC Spicy Turkish scrambled eggs (page 40)
SNACK 1	30g nuts and seeds	Hummus on a cracker	An apple	Dark chocolate, almond and sea salt clusters (page 142)	75g blueberries	An apple	30g nuts and seeds
LUNCH	RC Manchego, chilli jam and olive frittata (page 38)	RC Sesame cauliflower, pomegranate and mixed herb salad with tahini dressing (page 48)	RC Creamy coconut, carrot and sweet potato soup with chilli paneer croutons (page 131)	RC Poached salmon with cream cheese and scrambled eggs (or to be veggie swap salmon for asparagus; page 63)	PW Black bean, quinoa and sweet potato chilli (page 170)	RC Salt and pepper prawns with sweet chilli (or to be veggie swap prawns for tofu; page 100)	RC Coronation chicken salad (or to be veggie, swap chicken for cauliflower; page 115)
SNACK 2	An apple	75g blueberries	Walnut and roasted red pepper dip with crudités (page 140)	30g nuts and seeds	Boiled egg protein pot with spinach and tahini (page 134)	30g nuts and seeds	An apple
DINNER	RC Beetroot and feta patties with molasses and tomato salad (page 120)	PW Bombay potato hash with halloumi (page 178)	RC Tuna, white bean, marinated feta and salsa verde (or to be veggie swap tuna for courgette; page 52)	RC Saag paneer with cauliflower 'rice' (page 94)	RC Turkey and red pepper panang curry (to be veggie swap turkey for tofu; page 122)	PW Leftover black bean, quinoa and sweet potato chilli (page 170)	RC Mediterranean halloumi traybake (page 110)

VEGGIE WEEK: All recipes this week are either veggie, or feature a simple veggie swap (see specific recipe pages for details).

WEEK 3	DAY 15	DAY 16	DAY 17	DAY 18	DAY 19	DAY 20	DAY 21
EXERCISE	MORNING WORKOUT	REST	EVENING WORKOUT	MORNING WORKOUT	REST	MORNING WORKOUT	LUNCHTIME WORKOUT
BREAKFAST	**PW** Parma ham and pesto poached egg bagel *(page 190)*	**RC** Blueberry smoothie *(page 35)*	**PW** Poached salmon with cream cheese and chive scrambled eggs *(page 63)*	**PW** Overnight oats/porridge	**RC** Golden smoothie *(page 35)*	**PW** Overnight oats/porridge	**RC** Manchego, chilli jam and olive frittata *(page 38)*
SNACK 1	75g blueberries	An apple	30g nuts and seeds	Hummus on a cracker	30g nuts and seeds	An apple	75g blueberries
LUNCH	**RC** Salt and pepper prawns with sweet chilli *(page 100)*	**RC** Steak fajita fried eggs *(page 67)*	**RC** Sesame cauliflower, pomegranate and mixed herb salad with tahini dressing *(page 48)*	**PW** Leftover beef cobbler with chive and horseradish dumplings *(page 148)*	**RC** Paprika prawn, corn and cheddar chowder *(page 68)*	**RC** Wasabi tuna mayo 'poke bowl' *(page 50)*	**PW** Lancashire hotpot *(page 152)*
SNACK 2	30g nuts and seeds	Walnut and roasted red pepper dip with crudités *(page 140)*	75g blueberries	An apple	Dark chocolate, almond and sea salt clusters *(page 142)*	Walnut and roasted red pepper dip with crudités *(page 140)*	30g nuts and seeds
DINNER	**RC** Seared steak, blue cheese, pear and watercress *(page 62)*	**RC** Grilled lamb chops with warm hummus, quick pickled red onions and pistachios *(page 86)*	**PW** Beef cobbler with chive and horseradish dumplings *(page 148)*	**RC** Sea bass with pesto and charred courgette, chilli and mint *(page 112)*	**RC** Steak haché *(page 102)*	**PW** Almond butter satay chicken with Asian slaw *(page 98)*	**RC** Lamb and pea keema *(page 105)*

THE 30 DAY PLAN

WEEK 4-5	DAY 22	DAY 23	DAY 24	DAY 25	DAY 26	DAY 27	DAY 28	DAY 29	DAY 30
EXERCISE	MORNING WORKOUT	EVENING WORKOUT	LUNCHTIME WORKOUT	REST	MORNING WORKOUT	EVENING WORKOUT	LUNCHTIME WORKOUT	REST	EVENING WORKOUT
BREAKFAST	PW Overnight oats/porridge	RC Carrot, orange and ginger smoothie (*page 35*)	RC Chai spiced banana smoothie (*page 32*)	RC Blueberry smoothie (*page 35*)	PW Overnight oats/porridge	RC Elvis pancakes (*page 36*)	RC Sausage shakshuka (*page 76*)	RC PBJ smoothie (*page 32*)	RC Golden smoothie (*page 35*)
SNACK 1	30g nuts and seeds	75g blueberries	Hummus on a cracker	An apple	Boiled egg protein pot with spinach and tahini (*page 134*)	30g nuts and seeds	An apple	75g blueberries	Hummus on a cracker
LUNCH	RC Wasabi tuna mayo 'poke bowl' (*page 50*)	RC Thai green pork lettuce cups (*page 90*)	PW Soy mushroom banh mi (*page 172*)	RC Cumin-spiced lamb and feta fattoush (*page 61*)	RC Grilled chicken cobb salad (*page 69*)	RC Blackened cod with pico de gallo salsa and smashed avo (*page 45*)	PW Leftover chicken and chorizo filo pie (*page 162*)	RC Parma ham and sundried tomato parmigiana (*page 126*)	RC Coronation chicken salad (*page 115*)
SNACK 2	An apple	Hummus on a cracker	75g blueberries	30g nuts and seeds	75g blueberries	An apple	Dark chocolate, almond and sea salt clusters (*page 142*)	30g nuts and seeds	Boiled egg protein pot with spinach and tahini (*page 134*)
DINNER	RC Chipolatas in onion gravy with buttery carrot and parsnip smash (*page 56*)	PW Lamb rogan josh (*page 165*)	RC Parma ham and sundried tomato parmigiana (*page 126*)	RC Prawn and lemongrass coconut curry with mange tout (*page 58*)	RC Tomato-baked cod with capers and pine nuts (*page 124*)	PW Chicken and chorizo filo pie (*page 162*)	RC Tikka masala, halloumi and chickpea kachumba (*page 129*)	RC Seared steak, blue cheese, pear and watercress (*page 62*)	PW Kale and walnut pesto gnocchi (*page 150*)

INDEX

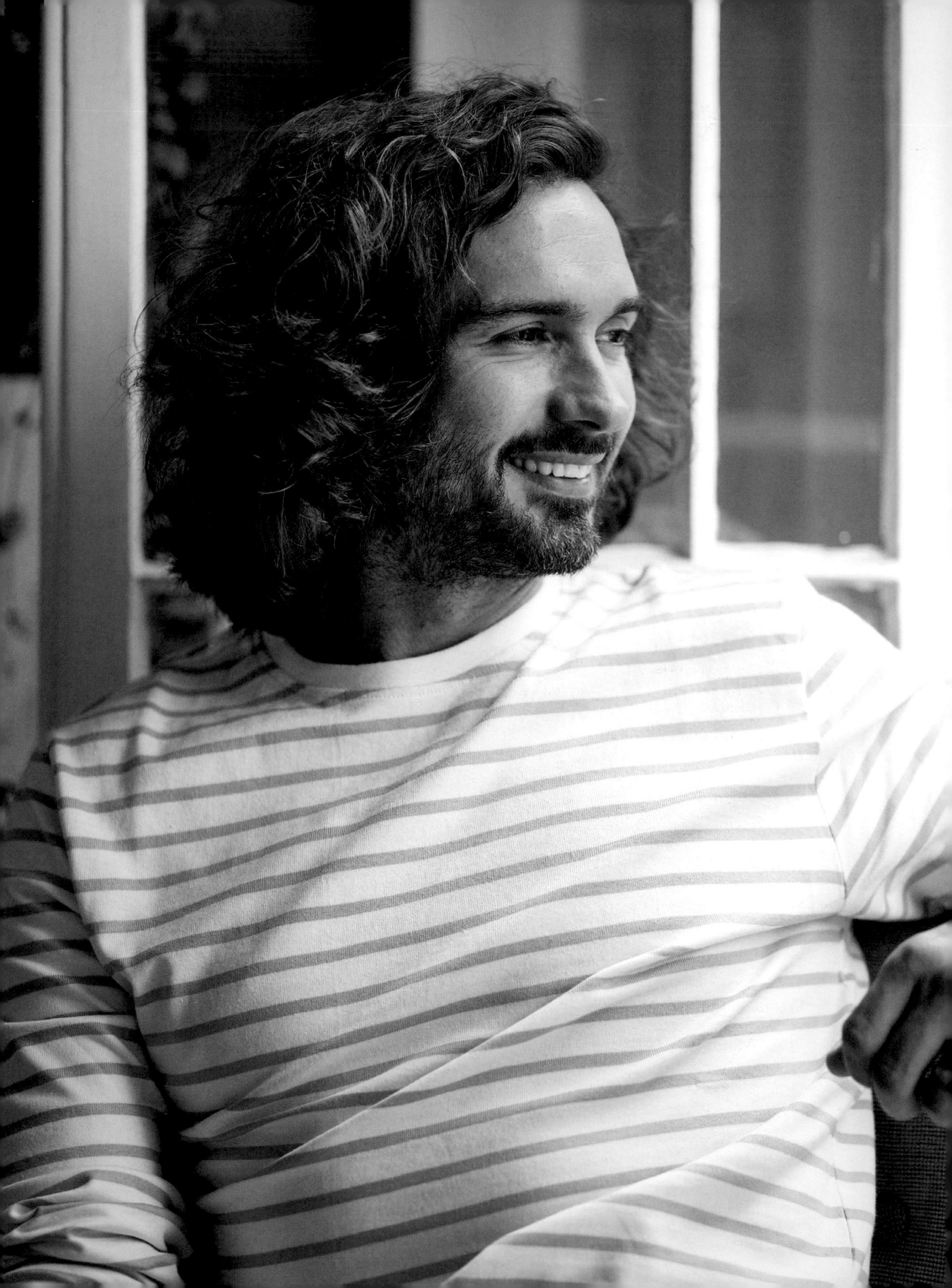

ACKNOWLEDGEMENTS

I'd like to start by saying a big thank you to my team at Bluebird for helping me create yet another book I'm really proud of. This is my ninth book in five years and I feel so fortunate to have been able to work with you all and have your support.

I also love every single photo in the book and would like to say thank you to the team who created all the images. Andrew, Natalie, Charlie, Nikki and Emma: you smashed it.

Finally I'd like to say a big thank you to you for picking up this book. I hope it brings you lots of joy, energy and happiness. Good luck.

ABOUT JOE

Joe Wicks, aka **The Body Coach**, is Britain's favourite healthy cook and PE teacher. He has helped millions of people achieve new levels of fitness and fat loss with his lockdown PE lessons, bestselling recipe books and 90 Day Plans, as well as through his online social media community and YouTube channel.

Joe was appointed **Children in Need's first Schools Ambassador** in 2019 with the aim of encouraging UK schoolchildren to become more active and have fun in the process. During his UK Schools HIIT Tour in 2019, he travelled the length and breadth of the UK, helping to show young people that exercising is enjoyable as well as hugely beneficial.

Joe lives in London with his wife Rosie and two young children.

[instagram] **@thebodycoach**

[twitter] **@thebodycoach**

[facebook] **@JoeWicksTheBodyCoach**

[youtube] **The Body Coach TV**

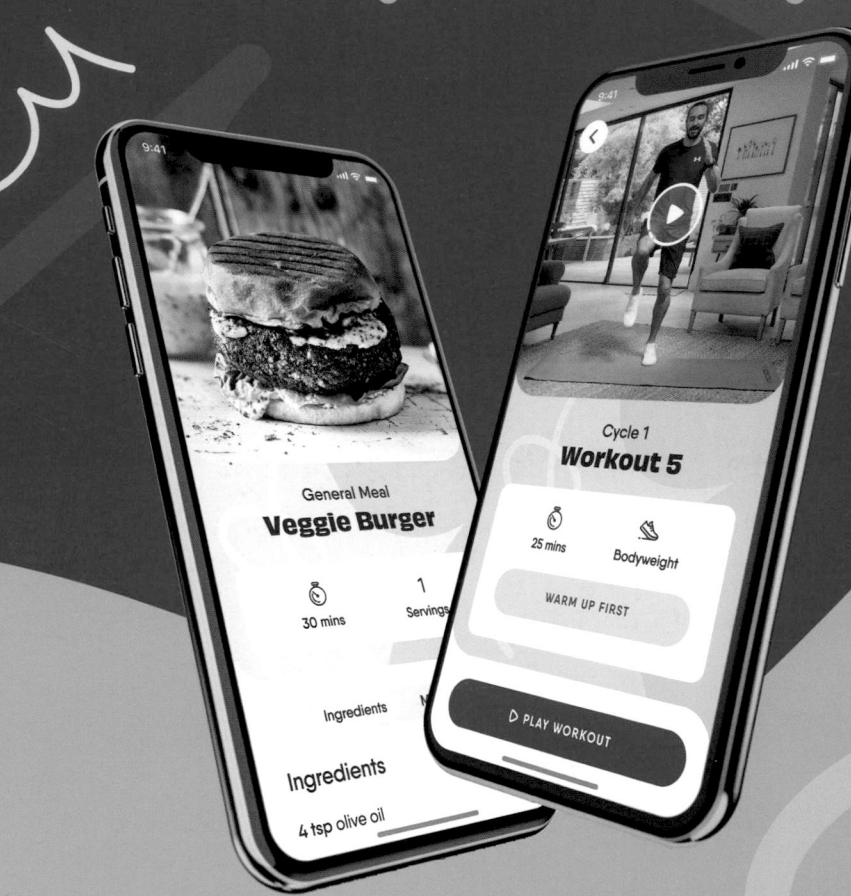

the body coach

SAY HELLO TO A REAL GAME CHANGER

THE BODY COACH APP
launching early 2021

Continue your journey at **thebodycoach.com**